ATLAS of
SUTURING
TECHNIQUES

ATLAS of SUTURING TECHNIQUES

Approaches to Surgical Wound, Laceration, and Cosmetic Repair

Second Edition

Jonathan Kantor, MD, MA, MSt, MSc, MSCE

Department of Dermatology
Center for Global Health
Center for Clinical Epidemiology and Biostatistics
University of Pennsylvania Perelman School of Medicine
Philadelphia, Pennsylvania

Florida Center for Dermatology, PA
St. Augustine, Florida

New York Chicago San Francisco Athens London Madrid Mexico City
Milan New Delhi Singapore Sydney Toronto

Atlas of Suturing Techniques: Approaches to Surgical Wound, Laceration, and Cosmetic Repair, Second Edition

1 2 3 4 5 6 7 8 9   DSS   27 26 25 24 23 22

ISBN 978-1-264-26439-1
MHID 1-264-26439-9

This book was set in Stempel Schneidler Std by KnowledgeWorks Global Ltd.
The editors were Leah Carton and Christie Naglieri.
The production supervisor was Richard Ruzycka.
Project management was provided by Nitesh Sharma, KnowledgeWorks Global Ltd.
The cover designer was W2 Design.

This book was printed on acid-free paper.

Library of Congress Cataloging-in-Publication Data

Names: Kantor, Jonathan, 1976- author
Title: Atlas of suturing techniques : approaches to surgical wound,
    laceration, and cosmetic repair / Jonathan Kantor.
Description: Second edition. | New York : McGraw Hill Education, [2021] |
    Includes bibliographical references and index. | Summary: "Everything
    you need to know about the fundamental principles of suturing and wound
    repair in an accessible, meticulously illustrated atlas"– Provided by
    publisher.
Identifiers: LCCN 2021019633 | ISBN 9781264264391 (trade paperback ; alk.
    paper) | ISBN 1264264399 (trade paperback ; alk. paper) | ISBN
    9781264264407 (ebook)
Subjects: MESH: Suture Techniques | Sutures | Lacerations–surgery |
    Cosmetic Techniques | Atlas
Classification: LCC RD73.S8 | NLM WO 517 | DDC 617.9/178–dc23
LC record available at https://lccn.loc.gov/2021019633

For Bella, who found me wandering and pointed me on the road to Dotan.

CONTENTS

 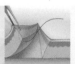

CHAPTER 5

SUTURE TECHNIQUES FOR SUPERFICIAL STRUCTURES: TRANSEPIDERMAL APPROACHES   197

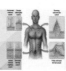

CHAPTER 6   SUTURING TIPS AND APPROACHES BY ANATOMICAL LOCATION   365

CHAPTER 7   APPROACH TO TECHNIQUE SELECTION BY CLOSURE TYPE   391

Videos are available by accessing QR codes that can be found throughout the book. Videos are also accessible via mhprofessional.com/atlasofsuturingtechniques2e

The minute you get away from fundamentals—whether its proper technique, work ethic or mental preparation—the bottom can fall out of your game, your schoolwork, your job, whatever you're doing.

Get the fundamentals down and the level of everything you do will rise.
—Michael Jordan

Only the very lucky discover the keystone.
—Wallace Stegner, *Angle of Repose*

Cutaneous reconstructive and aesthetic surgery has experienced a meteoric evolution. Intricate flap and graft procedures have been developed to restore surgically affected patients to a normal, unoperated appearance. These techniques have enjoyed wide exposure in manuscripts, textbooks, and professional meetings. And yet, as innovative as these procedures may be, their ability to re-create normalcy will fail dramatically unless meticulous attention is paid to the keystone of surgical fundamentals—suture technique. Unless the scars are intrinsic to tissue movement and transfer approach, the ideal of invisibility, a reconstructive procedure will not be fully restorative, only partially corrective. Whatever marvels of repair have been achieved, all the patient and the outside observer will see and appreciate is the visibility or lack thereof in the resultant scar. Without meticulous attention to this fundamental, the optimal end point will not be achieved. Sadly, attention to the details of suture technique

has to date taken a backseat to the glitz and appeal of flap and graft dynamics and aesthetic procedures. Only single chapters in textbooks and rare journal articles are available to detail the broad suturing armamentarium available to the surgeon. Fortunately, with this atlas, Dr. Kantor has superbly filled a void that has not yet been addressed—the keystone of cutaneous surgery—suture technique.

Dr. Kantor's passion for this topic is readily apparent. Techniques that are familiar to most and some with which many are unacquainted are equally explored in comprehensive detail. All methods include discussion of application, suture material choice, and procedure mechanics. Unique to this atlas are Dr. Kantor's tips and pearls for each technique as well as the caveats of drawbacks and cautions. Each method is diagrammatically illustrated and supplemented by online videos.

It is not an exaggeration to say that this atlas is unique and innovative. There is no other reference that explores this topic with such detail, clarity, and comprehension. For those of us attempting to provide our patients with the very best that reconstructive and aesthetic surgery can offer, this atlas is invaluable. We owe Dr. Kantor a huge debt of gratitude for sharing his expertise and passion.

Leonard Dzubow, MD
Former Professor and Director of Mohs
and Dermatologic Surgery
University of Pennsylvania
Philadelphia, Pennsylvania
Private Practice, Media, Pennsylvania

FOREWORD TO THE SECOND EDITION

Comprehensive surgery textbooks are important references, but also, by necessity, often derivative and duplicative. There are only so many pages that can be compressed into even the most enormous book, and each such textbook attempts to fill its thousands of pages with the full range of the same broadly relevant topics. Hence it is necessary to own only one or two comprehensive texts.

Paradoxically, despite their heft, the heavy and imposing encyclopedic volumes that purport to cover all of dermatologic surgery are still not long enough to address every topic in detail. To stay of a size that can be handled, they must summarize and sift.

This means that there remains a role for specialized texts that address only a single topic in cutaneous surgery. Unitary focus allows such books to be constructed in such a way to be maximally useful. They are relatively short, clearly organized, and proud of their depth rather than their width. Needless to say, even among such specialized slim books, some address more useful topics, and some are better written.

The book you are holding is among the best—well written, well organized, extremely complete, and overall indispensable. Why indispensable? Well, this book is unusual and unusually valuable in that collates and conveys a type of practical information, all the many ways in which skin can be sutured, that is not available in any other single reference. Kantor has done careful detective work to uncover every suture technique and variant buried in a research paper, chapter, unpublished manuscript, poster, or presentation. Then, instead of just copying and pasting with minimal paraphrasing, he has gleaned the essential elements of each technique, illustrated the associated hand motions with clear and consistently drawn diagrams, and served up readable morsels in an extremely digestible format.

Unlike some other specialized textbooks, this is for beginners and experts alike. No matter how exalted the expert, it is unlikely that they know every technique described herein, and more or less inconceivable that they *use* each such method routinely. For the beginner, there is an abundant landscape to explore, and choices to be made.

Given the outstanding editor and author that he is, Kantor has not rested, but instead has produced a yet more complete second edition. New techniques have been added, and previously included methods have been updated with the latest findings.

Suturing is probably the single most important skill in the dermatologic surgeon's toolkit. It is certainly what allows us to restore structure and function, to patients' delight and relief. This important book tells us all we need to know. With it, we can be maximally versatile and prepared, benefit from the collective experience of many others, and be guided to select the suture techniques best suited for each patient and clinical circumstance.

Murad Alam, MD, MBA, MSCI
Chicago, July 2021
Professor or Dermatology, Medical Social Sciences, and Otolaryngology-Head & Neck Surgery
Northwestern University Feinberg School of Medicine

CHAPTER 1

Introduction

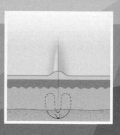

All desirable scars are alike; all undesirable scars are undesirable in different ways. For millennia, surgical and traumatic wounds have been closed with sutures and similar materials, yet it was only with the introduction of local anesthesia 130 years ago that surgeons were able to move from focusing on the most rapid suture placement technique to the most effective. From William Halsted's promotion of the buried suture technique in the late nineteenth century to contemporary articles on the subtleties of suture placement and tissue handling, a paradigm shift has taken place, with an increasing appreciation that not only are there multiple available approaches for any single suture placement, but that this choice may impact outcomes.

Shifting tension as deep as possible in the surgical wound is the key principle of suture placement, and indeed, adhering to this approach leads directly to improved patient outcomes, both functionally and aesthetically. Tension across the superficial dermis leads to increased scarring; shifting this tension to the deep dermis or even the fascia and suturing in a fashion that keeps the tension deep permit wounds to heal with the subtlest of scars.

The surgical literature is rife with myriad techniques with flashy names and multiletter acronyms. While sexy and catchy technique names and acronyms are sometimes appealing, they do little to describe a technique or place it within the larger context of other fundamental and well-established approaches. Moreover, this tendency increases the risk that previously described approaches could simply be shined off, dressed up, and renamed as ostensibly novel approaches—something that only serves to increase confusion for the novice and expert alike, since developing a common language is an important step in improving techniques and therefore outcomes. When possible, the second edition of *Atlas of Suturing Techniques: Approaches to Surgical Wound, Laceration, and Cosmetic Repair* utilizes descriptive names for suture techniques so that the nature of the technique is, at least somewhat, described by its name. Furthermore, when possible, techniques are explained in the context of the existing literature; for example, the "running looped suture" does not tell the reader what the technique entails, but referring to it as a "running locking horizontal mattress suture" suddenly allows the reader to understand the fundamental approach, even in the absence of a multipage description.

In the interest of consistency and developing a meaningful and translatable nomenclature, some liberty has been taken in (re)naming techniques so that they make intuitive sense. Therefore, for example, what was described in the literature as the "modified tip stitch" is referred to as the "modified vertical mattress tip stitch," and what was originally named as the "vertical mattress tip stitch" is instead referred to as the "hybrid mattress tip stitch." Once the reader has an understanding of the techniques on which these approaches are based, the value of the slight shift in nomenclature should become obvious. This shift in terminology is not meant as a slight to those who have named techniques in the past, but rather as an aid to those becoming increasingly familiar with myriad suture technique variations.

Throughout the text, certain terms are used regularly. As there is significant regional variability in training and terminology, it may be worthwhile to clarify some terms. Each "bite" refers to a pass of the needle through tissue; thus, a simple interrupted suture could be performed by taking a single large bite (assuming the needle is sufficiently large), starting by entering the skin on one wound edge and ending by exiting the skin on the contralateral wound edge, but it may also be closed with two separate bites, with the transition between the two bites consisting of the needle's exit and subsequent reloading and reentry between the incised wound edges. Similarly, each "throw" refers to a single half knot, formed by the loop of the suture material around the needle driver in the case of an instrument tie.

Suture techniques are divided largely between two sections: (1) those used for deeper structures, such as the dermis or fascia, and (2) those used for superficial structures that are placed through the outside of the skin. These sections could also easily be differentiated as (1) techniques that largely employ absorbable suture material and (2) techniques that generally utilize nonabsorbable suture material. Ideally, since wounds heal better with tension shifted deep to the deep dermis and fascia, all closures would only be in the first category, though in real-world situations, often a layered combination of approaches is utilized.

The term "percutaneous" as used in this text refers to techniques that are largely buried but that have a small component that traverses the epidermis. Thus, the percutaneous set-back dermal suture is a buried technique wherein the suture material briefly exits and reenters the skin. While this nomenclature is generally accepted, the literature includes some publications where this term is used to mean a technique that is performed entirely through the outside of the skin, and therefore, clarifying this point is necessary.

The fundamental principle of all suture techniques is simple: finely coapt the wound edges, preferably with eversion, while shifting the tension deep, away from the surface of the skin. For wounds under tension—and this would include all wounds due to excisional surgery—repairing the deeper structures, whether muscle, fascia, or deep dermis, and placing sutures in these structures permit the wound edges to drape together under minimal tension. While it is certainly easy to close many wounds using transepidermal sutures alone, such as the simple interrupted suture, this technique alone means that the tension of the closure is held by a suture that crosses over the surface of the skin. There are two important disadvantages to such a technique: (1) once the sutures are removed, there is no residual support for the wound, leading to an increased risk of dehiscence (and if the sutures are left in place for too long, this all but guarantees that suture track marks will be present), and (2) since a high-tension closure is effected directly across the wound edge, the scar will have a tendency to spread and may be more likely to become hypertrophic and unsightly.

Shifting tension to the deep dermis or fascia permits the epidermal and superficial dermal closure to occur under minimal to absent tension. Since the scar response results from, and is exacerbated by, tension, this approach permits not only a functional closure but also an aesthetically pleasing one.

The accomplished surgeon should move from simply attempting to coapt wound edges to designing closure techniques that will maximize the chance of outstanding healing and a return to "normal" as much as possible. For example, suture material left between the incised wound edges may serve as a barrier to healing; this may be conceptualized as an iatrogenic eschar phenomenon. The importance of debriding eschar that rests between wound edges is clear to most surgeons, as the mechanical blockade of tissue healing cofactors by the mass of eschar clearly impairs the rapidity with which a wound can heal and, ultimately, its functional and cosmetic outcome. Therefore, buried suture techniques that minimize the placement of suture material between the incised wound edges, such as the set-back suture and its variants, may confer a clinical advantage. Since no suture material is present between the incised wound edges, nothing impedes the cellular migration necessary for healing.

The goal of surgical procedures on the skin and soft tissues is to return the skin as close to "normal" as possible. By definition, every wound heals with a scar. Wound edges should in most cases be smooth and perpendicular to the surface (some repairs, such as the butterfly suture, call for a beveled edge). Tissue must be handled as atraumatically as possible. Careful attention to hemostasis is a must. A thorough understanding of anatomy, tissue mechanics, flap mechanics and geometry, and other considerations is imperative before approaching complex repairs. The cornerstone of every closure, however, is simple. If there is minimal tension across the surface of a wound—if the wound is splinted or cast in place by the presence of precisely placed, meticulously designed sutures through the deep dermis—then it will heal with a nearly imperceptible scar.

Since all tissues are not created equal, all body sites do not respond to the same techniques, and technical challenges in suture placement are a reality, there is no single suture technique that will be appropriate in every situation. Certain workhorse techniques that effectively reduce tension across the surface of the wound, such as the set-back dermal suture or buried vertical mattress suture, may be used in almost every surgical case. Others, such as the pulley versions of the previously mentioned techniques, may be used occasionally, while still others, such as percutaneous running suturing techniques, may be niche approaches that are used only infrequently by most surgeons.

Lacerations in the context of the emergency department, urgent care center, or primary care office may be addressed in a number of ways. All of the techniques described in this book may be used for any repair, from a simple laceration to a multilayered flap. That said, approaches to a laceration—as opposed to a surgical wound purposely caused by the surgeon—may differ subtly from iatrogenic incision repairs. First, lacerations, of course, need to be properly prepped via debridement and irrigation, as appropriate. Second, lacerations, like skin incisions (but unlike excisional defects), generally do not involve removal of skin, and therefore, the wound is under only modest tension, as tissue does not need to be recruited in order to effect a closure. Thus, suturing techniques designed for high-tension closures (such as pulley techniques) may be needed only infrequently. Third, undermining is often not performed when closing lacerations, so that certain techniques predicated on a well-undermined dermis (such as the butterfly suture) may be less appropriate, though select lacerations may benefit from undermining in order to reduce final closure tension.

Many practitioners close lacerations with only transepidermal sutures, whether for presumed ease of placement, minimization of infection risk by avoiding the theoretical risk of bacterial contamination of absorbable suture material, or a sense that deep sutures are only needed in wounds under marked tension. Still, as with any wound, closing a laceration so that there is minimal tension across the wound's surface will yield the most cosmetically acceptable scar in the long run. Therefore, placing deep sutures, such as the buried vertical mattress suture or set-back dermal suture, may both reduce the tension across the surface of the wound and (when used as a single-layer closure without transepidermal sutures) allow for avoidance of suture removal visits. Other frequently used techniques in laceration repair include the simple interrupted suture, simple running suture, running locking suture, depth-correcting simple interrupted suture, horizontal mattress suture, running subcuticular suture, and the various iterations of the tip stitch.

Half-buried variations of the horizontal or vertical mattress suture are also occasionally used adjacent to hair-bearing areas, so that the non–hair-bearing edge is not marred by the presence of transepidermal sutures. The full range of suture techniques are available to those involved in laceration repair; given the substantial clinical variation seen in these wounds, familiarity and comfort with high-level suturing techniques may yield markedly improved outcomes for patients in the acute setting.

All of surgery is both art and science; it is the goal of this text to break down some of the art of surgical technique, distil it to its essence, and convey this information in as straightforward a way as possible. This second edition of the *Atlas* also serves to catalogue some fundamental techniques that may be useful to both the novice and virtuoso surgeon alike. Perspective is simplified when standing on the shoulders of giants, and indeed, while there is nothing new under the sun, it may be helpful to shine its rays on a variety of approaches that may serve to expand the armamentarium of all of those involved in improving outcomes for the individual who is always the most important person in the surgical suite—the patient. Caring for patients in the *best* possible way—and suturing technique may translate directly into improved outcomes—is both our responsibility and our privilege.

CHAPTER 2

The Surgical Tray

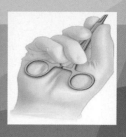

The range of available options for suture materials, instruments, and durable medical equipment can be bewildering. Before approaching a surgical repair, it is very helpful to have a working knowledge and appreciation of the appropriate surgical instruments and options for suture material and needle choice. As with any endeavor, organized and meticulous preparation will help foster a smooth, rapid, and elegant surgical closure.

Some prerequisites to performing skin and soft tissue surgery include an appreciation of surgical anatomy, basic operative technique, and an understanding of tissue movement and mechanics.

Attention to effective patient positioning is also helpful in creating a comfortable and ergonomically sensible environment. When possible, the surgical site should be level and at a comfortable working height for the surgeon. Surgical loops may be helpful in maintaining an ergonomically correct operating position. Time ostensibly saved by the assistant in failing to adequately prepare the surgical site is invariably lost intraoperatively as improper patient positioning or preparation leads to increased operative time and an ensuing increased risk of surgical site complications.

Surgeons are widely known for their particularity regarding surgical instruments. This is not without reason, as an experienced surgeon expects their surgical instruments to function flawlessly, functioning as an extension of the surgeon's hands for precisely and accurately handling tissues and all aspects of the surgical field.

Surgical trays used for skin and soft tissue reconstruction may range from a simple set of four or five instruments to highly specialized instrument arrays consisting of dozens of finely calibrated surgical instruments. While larger surgical cases may require a larger quiver of instruments, most straightforward cases can be completed safely and efficiently with a few discrete components: the scalpel; the needle driver, used for holding the needle securely (and for knot tying); the surgical pickups or forceps, used for securely holding the tissue; the skin hook, used for atraumatically improving visualization of the deeper tissues and, in some hands, for wound edge control during suturing; tissue scissors, for delicately and accurately trimming the skin and soft tissues; and suture scissors, used for cutting and trimming suture material. Most surgical trays also include an electrosurgical device to aid in hemostasis as well as gauze. Nonwoven gauze is preferred as it has excellent wicking properties and does not tend to unravel, which could potentially introduce foreign-body material into the wound (Figure 2-1).

Surgical instruments may include tungsten carbide inserts to increase their longevity (and cost), as this material is both stiffer and denser than the stainless steel out of which most modern instruments are constructed.

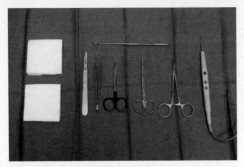

Figure 2-1. A very basic surgical tray.

The Surgical Blade

Most modern scalpel blades are made from stainless or carbon steel. Stainless steel blades are very sharp and resist dulling from repetitive friction across tissue. Carbon steel blades, while marginally sharper than their stainless equivalents, are more susceptible to dulling. Disposable scalpel handles, with the blade permanently affixed, are sometimes used in settings where small volumes of procedures are performed or where access to an autoclave is limited but are generally not used in busy surgical practices.

While a variety of scalpel handles are available, most skin and soft tissue surgery is performed using a no. 3 Bard-Parker flat handle. This permits the use of various scalpel blades, including the 15 blade, by far the most frequently used surgical blade in cutaneous surgery. Other scalpel handles include the no. 7 scalpel handle, which accepts the same blades as the no. 3, and the Beaver handles, for which special blades must be used. In addition to the 15 blade, the smaller 15c is sometimes used for delicate excisions around the eyelids and ears (and, by some, on all facial cases), while the larger 10 blade is used for areas with a more robust dermis, such as the back. Despite the plethora of available options, it is possible to use a simple no. 3 handle and 15 blade for essentially all skin and

soft tissue surgery without any compromise in outcome.

The Needle Driver

The needle driver is used for grasping and manipulating the needle and suture. A variety of options exist, many named for esteemed surgeons of the past, including the Webster, Halsey, or Mayo-Hegar needle drivers. While some surgical trays include an array of needle drivers, a minimalist approach could include a single 4¾-inch Webster needle holder for grasping all but the largest CP-2 needles, perhaps with the addition of a 5-inch Mayo-Hegar needle holder for grasping these larger needles. Smooth jaws are generally preferred when instrument ties will be used, as serrated jaws may damage the grasped suture, though serrations concomitantly add stability for securing larger needles.

A single click is sufficient for locking the needle, and indeed, cranking down on the needle driver excessively will result in a loosening of the locking mechanism, leading to inadvertent suture needle slippage in the future. The needle driver may be palmed, where it is locked or released via gentle pressure from the thenar eminence, or may be held with the thumb and fourth finger (Figures 2-2 through 2-4). When delicately placing fine-gauge sutures in the face, the body of the needle driver may be held with the thumb and first and second fingers and delicately rotated through the skin, permitting precise placement of fine sutures (Figure 2-5).

 Video 2-1. Options for grasping the needle driver
Access to video can be found via mhprofessional.com/atlasofsuturingtechniques2e

When grasping the needle body with the needle driver, the default position is to grasp the needle with the end of the

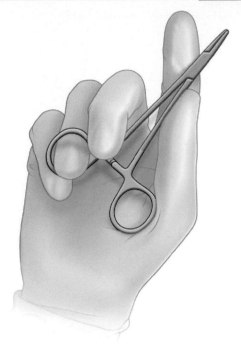

Figure 2-3. Palming the needle driver. This is the default position for many surgeons. The fourth finger may rest slightly on the inside of the ring.

Video 2-2. Loading the needle driver
Access to video can be found via mhprofessional.com/atlasofsuturingtechniques2e

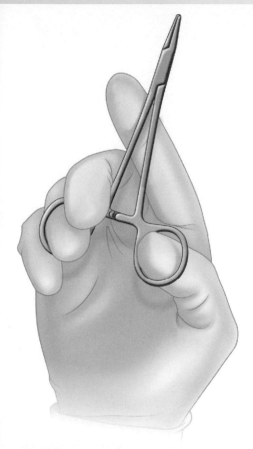

Figure 2-2. The basic needle driver grasping position, with thumb and fourth finger in the rings.

needle driver perpendicular to the body of the needle approximately one-third of the distance from the swage where the suture material is bonded to the needle. When first loading a needle, this may be executed by gently pressing the slightly open jaws of the needle driver perpendicularly against the needle and closing the needle driver with a single click. For closures in tight spaces, the needle may be grasped toward the middle or even slightly distally so that the arc of needle placement is relatively shallow, while for other select closures, such as the running subcuticular technique, the needle may be held at an angle relative to the jaws of the needle driver.

Forceps

The surgical pickups permit easy tissue handling and manipulation, and to the experienced surgeon, they function as a delicate and precise extension of the non-dominant hand for tissue manipulation and wound edge handling (Figures 2-6 and 2-7).

Numerous iterations of forceps are available, from fine Bishop-Harmon forceps that, when used with a tying platform, are effective for delicate closures on the nose, lips, ears, and eyelids, to toothed Adson forceps that, when used with a tying platform, are the workhorse for most skin and soft tissue closures.

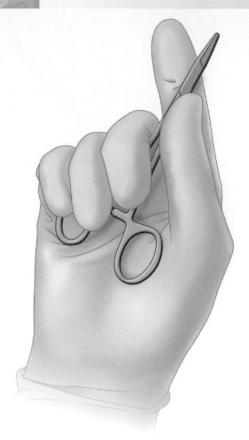

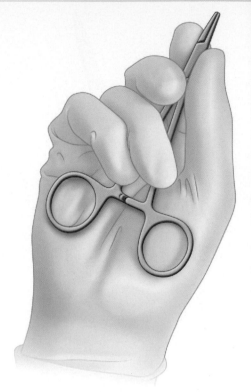

Figure 2-5. Needle driver grasping position when performing fine suturing.

Figure 2-4. Palming the needle driver with no fingers in the rings.

While some trays include a wide variety of forceps, a single Adson forceps with teeth and a tying platform is likely sufficient for most cases, while a Bishop-Harmon forceps, with its delicate teeth more akin to a set of skin hooks, is a nice addition for smaller closures.

 Video 2-3. Grasping the forceps
Access to video can be found via
mhprofessional.com/atlasofsuturingtechniques2e

Skin Hooks

Skin hooks are most useful when utilized in pairs, as the assistant provides traction and lift to the wound edges, permitting easy visualization of the deeper structures

for electrocautery, vessel ligation, and inspection. They are available in numerous formats, from a single hooked Frazier skin hook to larger, multipronged

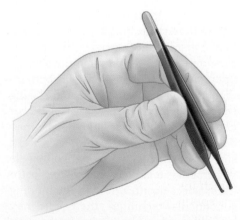

Figure 2-6. Holding the forceps for tissue or needle handling.

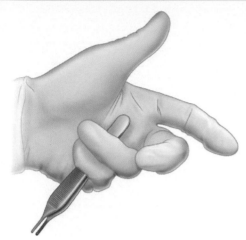

Figure 2-7. Palming the forceps to free up the fingers for grasping suture material and knot tying.

varieties designed for retraction of larger tissues. While a large array of hooks could be included on the tray, a reasonable approach is to utilize a set of single-pronged skin hooks, though double-pronged hooks may marginally decrease the risk of a stick injury and are preferred by some surgeons.

Tissue Scissors

Scissors used for cutting tissue should be extremely sharp; dulling of the surgical scissors not only makes their use frustrating for the surgeon but also leads to unnecessarily increased tissue trauma from crush injury as the tissue is forced between the blades of the scissors. Some surgical trays contain a plethora of skin scissors for different purposes, such as fine, straight, and curved iris scissors for cutting dog ears, dull-tipped blepharoplasty scissors for undermining, Metzenbaum scissors for broader undermining, and others. If a minimalist approach is desired, for most small skin surgeries, 4-inch iris scissors are adequate. Tissue scissors may utilize a SuperCut edge designed for exceptionally sharp and precise tissue cutting. Its disadvantage is that it is very easily dulled if used on anything but tissue, so that cutting suture material or sliding the sharp edge against other surgical instruments must be absolutely avoided. Tungsten carbide inserts, as well as their SuperCut variations, are also available.

Suture Scissors

Suture-cutting scissors should be sharp and, most importantly, should be differentiated from scissors used for cutting tissue. Since surgical assistants are often tasked with cutting sutures, it is important to adequately train them in utilizing only the tips of the scissors to cut tissue. The tendency is to focus on the area being actively cut; therefore, if surgical assistants are in the habit of cutting suture material with the center of the scissors, they may not attend to the location of the scissor tips that could be in a sensitive location such as the canthus. For most applications, a single 4-inch set of suture scissors is adequate. Needle drivers incorporating a cutting component are also available, permitting the surgeon to cut their own suture without switching instruments.

Hemostats

Hemostats are used for grasping vessels and permitting either suture ligation (which is generally preferred for larger vessels) or electrocautery. A variety of small hemostats, with both curved and straight tips, are available, such as the Halsted mosquito hemostat. A minimalist approach would also permit a needle holder to be used as a hemostat, though given the cost differential between these instruments, with hemostats being less expensive than needle holders, this is generally not necessary.

CHAPTER 3

Suture Materials, Knot Tying, and Postoperative Care

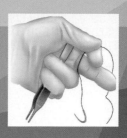

A wide variety of suture materials are available, all with variable handling characteristics, tissue reactivity, absorption characteristics, and costs. While much attention is paid to suture material, the needle may be as or more important than the suture material itself in promoting an ideal surgical outcome. Needles vary by manufacturer and even by suture material, and utilizing the most appropriate needle for the task is critical. Even the most accomplished surgeon will perform in a less-than-ideal fashion if their instruments or needle choices are flawed.

Most needles used for skin and soft tissue reconstruction are 3/8 circle in diameter, and most needles used for skin and soft tissue reconstructions are reverse cutting in nature (Figure 3-1). There are, however, important exceptions to this rule. For example, a semicircular P-2 needle may be used for narrow closures, such as those sometimes encountered on the nose, and a cutting needle, with the sharp edge on the inside of the curve, may be useful for nasal reconstruction where the thin atrophic dermis may be cut by the superficially coursing outside of the needle.

The two largest manufacturers of suture material used in cutaneous surgery are Ethicon and Covidien. While suture size is governed by USP guidelines (the larger the number of zeros, the smaller the suture), needle size and configuration are largely proprietary. Thus, the surgeon must be comfortable understanding the various needle sizes and configurations of the various manufacturers. Suture material packaging does include a cross-sectional image of the needle, permitting some comparison between companies. Of note, Covidien does not (except on its website) refer to any of its needles as reverse cutting; instead, they label cutting needles as conventional cutting and reverse cutting needles as cutting (Table 3-1). These distinctions are important when choosing suture, though many suture type and needle combinations are only available with a finite number of permutations. Since cutting and reverse cutting needles have a triangular tip, the orientation of the cutting end is indicated by whether the triangle on the box is pointing up (cutting) or down (reverse cutting).

The material used to make the needles themselves also varies considerably

Point   Body   Swage

Grasp here with needle driver for most applications.

Grasp here with needle driver when suturing in tight spaces or through dense tissue.

Figure 3-1. The suture needle.

TABLE 3-1 COMPARISON OF FREQUENTLY USED REVERSE CUTTING NEEDLES FROM ETHICON AND COVIDIEN

Ethicon	Covidien
P-1	P-10
P-3	P-13
PS-1	P-14
PS-2	P-12
CP-2	GS-10
FS-1	C-14
FS-2	C-13
P-2	P-21

Comparison does not imply equivalency, as the alloy and finish quality within and between companies will vary. All are 3/8 circle in diameter except the P-2/P-21, which are 1/2 circle.

between manufacturers, as proprietary alloys are used to maximize strength and durability. While Ethicon and Covidien products are used most often in skin and soft tissue reconstruction, many other reputable companies manufacture suture material, and individual preferences may vary widely (Table 3-2).

Any monofilament suture, including absorbable sutures, may be used for transepidermal suture placement. Thus, utilizing a monofilament absorbable suture may permit the use of a single suture pack for both buried and epidermal sutures.

Many suture characteristics are commonly discussed, including handling, memory, pliability, knot security, tissue reactivity, and others. Although there are subtle differences between the handling characteristics of different suture materials, most modern options fall well within the realm of utility, so that while the handling of silk, for example, is clearly superior to the handling of nylon, even nylon handles very well. Similarly, certain materials, such as catgut, may be highly reactive, though the more frequently used formulations, such as chromic gut and fast-absorbing gut, do not lead to enough inflammation to make a marked clinical difference in most situations. For the most part, monofilament sutures lead to less tissue drag and, therefore, are useful with running techniques, while braided sutures provide excellent handling and knot security and are therefore useful for interrupted buried sutures. With improvements in materials, the distinction between outcomes now likely relates more to suturing technique than to choice in suture materials.

TABLE 3-2 COMPARISON OF FREQUENTLY USED SUTURE MATERIALS FROM ETHICON AND COVIDIEN

Ethicon	Covidien	Application
Vicryl	Polysorb	Standard for buried sutures
VicrylRapide	Velosorb Fast	Alternative to fast-absorbing gut; excellent for skin grafts or when suture removal is not an option
Monocryl	Biosyn	Monofilament alternative for buried sutures; support is lost faster than Vicryl/Polysorb
PDS I/II	Maxon	Monofilament alternative for buried sutures; support lasts longer than Vicryl/Polysorb
Prolene	Surgipro I/II	Smooth monofilament nonabsorbable suture; excellent choice for running subcuticular sutures if suture removal is planned
Ethilon	Monosof	Standard nonabsorbable monofilament nylon suture for epidermal approximation

Note that this table does not imply equivalency; it is designed to outline suture materials that are roughly equivalent in terms of application to skin and soft tissue reconstruction.

Commonly Used Absorbable Suture Materials

Vicryl (polyglactin 910)

Vicryl is one of the most frequently used suture materials in skin and soft tissue reconstruction. It is a braided, coated suture material that retains its strength for approximately 3 weeks and is completely absorbed in less than 3 months. It has excellent handling characteristics and only mild tissue reactivity. Recently, a faster-absorbing variation, VicrylRapide, was developed, which loses its strength entirely in less than 2 weeks and may be seen as an alternative to fast-absorbing gut suture when suture removal is not desired. An antibacterial-coated variation is now also available in the market.

Polysorb (glycolide/lactide copolymer)

This is a braided absorbable suture, similar to Vicryl. It provides similar handling and knot security while ostensibly providing slightly improved initial tensile strength when compared with Vicryl. Its absorption characteristics are also similar to Vicryl. Velosorb Fast has also been developed as an alternative to VicrylRapide.

Monocryl (poliglecaprone)

Monocryl, often seen as a monofilament alternative to Vicryl, is another popular suture material choice. It is more expensive than Vicryl, has excellent handling characteristics for a monofilament suture, and loses its strength in less than 1 month, though complete absorption takes 3-4 months. As with Vicryl, an antibacterial option is also now available.

Maxon (polyglyconate)

Maxon is a long-lasting monofilament absorbable suture; while it loses some strength already after 3 weeks, it takes 6 months or more for the suture material to be entirely absorbed, making this a good choice when long-term strength retention may be helpful. It has good handling characteristics, though the slow absorption times should be taken into account if dyed suture material is used, as the suture may be visible if placed in a running subcuticular pattern.

Polydioxanone (PDS)

Polydioxanone I and II are very-long-lasting monofilament absorbable sutures. They are useful when long-term strength retention is critical. PDS II was developed as a better-handling alternative to PDS I, which was criticized for its less-than-ideal handling characteristics. It retains strength for an extended period of time, with 50% strength retention at 5 weeks, and may take more than 6 months to absorb.

Biosyn (glycomer 631)

Biosyn is another monofilament absorbable suture. It has very good handling characteristics and outstanding initial tensile strength. It retains its strength for at least 3 weeks and takes up to 4 months to absorb completely. If Biosyn is used for superficial closures, the undyed version may be preferable.

Caprosyn (polyglytone 6211)

Caprosyn is a fast-absorbing monofilament suture, often seen as an alternative to Monocryl. It absorbs completely in 8 weeks, while retaining tensile strength for 7-10 days postoperatively. It is therefore useful in low-tension closures, such as those on the face, where rapid suture material breakdown is an advantage.

Catgut

Plain gut is derived from bovine or sheep intestines and therefore breaks down by enzymatic degradation, rather than the hydrolysis that breaks down synthetic absorbable sutures. Chromic gut is a longer-lasting version of gut, while fast-absorbing gut is heat treated to speed up absorption. On a practical level, fast-absorbing gut may be useful for closures when transepidermal sutures are desired for wound-edge apposition but where suture removal is impractical or inconvenient. Gut does lead to more tissue reactivity than other absorbable sutures and has a tendency toward breakage after multiple passes through tissue (Table 3-3).

Commonly Used Nonabsorbable Suture Materials

Nylon

This is a frequently used nonabsorbable suture and provides minimal tissue reactivity coupled with very good handling. While a very good choice for most closures, it does not move through tissue as smoothly as polypropylene, so if buried subcuticular sutures are placed with nonabsorbable suture, the latter would be preferred. Nylon is available either braided or as monofilament; the former may confer slightly better handling, though this is outweighed by the ability of monofilament nylon to move easily through tissue.

Polypropylene (Prolene, Surgipro)

This is a minimally reactive suture that has the ability to move smoothly through tissue. It does have a fair amount of memory and, therefore, may be slightly more challenging to work with than nylon. Extra throws are often advisable during knot tying as well, though this does represent a good option for nonabsorbable subcuticular suturing.

TABLE 3-3 FREQUENTLY USED SUTURE MATERIALS IN SKIN AND SOFT TISSUE RECONSTRUCTION

Suture Material Name	Configuration	Handling	Tissue Reactivity	Loss of 50% Strength	Time to Complete Absorption
ABSORBABLE SUTURES					
Vicryl (polyglactin 910)	Braided, coated	Very good	Moderate	21 days	75 days
Polysorb (glycolide/lactide polymer)	Braided, coated	Very good	Moderate	21 days	75 days
Monocryl (poliglecaprone)	Monofilament	Very good	Moderate	7 days	60 days
Maxon (polyglyconate)	Monofilament	Very good	Moderate	21 days	6 months
PDS I/II (polydioxanone)	Monofilament	Good	Moderate	30 days	6 months
Biosyn (glycomer 631)	Monofilament	Very good	Moderate	21 days	60 days
Caprosyn (polyglytone 6211)	Monofilament	Very good	Moderate	7 days	60 days
Catgut	Braided	Very good	High	Plain: 7 days Chromic: 10 days Fast absorbing: 5 days	Plain: 70 days Chromic: 84 days Fast absorbing: 35 days
VicrylRapide	Braided, coated	Very good	Moderate	5 days	42 days
Velosorb Fast	Braided	Very good	Moderate	5 days	42 days
NONABSORBABLE SUTURES					
Monofilament nylon	Monofilament	Very good	Low		
Prolene, Surgipro (polypropylene)	Monofilament	Good	Low		
Novafil (polybutester)	Monofilament	Very good	Low		
Silk	Braided	Excellent	Moderate		

Novafil (polybutester)

This is a very well-handling suture material that also provides significant elasticity. Though not as widely used as some other materials, it provides excellent pliability. The elasticity may be helpful in areas where significant wound edema is anticipated, as it will accommodate tissue swelling while maintaining wound-edge apposition.

Silk

This is the most highly reactive of the nonabsorbable sutures. However, it is also the gold standard for suture material handling. Its natural softness makes it useful in closures along the lips, where synthetic suture has a tendency to poke against the delicate tissues. Its reactivity, however, makes it less useful on a daily basis for most other surgical sites.

Surgical Knot Tying

Most surgical knots in skin and soft tissue reconstruction are tied using an instrument tie. This is generally the fastest approach and also affords the least amount of suture material waste. Hand tying, using either one- or two-handed ties, may be used rarely in cutaneous surgery and reconstruction and will not be addressed here in detail.

The distinction in knot tying between transepidermal sutures, where pulling suture tight may lead to strangulation, and buried sutures, where the goal of suture placement is developing directly opposed dermal, muscle, or fascial structures, is critical. When tying a deep suture, it is generally desirable to pull the suture strands together as tightly as possible, secured with a stable knot. For transepidermal sutures, since the goal of suture placement is wound-edge apposition, placing the minimal necessary tension across of the surface of the wound is a must; overtightening these sutures will lead directly to strangulation, necrosis, and—at a minimum—track mark formation. Indeed, while dermal suture placement should be performed as tight as possible, transepidermal sutures should be secured with the minimal possible tension, and some additional give may be provided by permitting laxity between the first and second throws of the knot, anticipating tissue edema.

Generally, most surgical knots are tied as square knots, so that the two throws occur in opposite directions, locking the knot in place. Sometimes, a granny knot is desirable, where the first two throws are in the same direction, as this allows the suture material to be cinched down and tightened. It is critical, however, to follow the granny knot with a throw in the opposite direction so that once the knot is in place it is secured and cannot slip.

Each throw refers to one half knot, that is, a complete twisting of two strands. Thus, to secure a knot, by definition, a minimum of two throws are necessary, and for practical purposes, three throws are used for most braided sutures, while four throws are used for some sutures with a higher risk of knot slippage.

After placement of the suture itself, when beginning an instrument tie, the leading end of suture must be grasped with the nondominant hand. In order to minimize the risk of needle-stick injury, it is possible to grasp the suture material approximately 6-10 cm from the needle swage between the thumb and index finger of the left hand, allowing the needle to drop down below the hand. Since the needle is hanging freely and is not under tension, there is little chance for a needle-stick injury. Excess suture material may be wrapped around the nondominant hand with a gentle turn of the wrist. Some surgeons prefer to hold the needle itself in the nondominant hand.

Technique for Performing an Instrument Tie with Nonabsorbable Sutures

Video 3-1. Technique for performing an instrument tie with nonabsorbable sutures
Access to video can be found via mhprofessional.com/atlasofsuturingtechniques2e

1. The leading end of suture material is grasped between the thumb and index finger of the left hand, approximately 6 cm from the needle swage. The needle driver is brought between the leading and trailing strands of the suture, and the leading end of the suture is wrapped twice around the needle driver. This should be done by moving the needle driver around the suture, not moving the suture material around the needle driver, as this will permit better precision and economy of movement.

2. The needle driver then grasps the trailing end of the suture material.

3. The hands are pulled in opposite directions, perpendicular to the incised wound edge, so that the right hand moves to the left (where the leading end of the suture began) and the left hand moves to the right (where the trailing end of the suture began). This should form a surgeon's knot that will be resistant to slippage.

4. The trailing end of the suture is released by the needle driver, and the needle driver is then brought from the inside, between the two ends of the suture, and the leading end of the suture is wrapped once around the needle driver.

5. The needle driver grasps the trailing edge of the suture, and the hands again move in opposite directions, so that now the right hand moves to the right and the left hand moves to the left. The knot is now locked.

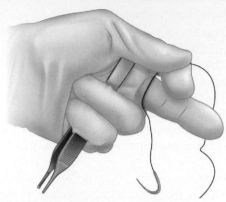

Figure 3-2. Grasping the suture material during knot tying; the suture material may be looped around the left hand if needed. Note that the needle hangs freely, without tension.

6. For the third (and often final) throw, steps (1) through (3) are then repeated, except that now the suture is wrapped only once around the needle driver. Additional throws may be placed if needed (Figures 3-2 through 3-11).

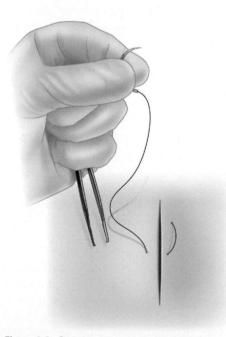

Figure 3-3. Grasping the needle during knot tying.

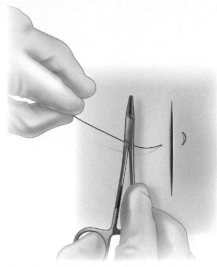

Figure 3-4. The instrument tie for nonabsorbable suture material, step 1: the needle driver is brought between the leading and trailing strands of suture.

Technique for Performing an Instrument Tie with Buried Sutures

Video 3-2. Technique for performing an instrument tie with buried sutures
Access to video can be found via mhprofessional.com/atlasofsuturingtechniques2e.

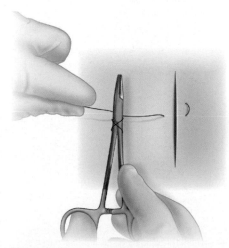

Figure 3-5. The instrument tie for nonabsorbable suture material, step 2: the suture material is looped twice around the needle driver by rotating the needle driver around the suture material.

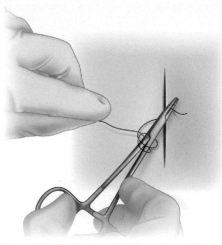

Figure 3-6. The instrument tie for nonabsorbable suture material, step 3: the needle driver is then used to grasp the tail of the suture material.

1. The leading end of the suture material is grasped between the thumb and index finger of the left hand, approximately 6 cm from the needle swage. The needle driver is brought between the leading and trailing strands of the suture, and the leading end of the suture is wrapped twice around the needle driver. This should be done by moving the needle driver

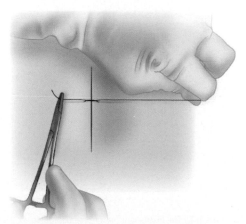

Figure 3-7. The instrument tie for nonabsorbable suture material, step 4: the two ends of the suture are pulled in opposite directions, perpendicular to the wound, allowing the knot to lay flat.

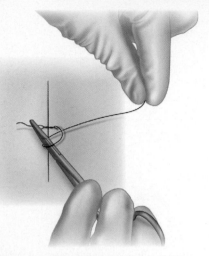

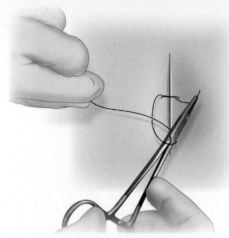

Figure 3-8. The instrument tie for nonabsorbable suture material, step 5: the needle driver is then again brought between the ends of the suture, and the leading end of the suture material is wrapped once around the needle holder, and the trailing tail is grasped.

Figure 3-10. The instrument tie for nonabsorbable suture material, step 7: for the third throw, the procedure is repeated again with the needle driver brought between the two strands; the needle driver wraps the leading end of the suture around itself once, and the trailing end is grasped.

around the suture, not moving the suture material around the needle driver, as this will permit better precision and economy of movement.

2. The needle driver then grasps the trailing end of the suture material.

3. The hands are pulled in opposite directions, parallel to the incised wound edge, so that the right hand moves in the direction of where the leading end of the suture began, and the left hand moves in the direction

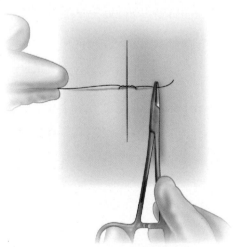

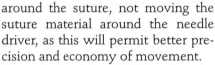

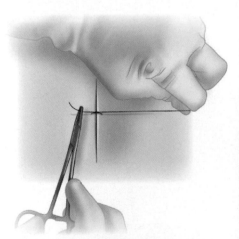

Figure 3-9. The instrument tie for nonabsorbable suture material, step 6: the two ends of the suture are again pulled apart, now moving in the direction opposite the prior throw, again perpendicular to the wound edge.

Figure 3-11. The instrument tie for nonabsorbable suture material, step 8: the hands are then pulled in opposite directions, pulling the throw tight and securing the knot. For most braided suture materials, three throws are adequate, while for some monofilament sutures, a fourth throw may be added.

of where the trailing end of the suture began. This should form a surgeon's knot that will be resistant to slippage.

4. The trailing end of the suture is released by the needle driver, and the needle driver is then brought from the inside, between the two ends of the suture, and the leading end of the suture is wrapped once around the needle driver.

5. The hands again move in opposite directions parallel to the wound, so that the right hand moves in the direction of where the leading strand began and the left hand moves in the direction of where the trailing strand began. The knot is now locked.

6. For the third (and often final) throw, steps (1) through (3) are then repeated, except that now the suture is wrapped only once around the needle driver. Additional throws may be placed if needed (Figures 3-12 to 3-19).

Absorbable suture material is generally trimmed either at the knot (for braided suture material) or with a 1- to 2-mm tail of suture (for monofilament suture material). Nonabsorbable sutures are generally left with a 3- to 6-mm tail, depending on

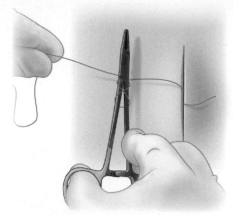

Figure 3-13. The instrument tie for absorbable suture material, step 2: the suture material is looped twice around the needle driver by rotating the needle driver around the suture material.

surgeon preference, suture material size, and the anatomic location.

When tying knots with nonabsorbable suture, if there is only minimal tension across the surface of the wound, it is sometimes desirable to leave a gap between the initial surgeon's knot and the square knot. To execute this maneuver, the first throw is placed as a surgeon's knot. The next throw is not tightened to lock the surgeon's knot, but rather leaves

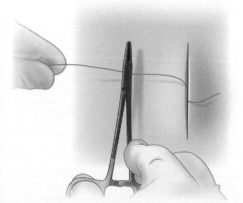

Figure 3-12. The instrument tie for absorbable suture material, step 1: the needle driver is brought between the leading and trailing strands of the suture.

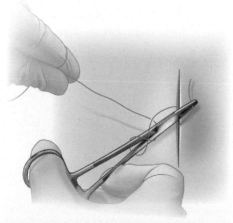

Figure 3-14. The instrument tie for absorbable suture material, step 3: the needle driver is then used to grasp the tail of the suture material.

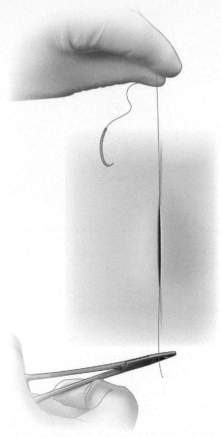

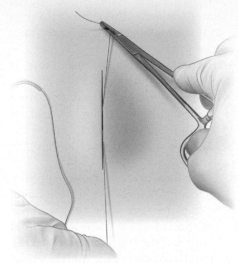

Figure 3-17. The instrument tie for absorbable suture material, step 6: the two ends of the suture are again pulled apart, now moving in the direction opposite the prior throw, again parallel to the wound edge.

1-2 mm of space between the surgeon's knot throw and the subsequent throws. This allows for some give so that tissue edema does not cause the suture material to overly constrict the wound edges.

Figure 3-15. The instrument tie for absorbable suture material, step 4: the two ends of the suture are pulled in opposite directions, parallel to the wound, allowing the knot to lay flat.

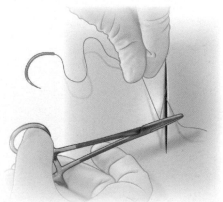

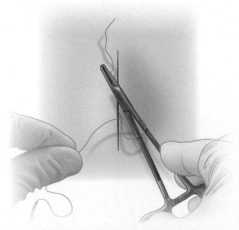

Figure 3-18. The instrument tie for absorbable suture material, step 7: for the third throw, the procedure is repeated again, with the needle driver brought between the two strands, the needle driver wrapping the leading end of suture around itself once, and grasping the trailing end.

Figure 3-16. The instrument tie for absorbable suture material, step 5: the needle driver is then again brought between the ends of the suture, the leading end of the suture material is wrapped once around the needle holder, and the trailing tail is grasped.

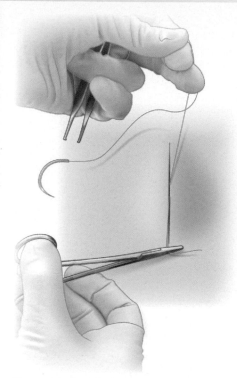

Figure 3-19. The instrument tie for absorbable suture material, step 8: the hands are then pulled in opposite directions, parallel to the wound axis, pulling the throw tight and securing the knot. For most braided suture materials, three throws are adequate, while for some monofilament sutures, a fourth throw may be added.

Postoperative Care

After suturing a wound, the surgeon must decide on the most appropriate dressing. In general, wounds heal best in a moist environment, and therefore, an occlusive film dressing is often appropriate.

Such dressings are also helpful in providing a protectant film over the nascent wound in order to minimize the risk of bacterial colonization. Film dressings are usually adequate for most surgical wounds, since these wounds are generally not highly exudative, as the wound margins have already been adequately approximated. Dressings can usually be left in place for at least 48 hours, and leaving a film dressing in place for a week or more is often a reasonable choice for many wounds, as this also improves the convenience for the patient.

Adhesive strips are sometimes used to help with wound-edge approximation. That said, the degree of gain achieved by adding adhesive strips to an already well-sutured wound is minimal, and these strips may sometimes become covered in serous fluid or serve as a magnet for bacterial colonization.

Suture removal timing remains more of an art than a science. In general, the sooner sutures are removed, the better. Since nonabsorbable sutures generally should not be holding significant tension across the wound and ideally are used for fine-tuning wound-edge approximation only, they may be removed as early as 5 days postoperatively. In the rare event that these sutures are carrying significant tension, sutures may be left in place for 7-14 days or even longer, though patients should be warned of the high risk of leaving significant track marks.

Suture Techniques for Deeper Structures: The Fascia and Dermis

The Simple Buried Dermal Suture

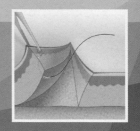

Synonyms

Buried suture, subcuticular suture

Video 4-1. Simple buried dermal suture
Access to video can be found via
mhprofessional.com/atlasofsuturingtechniques2e

Application

This technique is best used in areas under moderate tension, and it is the standard technique discussed in many plastic surgery textbooks. Its use in dermatologic and plastic surgery has, however, fallen somewhat out of favor as other techniques, such as the buried vertical mattress and set-back dermal suture, have become increasingly popular. This straightforward technique is generally reported as useful in a broad array of applications, and it may be used in both facial and truncal skin, though it is particularly useful in areas where inversion is desired. This would include the nasolabial and melolabial folds as well as select areas along the antihelix and umbilicus, where restoration of anatomical inversion is desirable.

Suture Material Choice

Suture choice is dependent in large part on location, though because this technique leaves residual suture material both between the incised wound edges and in the superficial dermis, care should be taken to minimize the liberal use of larger-gauge suture material. On the face and ears, a 5-0 absorbable suture may be used, and on the distal extremities, a 4-0 suture is generally adequate. Using this technique, a 3-0 absorbable suture works well on the back. It may be advisable to eschew the use of 2-0 suture with this technique to minimize the risk of suture spitting.

Technique

1. The wound edge is reflected back using surgical forceps or hooks.
2. While reflecting back the dermis, the suture needle is inserted at 90 degrees into the underside of the dermis 2 mm distant from the incised wound edge.
3. The first bite is executed by following the curvature of the needle and allowing the needle to exit in the incised wound edge. The size of this bite is based on the size of the needle, the thickness of the dermis, and the need for and tolerance of eversion. The needle's zenith with respect to the wound surface should be between the entry and exit points.
4. Keeping the loose end of the suture between the surgeon and the patient, the dermis on the side of the first bite is released. The tissue on the opposite edge is then gently grasped with the forceps.
5. The second and final bite is executed by inserting the needle into the contralateral incised wound edge at the level of the superficial papillary dermis. This bite should be completed by following the curvature of the needle and avoiding catching

the undersurface of the epidermis, which could result in epidermal dimpling. It then exits approximately 2 mm distal to the wound edge on the undersurface of the dermis. This should mirror the first bite taken on the first side of the wound.

6. The suture material is then tied utilizing an instrument tie (Figures 4-1A through 4-1G).

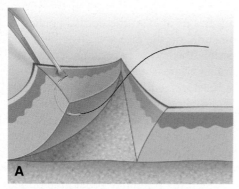

Figure 4-1A. First throw of the simple buried dermal suture. Note that the suture placement follows the curvature of the needle, exiting at the incised wound edge.

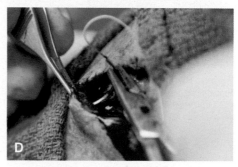

Figure 4-1D. Beginning of the first throw of the simple buried dermal suture. Note that the needle enters through the deep dermis.

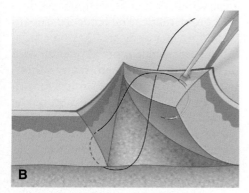

Figure 4-1B. The needle is then inserted at the incised wound edge on the contralateral side.

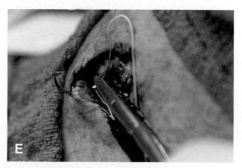

Figure 4-1E. Completion of the first throw of the simple buried dermal suture. Note that suture placement follows the curvature of the needle, exiting at the incised wound edge.

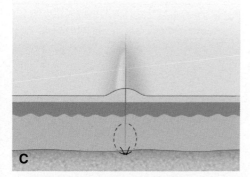

Figure 4-1C. Cross-sectional view depicting the essentially circular course of the suture through the dermis.

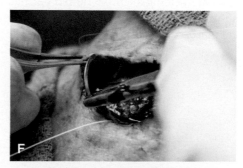

Figure 4-1F. Beginning of the second throw of the simple buried dermal suture. The needle enters at the incised wound edge.

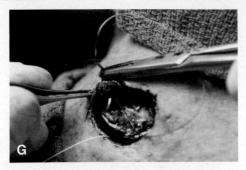

Figure 4-1G. Completion of the second throw of the simple buried dermal suture. Note that suture placement follows the curvature of the needle, exiting in the deep dermis.

Tips and Pearls

This technique is best utilized in areas where slight inversion is desirable, such as the nasolabial fold. It also may be useful toward the apices of elliptical incisions, where a slight inversion of the wound edges may reduce the tendency toward dog-ear formation by pulling the nascent dog ear down toward the subcutaneous tissue.

A particularly well-executed traditional simple buried dermal suture is very similar to the buried vertical mattress, since the placement of the suture following the curvature of the needle results in a slight eversion of the wound edge. Many experienced surgeons who believe that they are placing a simple buried dermal suture may be performing a buried vertical mattress suture.

Drawbacks and Cautions

The standard buried dermal suture, while seemingly a simple approach, can be difficult to execute properly. As with many buried techniques, epidermal dimpling may occur where the arc of the suture reaches its apex at the dermal-epidermal junction; on the face and areas with thin dermis, this should be assiduously avoided. Similarly, areas with sebaceous skin, such as the nose, require meticulous avoidance of dimpling, which has the potential to persist. In truncal areas or those with thick dermis, however, a small degree of dimpling will resolve with time as the absorbable sutures are gradually resorbed.

Given the tendency for simple buried dermal sutures to result in wound inversion, this technique should be avoided in areas where wound inversion is particularly problematic. The tendency toward wound inversion means that superficial sutures are needed more frequently with this technique than with many others, since the transepidermal sutures are utilized in order to effect eversion of the wound edges. Since obviating the need for superficial sutures may be desirable in terms of patient comfort and convenience as well as ultimate cosmetic and functional outcome, this should be considered before broadly applying this technique.

Reference

Straith RE, Lawson JM, Hipps CJ. The subcuticular suture. *Postgrad Med*. 1961;29:164-173.

The Set-Back Dermal Suture

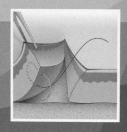

Synonyms

Kantor suture, set-back suture

Video 4-2. Set-back buried dermal suture

Access to video can be found via mhprofessional.com/atlasofsuturingtechniques2e

Application

This technique is often used in areas under significant tension. The back, shoulders, and thighs are particularly amenable to the set-back technique, though it may be used in almost any location, including the central face and ears. Areas prone to wound inversion, such as the cheek and forehead, may also be well served utilizing this technique.

Since it is easier to place than a buried vertical mattress suture, this technique may be used by budding surgeons, medical students, and residents as the workhorse technique for deep tension-relieving sutures.

Suture Material Choice

Suture choice is dependent in large part on location, though as this technique is designed to bite the deep dermis and remain buried well below the wound surface, the surgeon may choose to utilize a larger gauge suture than would be used for an equivalently placed buried simple or buried vertical mattress suture. Using a 2-0 absorbable suture on the back with this technique results in only vanishingly rare complications, since the thicker suture remains largely on the underside of the dermis, and suture spitting is an uncommon occurrence. On the extremities, a 3-0 or 4-0 absorbable suture material may be used, and on the face and areas under minimal tension, a 5-0 absorbable suture is adequate.

Technique

1. The wound edge is reflected back using surgical forceps or hooks. Adequate visualization of the underside of the dermis is required.
2. While reflecting back the dermis, the suture needle is inserted at 90 degrees into the underside of the dermis 2-6 mm distant from the incised wound edge.
3. The first bite is executed by traversing the dermis following the curvature of the needle and allowing the needle to exit closer to the incised wound edge. Care should be taken to remain in the dermis to minimize the risk of epidermal dimpling. The needle does not, however, exit through the incised wound edge, but rather 1-4 mm distant from the incised edge. The size of this first bite is based on the size of the needle, the thickness of the dermis, and the need for and tolerance of eversion.
4. Keeping the loose end of the suture between the surgeon and the patient, the dermis on the side of the first bite is released. The tissue on the

opposite edge is then reflected back in a similar fashion as on the first side, assuring complete visualization of the underside of the dermis.

5. The second and final bite is executed by inserting the needle into the underside of the dermis 1-6 mm distant from the incised wound edge. Again, this bite should be executed by following the curvature of the needle and avoiding catching the undersurface of the epidermis that could result in epidermal dimpling. It then exits further distal to the wound edge, approximately 2-6 mm distant from the wound edge. This should

mirror the first bite taken on the contralateral side of the wound.

6. The suture material is then tied utilizing an instrument tie (Figures 4-2A through 4-2H).

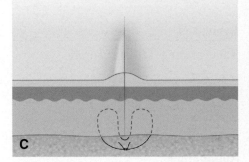

Figure 4-2C. Cross-sectional view demonstrating the path of the suture material through the dermis and the effect on wound eversion.

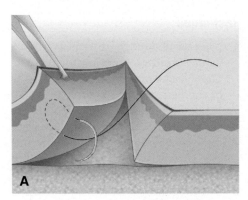

Figure 4-2A. The needle is inserted through the underside of the dermis, exiting again through the underside of the dermis set back from the wound edge.

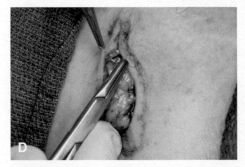

Figure 4-2D. The needle is inserted through the underside of the dermis, perpendicular to the wound edge.

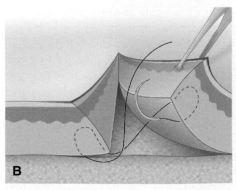

Figure 4-2B. This is repeated on the contralateral wound edge.

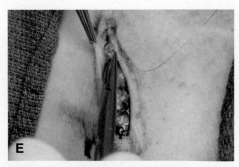

Figure 4-2E. The needle exits the undersurface of the dermis set back from the wound edge.

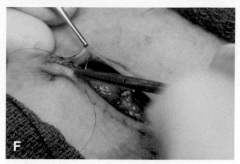

Figure 4-2F. On the contralateral wound edge, the needle is inserted set back from the wound edge.

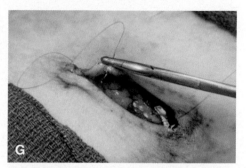

Figure 4-2G. The needle passes through the dermis, exiting further set back from the wound edge.

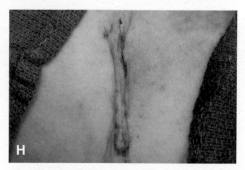

Figure 4-2H. Immediate postoperative appearance. Note the pronounced wound eversion, which will resolve with time.

Tips and Pearls

The set-back suture technique was found to be superior to the buried vertical mattress suture in terms of physician- and patient-rated cosmetic outcome and eversion in a randomized controlled trial.

One of the chief advantages of this technique is its ease of execution; since the suture follows the arc of the needle on the undersurface of the dermis, there is no need to change planes, effect a heart-shaped suture placement, or guarantee that the suture exit point is precisely at the inside edge of the lower dermis, as may be needed with the buried vertical mattress suture.

Accurate suture placement is predicated on having a sufficiently undermined plane, since the entire suture loop lays on the undersurface of the dermis. Therefore, broad undermining is a prerequisite for utilizing this technique, since the first throw of the needle begins 2-6 mm distant from the incised wound edge.

This technique may also be used to minimize dead space when excising a space-occupying lesion such as a cyst or lipoma. In this event, taking the first bite set back even further from the incised wound edge will translate into a larger ridge and will simultaneously minimize the laxity in the central portion of the wound as the dermis is pulled taut so that potential dead space is converted to a hyper-everted wound ridge that will absorb with time.

Finally, a recent study has demonstrated that treating chest keloids with a combination of the set-back suture and postoperative electron beam irradiation led to an almost 98% success rate. The authors posited that the combination of tension reduction across the wound surface coupled with deep suture placement and suture material placement away from the incised wound edge was responsible for this dramatic effect.

Drawbacks and Cautions

The set-back dermal approach creates significant wound eversion, and the degree of eversion elicited by this approach may, depending on how far set back the dermal bite is taken, elicit significantly more wound eversion than even the buried vertical mattress technique.

Patients should be cautioned that they might develop a significant ridge in the immediate postoperative period. Depending on the suture material used and the density of the sutures, this ridge may last from weeks to months. Explaining that the technique is akin to placing a subcutaneous splint may help the patient develop reasonable and realistic expectations and reduce anxiety regarding the immediate postoperative appearance of the wound.

A possible complication of overeversion and an overly broad bite is that the raised ridge may be too large or bulky to be supported by the deep sutures. In this event, the wound edges may paradoxically collapse centrally leading to the appearance of a dramatically raised ridge with a central valley approximately 1 week postoperatively. As the sutures absorb over time, this will yield a depressed or inverted scar line. This can generally be avoided by not setting back the sutures more than a few millimeters from the wound edge and by placing a sufficient number of sutures so that the body of the ridge may be easily supported.

Epidermal dimpling will occasionally occur where the arc of the suture reaches its apex at the dermal-epidermal junction; on the face and areas with thin dermis, this should be assiduously avoided. Similarly, areas with sebaceous skin, such as the nose, require meticulous avoidance of dimpling, which has the potential to persist. In truncal areas or those with thick dermis, however, a small degree of dimpling will resolve with time as the absorbable sutures are gradually resorbed.

References

Kantor J. The set-back buried dermal suture: an alternative to the buried vertical mattress for layered wound closure. *J Am Acad Dermatol.* 2010;62(2):351-353.

Kantor J. The subcutaneous splint: a helpful analogy to explain postoperative wound eversion. *JAMA Dermatol.* 2014;150(10):1122.

Trufant JW, Leach BC. Commentary: wound edge eversion: surgical dogma or diversion? *J Am Acad Dermatol.* 2015;72:681-682.

Wang AS, Kleinerman R, Armstrong AW, et al. Set-back versus buried vertical mattress suturing: results of a randomized blinded trial. *J Am Acad Dermatol.* 2015;72:674-680.

Wang LZ, Ding JP, Yang MYU, Chen B. Forty-five cases of chest keloids treated with subcutaneous super-tension-reduction suture combined with postoperative electron-beam irradiation. *Dermatol Surg.* 2014;40:1378-1384.

Yang X-Y, Zhou T-T, Cao L. A simplified positioning technique for the set-back suture. *J Am Acad Dermatol.* In press. https://doi.org/10.1016/j.jaad.2020.11.031

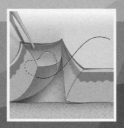

CHAPTER 4.3

The Buried Vertical Mattress Suture

Video 4-3. Buried vertical mattress suture

Access to video can be found via mhprofessional.com/atlasofsuturingtechniques2e

Application

This technique is a workhorse approach that is widely utilized by dermatologists and plastic surgeons. It is best used in areas under mild to moderate tension and is a highly effective approach that may be utilized on the face, as well as the extremities and trunk.

Because of the need to shift planes and the fact that the needle travels in the papillary dermis, this technique may not be particularly well suited to areas with atrophic skin. In areas with a very thick dermis or under extreme tension, the set-back suture may be easier to place and reduce the risk of bending a needle.

Suture Material Choice

Suture choice is dependent in large part on location, though since suture material traverses the papillary dermis and the incised wound edge, as always, the smallest gauge suture material appropriate for the anatomic location should be utilized. On the back and shoulders, 2-0 or 3-0 suture material is effective, though theoretically the risk of suture splitting or suture abscess formation is greater with the thicker 2-0 suture material. This needs to be weighed against the benefit of utilizing a larger CP-2 needle, which will almost never bend even

in the thickest dermis, and the benefit of adopting the 2-0 suture material, which is less likely to snap under tension or fail during tension-bearing activities, leading to attendant dehiscence. On the extremities, a 3-0 or 4-0 absorbable suture material may be used, and on the face and areas under minimal tension, a 5-0 absorbable suture is adequate.

Technique

1. The wound edge is reflected back using surgical forceps or hooks. Adequate visualization of the underside of the dermis is desirable.
2. While reflecting back the dermis, the suture needle is inserted at 90 degrees into the underside of the dermis, 4 mm distant from the incised wound edge.
3. The first bite is executed by following the needle initially at 90 degrees to the underside of the dermis and then, critically, changing direction by twisting the needle driver so that the needle exits in the incised wound edge. This allows the apex of the bite to remain in the papillary dermis while the needle exits in the incised wound edge at the level of the reticular dermis.
4. Keeping the loose end of the suture between the surgeon and the patient, the dermis on the side of the first bite is released. The tissue on the opposite edge is then reflected back in a similar fashion as on the first side.
5. The second and final bite is executed by inserting the needle into the

incised wound edge at the level of the reticular dermis. It then angles upward and laterally so that the apex

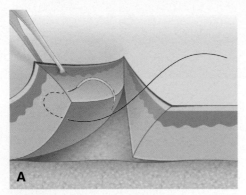

A

Figure 4-3A. The needle is inserted through the underside of the dermis and moves upward and outward in the dermis before returning to exit at the incised wound edge.

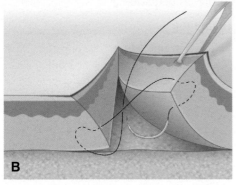

B

Figure 4-3B. The needle is then inserted through the incised wound edge before moving upward and outward away from the wound edge and exiting in the deeper dermis.

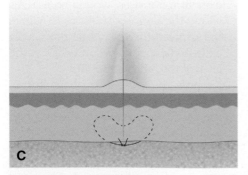

C

Figure 4-3C. Lateral view of the buried vertical mattress suture highlighting the heart-shaped path the suture material takes through the dermis.

of the needle is at the level of the papillary dermis. This should mirror the first bite taken on the contralateral side of the wound.

6. The suture material is then tied utilizing an instrument tie (Figures 4-3A through 4-3H).

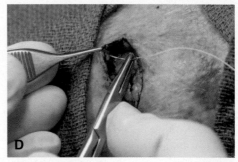

D

Figure 4-3D. The needle is inserted through the underside of the dermis and moves upward and outward in the dermis.

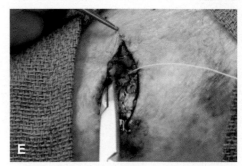

E

Figure 4-3E. The needle then exits at the incised wound edge.

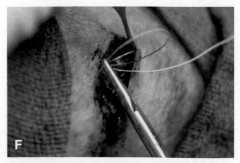

F

Figure 4-3F. The needle is then inserted through the contralateral incised wound edge before moving upward and outward away from the wound edge.

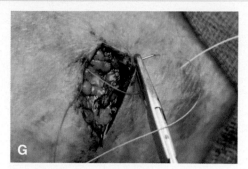

Figure 4-3G. The needle continues its rotation and exits in the deeper dermis.

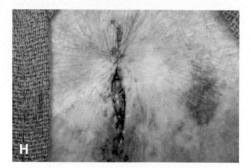

Figure 4-3H. Immediate postoperative appearance after placing a single buried vertical mattress suture in atrophic skin.

Tips and Pearls

This technique requires some practice to master, though once mastered it is straightforward to execute. The first bite may also be finessed by first reflecting the wound edge back sharply during needle insertion and then returning the edge medially after the apex has been reached. This approach helps lead the needle in the correct course without an exaggerated changed in direction with the needle driver and is often preferred by experienced surgeons.

A similar approach may be utilized by surgeons who favor skin hooks over surgical forceps; here again, the hook may be used to hyper-reflect the skin edge back during the first portion of the first bite and then similarly pull the incised wound edge toward the center of the wound during the second portion of the

first bite. This will encourage the needle to follow the desired heart-shaped path without necessitating a dramatic twist of the needle driver as the needle changes course. When suturing, the obviously active element (the needle and needle driver, held by the dominant hand) and the ostensibly passive element (the skin, held by forceps or a skin hook) have the potential to move in three dimensions. Thus, changing the way the needle moves through the skin can be accomplished by either adjusting the way the needle is moved through the skin with the dominant hand, adjusting how the skin is held or manipulated by the other hand, or a combination of the two. With experience, a combination is often more effective at implementing the vertical mattress suture in an elegant and efficient fashion.

The apex of the needle should be in the papillary dermis; if the needle courses too superficially, dimpling may occur. While such dimpling is sometimes almost unavoidable, such as in areas with a very thin dermis such as the eyelids, and generally resolves with time, it remains best to avoid it if possible since: (1) patients may sometimes have some concern regarding the immediate postoperative appearance, and (2) dimpling signifies that the suture material traverses very superficially, raising concern that it could be associated with an increased risk of suture spitting.

This technique, if executed appropriately, leads to both excellent wound eversion and outstanding wound-edge approximation, explaining the popularity of this approach among plastic surgeons and dermatologists.

A particularly well-executed traditional simple buried dermal suture is very similar to the buried vertical mattress, since the placement of the suture following the curvature of the needle results in a slight eversion of the wound edge.

This approach has also been described in the context of a modified buried vertical mattress suture, which relies on the same suture technique but assumes that the wound edges were incised with a reverse bevel, similar to a butterfly suture.

Drawbacks and Cautions

In areas under marked tension, such as the back, this technique should be executed with caution in order to minimize the risk of bending the needle especially when smaller needles, such as the FS and PS, are used.

While the eversion is less pronounced than is seen with other techniques, such as the set-back dermal suture, patients may still be left with a small ridge in the immediate postoperative period. While this is desirable, it is also important to warn patients of this outcome; explaining that the technique is akin to placing a subcutaneous splint may help the patient develop reasonable and realistic expectations and reduce anxiety regarding the immediate postoperative appearance of the wound.

References

Liu Z, Tang Z, Hao X, et al. Modified buried vertical mattress suture versus buried intradermal suture: a prospective split-scar study. *Dermatol Surg.* 2020. Epub ahead of print. doi:10.1097/DSS.0000000000002642

Straith RE, Lawson JM, Hipps CJ. The subcuticular suture. *Postgrad Med.* 1961;29:164-173.

Zitelli JA, Moy RL. Buried vertical mattress suture. *J Dermatol Surg Oncol.* 1989;15(1):17-19.

The Buried Horizontal Mattress Suture

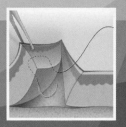

Synonym

Fully buried horizontal mattress suture

 Video 4-4. Buried horizontal mattress suture
Access to video can be found via mhprofessional.com/atlasofsuturingtechniques2e

Application

This is a niche technique, useful when closing narrow wounds or those where there is limited space to insert the needle driver and when placing a buried suture is desirable. It may be employed in a variety of locations, including the scalp, ears, and lower leg, though it has been applied broadly and may be utilized in any number of anatomic locations.

This technique results in adequate wound eversion; depending on how far back the bites are taken and whether the incised wound edge is cut with an inward bevel, it may result in only modest wound-edge approximation.

Suture Material Choice

As always, suture material choice depends on preference and location; while the suture material remains on the undersurface of the dermis, it does traverse the midpapillary dermis, and therefore, care should be taken to utilize the smallest caliber of suture that provides adequate tensile strength. Similarly, the knot remains relatively superficial at the level of the reticular dermis, confirming the need to utilize the finest suture available.

This approach should only rarely be used in areas with a thick dermis and under marked tension, such as the chest and back. On the extremities, a 4-0 absorbable suture material may be used, and on the face and areas under minimal tension, a 5-0 absorbable suture is adequate. A 3-0 caliber suture may be used on areas such as the lower legs if needed, though this should be utilized with caution as the larger caliber suture material has more of a tendency to spit or result in foreign-body reactions.

Technique

1. The wound edge is reflected back using surgical forceps or hooks. Adequate visualization of the underside of the dermis is desirable.
2. While reflecting back the dermis, the suture needle is inserted into the undersurface of the dermis parallel to the incision line just lateral to the incised wound edge.
3. The first bite is executed by placing gentle pressure on the needle so that it enters the papillary dermis and then relaxing pressure to permit the needle to exit on the undersurface of the dermis.
4. Keeping the loose end of suture between the surgeon and the patient, the dermis on the side of the first bite is released. The tissue on the opposite edge is then reflected back in a similar fashion as on the first side.

5. The second and final bite is executed by inserting the needle into the undersurface of the dermis on the contralateral side, with a backhand technique if desired, and completing a mirror-image loop, so that the needle exits directly across from its original entry point on the contralateral side.

6. The suture material is then tied utilizing an instrument tie (Figures 4-4A through 4-4F).

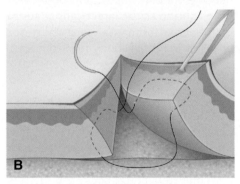

Figure 4-4A. The needle is inserted through the dermis running parallel to the incised wound edge.

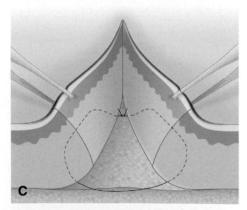

Figure 4-4B. This procedure is then reversed on the contralateral wound edge.

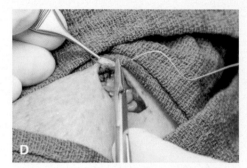

Figure 4-4D. The needle is inserted through the dermis, slightly set back from the wound edge, running parallel to the incised wound edge.

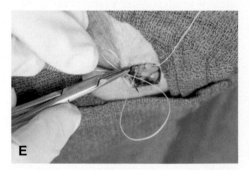

Figure 4-4E. This procedure is then reversed on the contralateral wound edge.

Figure 4-4C. Overview of the buried horizontal mattress suture technique.

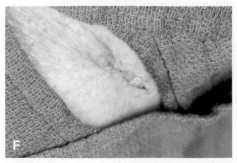

Figure 4-4F. Wound appearance after placement of a single buried horizontal mattress suture. Note the marked wound-edge eversion.

Tips and Pearls

This technique is useful for narrow or shallow wounds, such as those on the scalp and shins. It may also be used when adding an additional buried suture in an otherwise largely closed wound, where there is insufficient space to insert a vertically oriented buried suture in the narrow space between two other already-placed sutures.

As with the buried vertical mattress approach, the first bite may be finessed by first reflecting the wound edge back sharply during needle insertion and then returning the edge medially after the apex has been reached. This approach helps lead the needle in the correct course without an exaggerated change in direction with the needle driver, though the needle is oriented parallel to the incised wound edge, as opposed to the perpendicular approach utilized with the buried vertical mattress.

The needle driver may also be held like a pencil, and the needle may then be rotated through the dermis while reflecting back with the forceps to permit easy visualization.

As with any buried technique, the apex of the needle should be in or deep to the papillary dermis; if the needle courses too superficially, dimpling may occur.

Drawbacks and Cautions

While some have suggested this as a standard technique for excisional surgery, in general, this technique should not be adopted in all areas, and there are better options for use in areas with a robust dermis under moderate to marked tension, such as the back and shoulders. In those locations, the buried horizontal mattress approach should only be utilized for inserting additional sutures in between already-placed buried sutures, when there is insufficient space to place a set-back dermal suture or buried vertical mattress suture.

While the eversion is less pronounced than with other techniques, such as the set-back dermal suture, patients may still be left with a small ridge in the immediate postoperative period. While this is desirable, it is also important to warn patients of this outcome; explaining that the technique is akin to placing a subcutaneous splint may help the patient develop reasonable and realistic expectations and reduce anxiety regarding the immediate postoperative appearance of the wound.

Wound-edge necrosis has been raised as a potential risk of horizontally oriented suture placement, but in practice, this is only encountered very rarely and as a complication of tightly placed traditional horizontal mattress sutures, rather than with the buried equivalent. This is likely due to a constrictive effect on the incised wound edge, which is not typically seen with buried sutures.

The original description of this approach bears some resemblance to the butterfly suture; keeping in mind that the buried horizontal mattress suture should represent a buried version of the traditional horizontal mattress approach, however, the needle entry and exit points should both be in the undersurface of the dermis just lateral to the incised wound edge, as opposed to the butterfly suture where entry and exit occur at the juncture of the incised wound edge and the undersurface of the dermis and where the needle arcs on a diagonal.

References

Alam M, Goldberg LH. Utility of fully buried horizontal mattress sutures. *J Am Acad Dermatol.* 2004;50(1):73-76.

Nantel-Battista M, Murray C. Dermatologic surgical pearls: enhancing the efficacy of the traditional elliptical excision. *J Cutan Med Surg.* 2015;19(3):287-290.

The Butterfly Suture

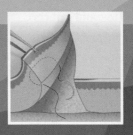

Video 4-5. Butterfly suture
Access to video can be found via
mhprofessional.com/atlasofsuturingtechniques2e

Application

The butterfly suture technique is a buried technique designed for wounds under moderate to marked tension. It is best utilized on the trunk and shoulders, where the combination of a thick dermis and the need for marked tension relief make it an occasionally useful approach.

Suture Material Choice

Suture material choice depends on preference and location. Though this technique is designed for wounds under significant tension on the trunk, it is commonly performed with a 3-0 suture. While adopting a 2-0 suture material is sometimes useful, especially to avoid bending smaller needles, the knot for this suture is buried in line with the incision and at the base of the dermis, and therefore, suture material spitting is a risk. Use of an absorbable monofilament (polydioxanone) has been proposed as providing superior outcomes over a braided absorbable suture.

Technique

1. This technique ideally requires that the wound edges be incised with a reverse bevel, allowing the epidermis to overhang the dermis in the center of the wound.

2. The wound edge is reflected back using surgical forceps or hooks. Adequate full visualization of the underside of the dermis is very helpful.

3. While reflecting back the dermis, the suture needle is inserted into the undersurface of the dermis near the junction of the base of the incised wound edge and the undersurface of the undermined dermis. The needle driver is held like a pencil at 90 degrees to the incised wound edge, and the needle may be held on the needle driver at an oblique angle to facilitate suture placement.

4. The first bite is executed by placing gentle pressure on the needle so that it moves laterally and upward, forming a horizontal loop that on cross section resembles the wing of a butterfly. The needle then exits the undersurface of the dermis after following its curvature, in the same plane as its entrance point.

5. Keeping the loose end of suture between the surgeon and the patient, the dermis on the side of the first bite is released. The tissue on the opposite edge is then reflected back in a similar fashion as on the first side.

6. The second and final bite is executed by inserting the needle into the undersurface of the dermis on the contralateral side, with a backhand technique if desired, and completing a mirror-image loop. The suture

material exits directly across from its initial entry point.

7. The suture material is then tied utilizing an instrument tie (Figures 4-5A through 4-5E).

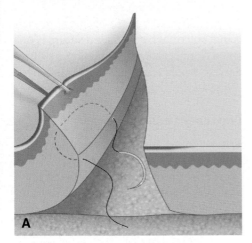

Figure 4-5A. First step of the butterfly suture technique.

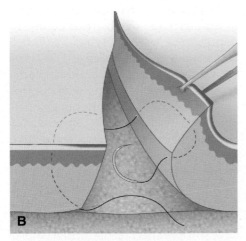

Figure 4-5B. Second step of the butterfly suture, presenting a mirror image of the first step.

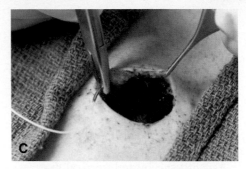

Figure 4-5C. First step of the butterfly suture technique. Note that the needle driver is held like a pencil and the needle is passed in a plane parallel to the incised wound edge, at an approximately 45-degree angle so that a more superficial bite of dermis is taken when the needle reaches its apex, leading to wound-edge eversion.

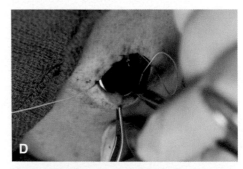

Figure 4-5D. Second step of the butterfly suture, presenting a mirror image of the first step.

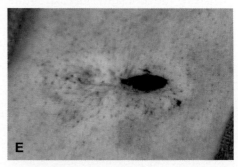

Figure 4-5E. Immediate postoperative appearance. Note the pronounced eversion.

Tips and Pearls

This technique is designed for areas under tension, though it may be used in any anatomic location. As such, utilizing a sufficiently robust needle may be very helpful in mitigating the risk of needle bending that can be seen when attempting to place the needle in the thick dermis of the back.

As with the buried vertical mattress approach, the first bite may be finessed by first reflecting the wound edge back sharply during needle insertion and then returning the edge medially after the apex has been reached. This approach helps lead the needle in the correct course without an exaggerated change in direction with the needle driver, though the needle is oriented parallel to the incised wound edge, and on a diagonal relative to the vertical axis, as opposed to the perpendicular approach utilized with the buried vertical mattress.

As with most approaches, the apex of the needle's pass should be in the papillary dermis or deeper; if the needle courses too superficially, dimpling may occur. This technique is unique in that it incorporates a large segment of dermis along the axis of the wound, theoretically increasing the robustness of each suture placement, and that it has the needle move on an upward and outward diagonal from the wound edge, facilitating wound eversion as well.

Proponents of this technique have advocated the use of a long-lasting nonabsorbable monofilament suture material, polydioxanone, since it retains its strength for an extended period of time and is therefore particularly amenable to use in high-tension closures.

Like the buried horizontal mattress suture, an advantage of this approach is the relatively generous section of dermis included in each suture. In areas of atrophy, the broader bite of dermis included in each suture may help mitigate the risk of tearing through the atrophic dermis that may be encountered when utilizing vertically oriented buried sutures in these circumstances.

An additional benefit of this approach is that since each completed suture is oriented horizontally, less individual sutures need to be placed to cover a given length of the wound.

Drawbacks and Cautions

The need to bevel the wound edges means that this technique requires a small degree of preplanning. The bevel may, however, be useful for other techniques as well, as it may help with wound-edge apposition in general, though there is also the theoretical risk of contracture leading to a small separation between the wound edges. If the butterfly suture is utilized without beveling the wound edges, a small amount of dermis may overhang in the incised wound edges, preventing wound-edge apposition. In this event, surgical scissors or a blade may be used to trim back the overhanging dermis to permit the epidermal wound edges to come together unimpeded.

Some authors have raised concerns regarding possible wound-edge necrosis associated with horizontally oriented suture placement. Advocates of this approach report that wound-edge necrosis has not been seen as a complication, and necrosis is generally only an issue with superficially placed horizontal mattress sutures, rather than with their buried counterparts. This is likely due to a constrictive effect on the incised wound edge, something not typically seen with buried sutures.

This technique should probably be avoided on the eyelids, as the dramatic eversion may not resolve with time with the thin dermis and minimal tension across the wound edges. Similarly, in areas where inversion is desirable, such as the nasolabial folds, this technique should similarly be avoided.

Given the marked eversion associated with this technique, patients may be left with a small ridge in the immediate postoperative period. While this is desirable, it is also important to warn patients of this outcome; explaining that the technique is akin to placing a subcutaneous splint may help the patient develop reasonable and realistic expectations and reduce anxiety regarding the immediate postoperative appearance of the wound.

References

Breuninger H, Keilbach J, Haaf U. Intracutaneous butterfly suture with absorbable synthetic suture material. Technique, tissue reactions, and results. *J Dermatol Surg Oncol.* 1993;19(7):607-610.

Breuninger, H. Intracutaneous butterfly suture: a horizontal buried interrupted suture for high tension. *Eur J Plast Surg.* 1998;2(8):415-419.

The Fascial Plication Suture

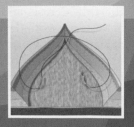

Video 4-6. Fascial plication suture

Access to video can be found via mhprofessional.com/atlasofsuturingtechniques2e

Application

This technique is designed for wounds under marked tension, especially those on the back and shoulders. It is a deep technique, permitting the tension of wound closure to shift from the dermis to the fascia, concomitantly creating a lower tension closure that is associated with less scar spread. In addition to tension reduction, this approach also leads to an increase in the apparent length-to-width ratio of an excised ellipse and improved dead-space minimization.

Suture Material Choice

Suture choice is dependent in large part on location. As this technique is designed to bite the fascia, generally a larger gauge suture can be utilized. Therefore, for the back and shoulders, a 2-0 or 3-0 absorbable suture may be used. Since suture material traverses the fascia, the incidence of suture abscess formation is vanishingly rare. If this technique is used on the scalp or forehead, a 4-0 absorbable suture may be used.

Technique

1. The wound edges are reflected back to permit visualization of the deep bed of the wound. In deep excisions,

such as those performed for melanoma or large cysts, the muscle fascia may be directly visible. Otherwise, visualizing the subcutaneous fat is appropriate as well.

2. The suture needle is inserted at 90 degrees through the deep fat 2-4 mm medial to the lateral undermined edge of the wound, running parallel to the incised wound edge.

3. The first bite is executed by entering the fascia and following the curvature of the needle. The suture material may be gently pulled to test that a successful bite of fascia has been taken.

4. Keeping the loose end of suture between the surgeon and the patient, attention is then shifted to the opposite side of the wound. The second bite is executed by repeating the procedure on the contralateral side, but with the needle entering in line with its initial exit point on the first side and exiting in line with its entry point on the first side.

5. The suture material is then tied utilizing an instrument tie. Hand tying may be utilized as well, particularly if the wound is deep and the instruments cannot be easily inserted to complete the tie (Figures 4-6A through 4-6F).

Tips and Pearls

This technique is very useful for wounds under marked tension, especially for large defects on the back and shoulders. Even

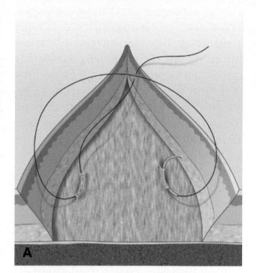

Figure 4-6A. Overview of the fascial plication suture technique. (Reproduced with permission from Kantor J. *Dermatologic Surgery and Cosmetic Procedures in Primary Care Practice.* New York, NY: McGraw Hill, 2021.)

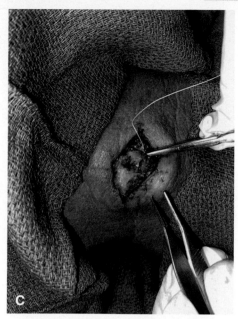

Figure 4-6C. Completed first throw of the fascial plication suture.

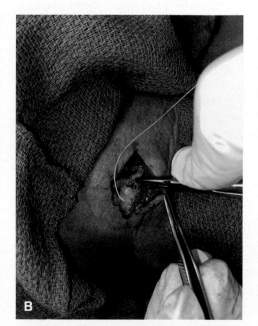

Figure 4-6B. Beginning of the first throw of the fascial plication suture. Note that the needle is inserted blindly through the subcutaneous fat at a 90-degree angle.

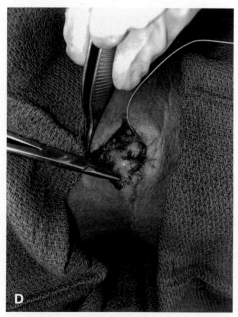

Figure 4-6D. Beginning of the second throw of the fascial plication suture. Note again that the needle entry occurs at 90 degrees to the fat and that the undermined dermis is reflected back, away from the center of the wound.

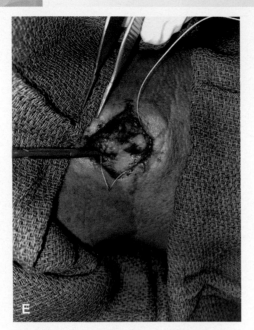

Figure 4-6E. Completed second throw of the fascial plication suture.

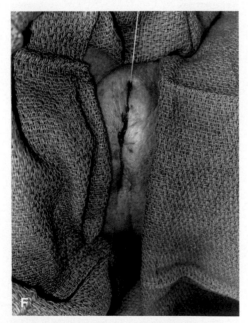

Figure 4-6F. Wound appearance after placing a single fascial plication suture. Note the more exaggerated fusiform appearance of the wound after suture placement.

a deep, gaping wound can be converted into a manageable fusiform defect with a single well-placed fascial plication suture. It can therefore be conceptualized as an alternative to pulley sutures that affords both a decrease in tension across the wound surface (by shifting tension from the dermis to the fascia) and an increase in the length-to-width ratio of the ellipse. This also makes the placement of standard buried sutures, such as set-back sutures, much easier since the wound edges are already brought close together under no tension through the single fascial plication suture.

Indeed, this approach often leads to a more fusiform defect, even when an oval-shaped excision has been performed. Therefore, it may be useful when attempting to keep a defect as short as possible without dog-ear formation. In cases where this approach is anticipated, it may be worthwhile to create a defect with a length-to-width ratio of less than 3:1, as is traditionally employed, as that may be sufficient to lead to a tapered ellipse.

A single fascial plication suture may be placed in the center of the wound. This balances the benefit of dead-space minimization and tension relief with the desire to minimize suture material piercing the muscle fascia, which may be associated with increased postoperative pain and a theoretical increase in infection rate.

In large wounds under marked tension, a series of spaced fascial plication sutures may be placed as well. Except for the largest wounds, typically no more than two or three sutures are needed to effectively plicate the underlying fascia.

This technique is also useful when large space-occupying lesions, such as cysts or lipomas, have been extirpated. In these cases, placing dermal sutures alone results in significant residual dead space that may be associated with a higher risk of hematoma or seroma formation, as well as subsequent infection. Fascial plication may serve to help minimize this dead space by pulling deeper structures centrally and thereby filling the potential space.

Drawbacks and Cautions

The chief drawback of this approach is the potential for increased postoperative pain when compared with utilizing dermal sutures alone. While this is not a typical occurrence, depending on how deep the suture material traverses through fascia—and the underlying muscle—pain may sometimes be experienced that is out of proportion to the defect size and depth. Generally this is felt at the time of needle insertion and resolves within 30 seconds; if it does not, the suture should be removed.

The other risk of this technique is plicating a nerve or vessel within the suture; therefore, this technique should be used with caution in danger zones or in areas where this is anticipated to represent a significant risk. While this technique is classically used on the back and chest, it can be very useful on the face as well, where even large defects can often be closed in a linear fashion as long as a judiciously placed fascial plication suture is used by surgeons with a well-developed appreciation of facial anatomy.

The lateral bites in the fascia should be taken no closer than 1-2 mm from the far lateral undermined edge of the tissue. Taking bites too far laterally, where there is no undermined plane between fascia and dermis, may result in dimpling at the lateral edges. This dimpling occurs when the bites of fascia are directly contiguous with the overlying dermis and epidermis, and the suture's lateral tension on the fascia also pulls on the dermis. While the dimpling may resolve with time, it is best avoided if possible.

References

Dzubow LM. The use of fascial plication to facilitate wound closure following microscopically controlled surgery. *J Dermatol Surg Oncol.* 1989;15(10):1063-1066.

Kantor J. The fascial plication suture: an adjunct to layered wound closure. *Arch Dermatol.* 2009;145(12):1454-1456.

The Running Subcuticular Suture

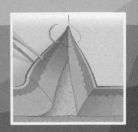

 Video 4-7. Running subcuticular suture
Access to video can be found via
mhprofessional.com/atlasofsuturingtechniques2e.

Application

This is an epidermal approximation technique suitable for wounds under minimal to no tension. This technique should almost never be employed in the absence of a deep dermal suture, since its strength is in fine-tuning epidermal approximation and it is less effective in the presence of significant tension. Its use is also predicated on the presence of a relatively robust dermis, since it is a primarily intradermal technique and therefore does not recruit any strength from the epidermis. Therefore, it should be avoided in the context of atrophic skin or in areas with a very thin dermis, such as the eyelids.

Suture Material Choice

As with any technique, it is best to utilize the thinnest suture possible for any given anatomic location. The subcuticular suture technique is not designed to hold tension irrespective of anatomic location. Since its utility is limited to fine-tuning epidermal approximation, 5-0 or 6-0 suture is often useful when adopting this technique.

Depending on the chosen technique variation, this technique may be used with either absorbable or nonabsorbable suture. If nonabsorbable suture is used, it is best to utilize a monofilament suture material to minimize the coefficient of friction when removing the suture. Since a relatively large amount of suture material will be left in the superficial dermis, if absorbable material is used, then utilizing a nonbraided monofilament suture may be best to minimize the risk of infection and foreign-body reaction.

Technique

1. The needle is inserted at the far right corner of the wound, parallel to the incision line, beginning approximately 2-5 mm from the apex. The needle is passed from this point, which is lateral to the incision apex, directly through the epidermis, exiting into the interior of the wound just medial to the apex. Note that this first pass may be finessed depending on the technique used for finishing the closure, as addressed in detail below.

2. With the tail of the suture material resting lateral to the incision apex and outside the wound, the wound edge is gently reflected back and the needle is inserted into the dermis on the far edge of the wound with a trajectory running parallel to the incision line. The needle, and therefore the suture, should pass through the dermis at a uniform depth. Bite size is dependent on needle size, though in order to minimize the risk of necrosis, it may be prudent to restrict the

size of each bite. The needle should exit the dermis at a point equidistant from the cut edge from where it entered.

3. The needle is then grasped with the surgical pickups and simultaneously released by the hand holding the needle driver. As the needle is freed from the tissue with the pickups, the needle is grasped again by the needle driver in an appropriate position to repeat the above step on the contralateral edge of the incised wound edge.

4. A small amount of suture material is pulled through, the skin of the contralateral wound edge is reflected back, and the needle is inserted into the dermis on the contralateral side of the incised wound edge and the same movement is repeated. The needle should enter slightly proximal (relative to the wound apex where the suture line began) to the exit point, thus introducing a small degree of backtracking to the snake-like flow of the suture material. This will help reduce the risk of tissue bunching.

5. The same technique is repeated on the contralateral side until the end of the wound is reached. At this point, the needle is inserted from the interior of the wound in line with the incision line and exits just lateral to the apex of the wound (Figures 4-7A through 4-7J).

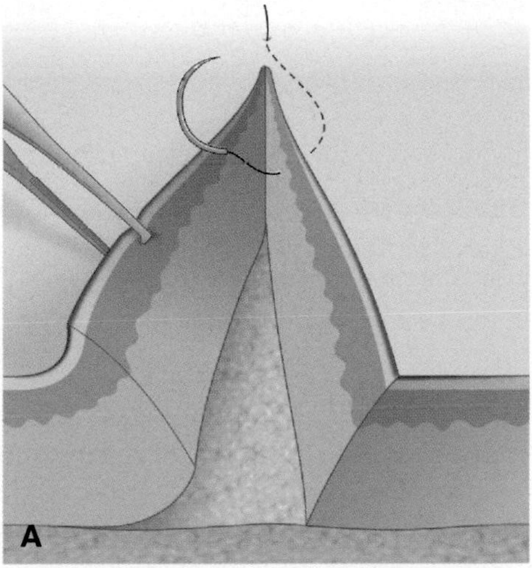

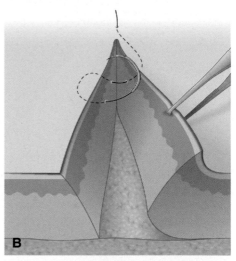

Figure 4-7B. This procedure is repeated on the contralateral wound edge.

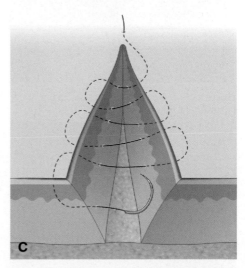

Figure 4-7C. Overview of the running subcuticular technique.

Figure 4-7A. After passing the needle from outside of the wound apex to the interior of the wound, the needle is rotated superficially through the dermis.

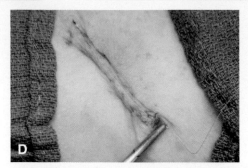

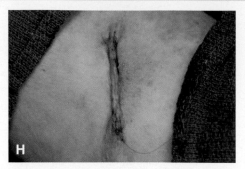

Figure 4-7D. The needle is passed from outside of the wound apex to the interior of the wound.

Figure 4-7H. Immediate postoperative appearance, with the leading and trailing suture material still visible.

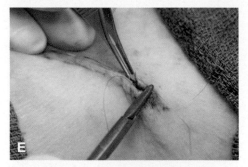

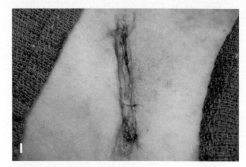

Figure 4-7E. The needle is then rotated superficially through the dermis on one side of the incised wound edge.

Figure 4-7I. Postoperative appearance when the suture is tied over top of the wound.

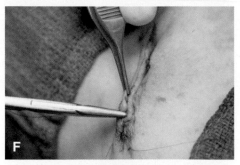

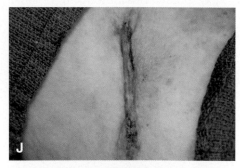

Figure 4-7F. This procedure is repeated on the contra-lateral wound edge.

Figure 4-6J. Postoperative appearance when the suture material is trimmed at the epidermis.

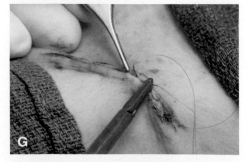

Figure 4-7G. The technique is repeated on alternating sides along the course of the wound.

Tips and Pearls

Body positioning can be very helpful in maintaining an efficient and comfortable subcuticular technique. Most surgeons are trained to work with the surgical site flat and perpendicular to their body. Since the motions associated with subcuticular suture placement are 90 degrees off from this, it may be useful to stand with the surgeon's body (shoulder to shoulder) parallel to the incision line. This allows for a flowing motion from right to left without the need to twist the shoulders or wrists.

One of the classic conundrums relating to this technique is how to start and finish the closure; there are myriad options available to the surgeon. Some of the available options for finishing this suture include the following:

1. Clipping the ends of the suture at the level of the epidermis: This technique is of maximal convenience to surgeon and patient and minimizes the risk of leaving any track marks whatsoever. Since the ends of the suture are not tacked down in any way, however, it does not have the potential to hold the epidermis in place in the face of stress. This is particularly true if an absorbable monofilament suture is used, as it can easily slip through the dermis and will naturally slip away from the areas under most tension.

2. Clipping the ends of the suture after leaving a long (3-6 cm) tail: The tails may be tacked down with adhesive strips, tissue glue, or surgical tape to minimize slippage over time. This approach is most suited if nonabsorbable monofilament will be used, as it may be left in place for 6 weeks or more. If the suture tails are not fixed in place, this may lead to some surface irritation where the suture material exits lateral to the apices of the wound.

3. Tying a single buried dermal suture or set-back dermal suture at each end of the running subcuticular loop: The first dermal suture is tied at the far end, and the end of the suture is trimmed either at the knot or slightly above the knot. The running subcuticular technique is then executed as noted earlier and a similar knot is tied at the other end. In this case, the first and last throws of suture do not begin and end outside of the wound (as outlined previously), but rather as dermal sutures at the apices of the repair.

4. The ends of the suture may be tied to each other in a bow over the top of the wound: This requires leaving sufficient laxity at the beginning as well as pulling through sufficient suture material so that the bow may be tied at approximately the center point of the wound. Risks associated with this approach include torque-induced tissue damage at the apices where the suture material exits the wound as well as the risk that the loose bow may be pulled by the dressing or an inattentive patient.

Attempting to execute this technique with fewer dermal bites occasionally results in crimping of the epidermis as the wound edges pleat together. This may be avoided by setting back each bite of the dermis slightly relative to the apex so that the pattern the suture makes in the dermis consists of wider U-shaped bites moving in a serpiginous pattern. Assiduous attention to detail in taking a sufficient number of bites should effectively mitigate the risk of epidermal crimping.

A smooth, flowing technique is of paramount importance in executing this technique effectively and efficiently. Some authors have advocated adjusting the angle used to hold the needle in the needle driver from the traditional 90 degrees to 135 degrees to increase the surgeon's comfort and minimize the need for physical contortion, though slightly adjusting the surgeon's body position helps significantly in this regard and obviates the need to adjust the needle loading angle.

Drawbacks and Cautions

While a central strength of the running subcuticular suture is its entirely intradermal placement, this may also represent one of its greatest drawbacks. This technique results in leaving a significant quantity of foreign-body material in the dermis in a continuous fashion. While this may not represent a major problem in areas with a thick dermis such as the back, in other anatomical locations, the large quantity of suture that is left in situ may result in concerns regarding infection, foreign-body reaction, and even the potential that the suture material itself could present a physical barrier that would impinge on the ability of the wound to heal appropriately—essentially an iatrogenic eschar phenomenon.

A similar concern relates to leaving a suture tunnel if nonabsorbable suture material is used and is then removed after a period of time. As one of the benefits of this approach is to permit the suture to remain in place for many weeks or months, it also means that removal of long-standing suture entails a theoretical risk that a potential space—albeit a thin and long one—is created on the removal of the suture material. Again, this theoretical risk may be mitigated by utilizing the thinnest possible suture material.

If nonabsorbable suture material is used, care should be taken to account for the eventual necessity of suture removal. Since the nonabsorbable monofilament will be removed by applying a continuous gentle pull on the free edge of the suture, it is imperative that the length of the continuous suture be kept to a reasonable maximum, to avoid the risk of suture snapping mid pull. In cases where a longer wound is closed using nonabsorbable suture material, a single simple interrupted suture may be placed as part of the course of the suture material every 4 cm or so, providing a site where the suture material may be snipped and pulled through at the time of suture removal.

In the event that slow-absorbing absorbable suture is used, consideration should be given to utilizing undyed suture material, since depending on the depth of suture placement and the degree of epidermal atrophy the suture material may sometimes remain visible.

Depending on the placement of the deep sutures, it is possible for this technique to lead to some mild inversion of the epidermal edges as they are pulled inward by the suture material. This is particularly the case when the suture is finished with a fixed knot holding the ends of the suture material in a fixed position. A randomized trial comparing running subcuticular sutures with nonabsorbable suture material (removed 1 week postoperatively) and simple interrupted sutures (also removed after 1 week) for the closure of facial wounds found no difference in cosmesis between groups, although hypo- and hyperesthesia were noted more frequently in the group closed with subcuticular sutures.

References

Ahmed AM, Orengo I. Surgical pearl: alternate method of loading needle to facilitate subcuticular suturing. *J Am Acad Dermatol*. 2007;56(5 suppl):S105-106.

Bickel KD, Gibbs NF, Cunningham BB. The subcuticular "spider" stitch: a simple solution to suture breakage and patient discomfort in long incisions. *Pediatr Dermatol*. 1998;15(6):480-481.

Clay FS, Walsh CA, Walsh SR. Staples vs subcuticular sutures for skin closure at cesarean delivery: a metaanalysis of randomized controlled trials. *Am J Obstet Gynecol*. 2011;204(5):378-383.

Figueroa D, Jauk VC, Szychowski JM, et al. Surgical staples compared with subcuticular suture for skin closure after cesarean delivery: a randomized controlled trial. *Obstet Gynecol*. 2013;121(1):33-38.

Genders RE, Hamminga EA, Kukutsch NA. Securing the subcuticular running suture. *Dermatol Surg.* 2012;38(10):1722-1724.

Lazar HL, McCann J, Fitzgerald CA, Cabral HJ. Adhesive strips versus subcuticular suture for median sternotomy wound closure. *J Card Surg.* 2011;26(4):344-347.

Liu X, Nelemans PJ, Frenk LDS, et al. Aesthetic outcome and complications of simple interrupted versus running subcuticular sutures in facial surgery: a randomized controlled trial. *J Am Acad Dermatol.* 2017;77(5):911-919.

Mashhadi SA, Loh CY. A knotless method of securing the subcuticular suture. *Aesthet Surg J.* 2011;31(5):594-595.

McKinley LH, Dorton DW. Modified intermediate running subcuticular technique with nonabsorbable suture. *Dermatol Surg.* 2012;38(6):924-925.

Onwuanyi ON, Evbuomwan I. Skin closure during appendicectomy: a controlled clinical trial of subcuticular and interrupted transdermal suture techniques. *J R Coll Surg Edinb.* 1990;35(6):353-355.

Retzlaff K, Agarwal S, Song DH, Dorafshar AH. The four-step subcuticular suture technique. *Plast Reconstr Surg.* 2010;126(1):50e-51e.

Sanders RJ. Subcuticular skin closure: description of technique. *J Dermatol Surg.* 1975;1(4):61-64.

Tuuli MG, Rampersad RM, Carbone JF, et al. Staples compared with subcuticular suture for skin closure after cesarean delivery: a systematic review and meta-analysis. *Obstet Gynecol.* 2011;117(3):682-690.

Watts GT. Modified subcuticular skin suture. *Br J Plast Surg.* 1956;9(1):83-84.

Williams IM, Wright DD, Hickman J. Subcuticular wound closure: alternative method of securing the suture. *Br J Surg.* 1994;81(9):1312.

The Backing Out Running Subcuticular Suture

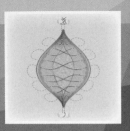

Synonyms

Backing out subcuticular suture, cross-running intradermal suture

Video 4-8. Backing out running subcuticular suture
Access to video can be found via
mhprofessional.com/atlasofsuturingtechniques2e

Application

This is a niche epidermal approximation technique suitable for wounds under minimal to no tension in areas with an excellent vascular supply. This technique should almost never be employed in the absence of a deep dermal suture, since its strength is in fine-tuning epidermal approximation and it is ineffective in the presence of significant tension.

Suture Material Choice

As with any technique, it is best to utilize the thinnest suture possible for any given anatomic location. Since the backing out subcuticular suture technique is not designed to hold tension and its utility is limited to fine-tuning epidermal approximation, 5-0 or 6-0 suture is generally adequate when adopting this technique. This is especially important since a large volume of suture material is left in situ when utilizing this approach. It is best to utilize a monofilament suture material to minimize the coefficient of friction at the time of suture removal.

Technique

1. The needle is inserted at the far right corner of the wound, parallel to the incision line, beginning approximately 2-5 mm from the apex. The needle is passed from this point, which is lateral to the incision apex, directly through the epidermis, exiting into the interior of the wound just medial to the apex.

2. With the tail of the suture material resting lateral to the incision apex and outside the wound, the wound edge is gently reflected back and the needle is inserted into the dermis on the far edge of the wound with a trajectory running parallel to the incision line. The needle, and therefore the suture, should pass through the dermis at a uniform depth. Bite size is dependent on needle size, though in order to minimize the risk of necrosis it may be prudent to restrict the size of each bite. The needle should exit the dermis at a point equidistant from the cut edge from where it entered.

3. The needle is then grasped with the surgical pickups and simultaneously released by the hand holding the needle driver. As the needle is freed from the tissue with the pickups, the needle is grasped again by the needle driver in an appropriate position to repeat the earlier mentioned step on the contralateral edge of the incised wound edge.

4. A small amount of suture material is pulled through and the needle is inserted into the dermis on the contralateral side of the incised wound edge and the same movement is repeated. The needle should enter slightly proximal (relative to the wound apex where the suture line began) to the exit point, thus introducing a small degree of backtracking to the snake-like flow of the suture material.

5. The same technique is repeated on the contralateral side of the incision line, and alternating bites are then taken from each side of the incision line, with continuing on until the end of the wound is reached. At this point, the needle is inserted from the interior of the wound in line with the incision line and exits just lateral to the apex of the wound.

6. A small roll of petrolatum gauze (or a dental roll) is then inserted in the space between the apex of the wound and the exit point of the suture material. The needle is then reinserted between the petrolatum gauze and the wound apex, securing the gauze in place and exiting at the interior of the wound.

7. Moving in the opposite direction, steps (1) through (5) are then repeated, with the suture material snaking an alternating course through the superficial dermis, using a backhand technique if desired.

8. After exiting lateral to the apex where the closure began, a roll of petrolatum gauze is again placed between the two ends of the suture and the suture material is tied off (Figures 4-8A through 4-8J).

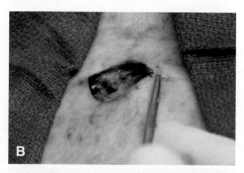

Figure 4-8B. The needle is inserted from outside of the apex of the wound into the wound interior.

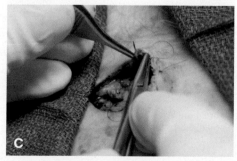

Figure 4-8C. The needle is then inserted through the superficial dermis, running parallel to the incised wound edge.

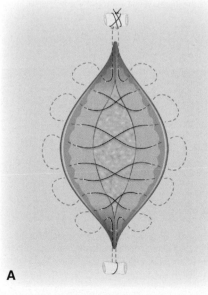

Figure 4-8A. Overview of the backing out running subcuticular suture technique.

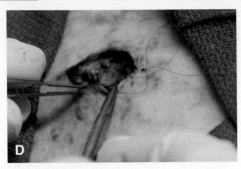

Figure 4-8D. This is sequentially repeated on opposite wound edges.

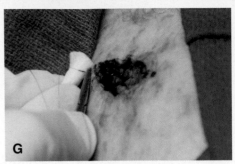

Figure 4-8G. A piece of rolled gauze may be placed as a bolster as the needle is loaded in a backhand fashion.

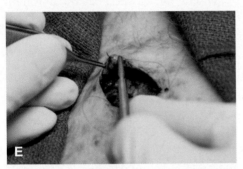

Figure 4-8E. The technique continues along the length of the wound.

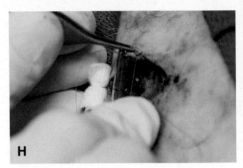

Figure 4-8H. The needle then follows along the superficial dermis in the opposite direction, heading toward the initial wound apex.

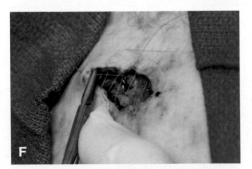

Figure 4-8F. When the opposite wound apex is reached, the needle is inserted from the deep dermis lateral to the apex directly outward through the skin.

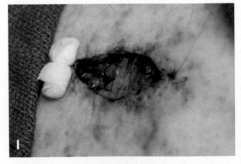

Figure 4-8I. Once the starting apex is reached, the needle again enters from the undermined deep dermis medial to the apex, exiting the skin medial to its initial insertion point.

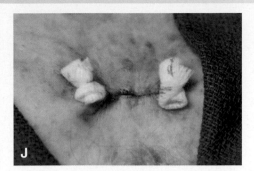

Figure 4-8J. Another piece of rolled gauze is placed as a bolster and the suture is tied. Note the slight gaping at the center of the wound where it is under the greatest tension.

Tips and Pearls

This is a niche technique, as the addition of a second row of subcuticular suture material in the wound probably does not add significantly to wound security while it doubles the amount of suture material that will ultimately need to be removed. Some authors have advocated its use since it provides more symmetrical pull on the wound edges and the central pull ostensibly leads to a reduction in wound length akin to a purse-string suture.

As with the standard running subcuticular suture, body positioning may be very helpful in maintaining an efficient and comfortable backing out subcuticular technique. Most surgeons are trained to work with the surgical site flat and perpendicular to their body. Since the motions associated with subcuticular suture placement are 90 degrees off from this, it may be useful to stand with the surgeon's body (shoulder to shoulder) parallel to the incision line. This allows for a flowing motion from right to left without the need to twist the shoulders or wrists.

Since this approach requires the surgeon to perform the second half of the closure moving in the opposite direction, it may be useful to use a backhand technique for many of the suture throws when moving back toward the original wound apex. This may add significantly to the time needed to complete this closure while facility with a backhand technique is improved.

As with the standard running subcuticular approach, a smooth, flowing technique is of paramount importance in executing this technique effectively and efficiently. Some authors have advocated adjusting the angle used to hold the needle in the needle driver from the traditional 90 degrees to 135 degrees to increase the surgeon's comfort and minimize the need for physical contortion, though adjusting the surgeon's body position may obviate the need for this adjustment.

Drawbacks and Cautions

Though it may be conceptualized as a bidirectional subcuticular closure, the extra row of sutures in this technique adds little to wound security, as the entire suture line is secured with a single knot. Therefore, it is not recommended as a solitary closure approach, but rather it is best utilized layered over the top of a deeper suturing technique.

This technique results in leaving a very significant quantity of foreign-body material in the dermis in a continuous fashion—essentially twice as much as the running subcuticular technique. While this may not represent a major problem in areas with a thick dermis such as the back, in other anatomical locations, the large quantity of suture that is left in situ may result in concerns regarding infection, foreign-body reaction, and even the potential that the suture material itself could present a physical barrier that would impinge on the ability of the wound to heal appropriately—an iatrogenic eschar phenomenon.

The extra row of subcuticular sutures used in this technique raises further concern regarding the possibility of tissue strangulation along the wound margin that could theoretically be associated with tightly placed subcuticular sutures. It, therefore, should be reserved for areas with an outstanding vascular supply, such as the face.

Removal of long-standing suture entails a theoretical risk that a potential space—albeit a thin and long one—is created on the removal of the suture material. This theoretical risk may be mitigated by utilizing the thinnest possible suture material, and this risk is higher in this approach than in the standard subcuticular suturing technique.

There is sometimes a tendency for the apices of the wound to develop exaggerated dog ears due to the tension vector created when looping and tying the suture material over the gauze bolsters lateral to the apices. Minimizing tension across this suture helps minimize this potential issue.

References

Huang L. The backing out subcuticular suture. *Br J Oral Maxillofac Surg.* 2011;49(5):e22-23.

Xiong L, Sun J, Pan Q, Yang J. The cross-running intradermal suture: a novel method for incision closure. *Facial Plast Surg.* 2012;28(5):541-542.

The Percutaneous Vertical Mattress Suture

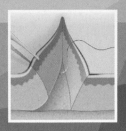

Synonyms

Haneke-Marini suture, modified buried vertical mattress suture

Video 4-9. Percutaneous vertical mattress suture

Access to video can be found via mhprofessional.com/atlasofsuturingtechniques2e

Application

This technique is designed to allow for excellent tension relief while concomitantly permitting easy suture placement in relatively tight spaces. It is best suited to areas with thicker dermis, though it may also be utilized in any body area when tension-relieving sutures must be placed and where insertion of the full needle is challenging.

Some authors have advocated this technique as a replacement for standard buried suture approaches and as an easy to implement alternative to the buried vertical mattress, while others prefer to think of this as a niche approach exclusively for areas where fully buried approaches are more challenging.

Suture Material Choice

Suture choice is dependent in large part on location. Because suture material travels percutaneously, exiting the epidermis and then reentering, the smallest gauge suture material appropriate for the anatomic location should be utilized. On the back and shoulders, 2-0 or 3-0 absorbable

suture material is effective, though theoretically the risk of suture spitting or suture abscess formation is greater with the thicker 2-0 suture material, particularly where the material has exited the epidermis entirely. On the extremities, a 3-0 or 4-0 absorbable suture material may be used, and on the face and areas under minimal tension, a 5-0 absorbable suture is adequate.

Technique

1. The wound edge is reflected back using surgical forceps or hooks. In areas under marked tension, or where full visualization is not possible, the needle may be blindly inserted from the undermined space without reflecting back the skin.
2. The suture needle is inserted at a 90-degree angle into the underside of the dermis 4 mm distant from the incised wound edge.
3. The first bite travels from the underside of the dermis in the undermined space, passes entirely through the dermis, and exits through the epidermis directly above the entry point.
4. The needle is then reloaded onto the needle driver with a backhanded technique and inserted through the epidermis either directly through the same hole as the suture followed during exit or just medial to it. A shallow bite is taken, and the needle exits on the lateral margin of the incised wound edge.

5. The needle is then reloaded, again in a backhanded fashion, and is inserted into the contralateral incised wound edge at the same depth as it exited on the first side. The needle again follows a mirror-image superficial course through the dermis, exiting through the epidermis again approximately 4 mm from the wound edge. Alternatively, this step may be combined with the prior step and the needle can be inserted into the contralateral edge while it is still loaded from the initial pass exiting the incised wound edge.

6. The needle is then loaded in a standard fashion and inserted either through the same hole or just lateral to it, following a deeper course and exiting the undersurface of the dermis into the undermined space.

7. The suture material is then tied utilizing an instrument tie (Figures 4-9A through 4-9K).

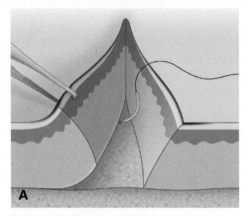

Figure 4-9A. The percutaneous vertical mattress suture is started by entering through the underside of the undermined dermis and exiting directly upward through the skin.

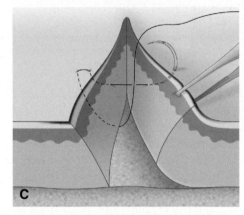

Figure 4-9C. The needle is then reinserted on the contralateral wound edge following a superficial course.

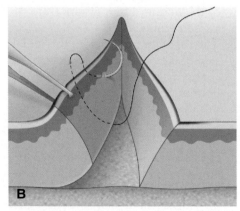

Figure 4-9B. The needle is then reinserted just medial to its exit point relative to the wound edge, or directly through the same hole, following a superficial course through the dermis and exiting at the incised wound edge.

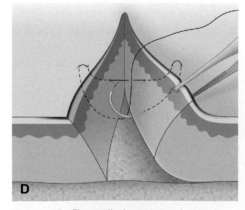

Figure 4-9D. The needle then reenters through the same hole or just lateral to it, following a deeper course and exiting through the underside of the dermis.

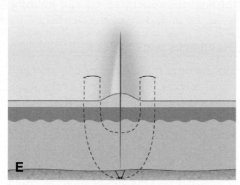

Figure 4-9E. Cross-sectional view of the percutaneous vertical mattress technique.

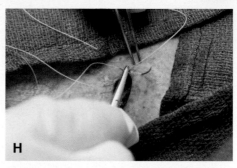

Figure 4-9H. The needle is then reinserted on the contralateral wound edge through the underside of the undermined dermis.

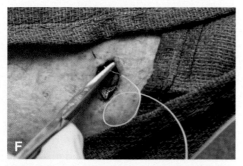

Figure 4-9F. The needle enters through the underside of the undermined dermis and exits directly upward through the skin.

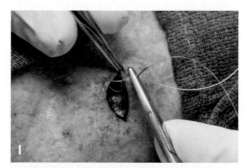

Figure 4-9I. The needle then reenters through the same hole or just lateral to it, following a deeper course and exiting through the underside of the dermis.

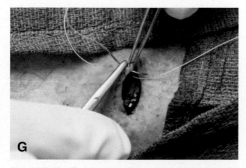

Figure 4-9G. The needle is then reinserted just medial to its exit point relative to the wound edge, following a superficial course through the dermis and exiting at the incised wound edge.

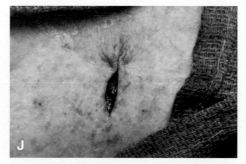

Figure 4-9J. Immediate appearance after placement of a single percutaneous vertical mattress suture. Note the dimpling, which will resolve as the suture material is absorbed.

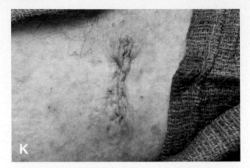

Figure 4-9K. Immediate postoperative appearance after a series of percutaneous vertical mattress sutures has been placed.

Tips and Pearls

This technique is ideal for use in areas where placement of a traditional buried suture is challenging due to limited space, such as the scalp and lower leg. Even using small semicircular needles and with extensive undermining, it may be difficult to insert the body of the needle into the undersurface of the dermis in these anatomic locations.

This technique may also be useful when placing an additional suture between two reasonably tightly set sutures, and where full retraction of the wound edge is, therefore, impossible.

This approach may also be used when it is difficult to visualize the undersurface of the dermis, since the needle throws may be placed in an almost blind fashion. The skin is grasped gently to make it taut and the needle is inserted through the undermined space, exiting on the outside of the skin. This may be executed by feel, an approach well suited to the scalp, where minimal dermal elasticity may preclude full exposure of the undersurface of the undermined dermis.

Finally, this technique may be utilized when a buried suture needs to be placed in an area that has not been undermined; the initial suture placement, entering from the underside of the dermis, can be performed blindly by sliding the needle through the superficial fat and entering from the underside of the dermis.

Drawbacks and Cautions

Since suture material exits the skin and then reenters, dimpling will likely occur. Patients should be warned that this is expected and will resolve with time. Reentering the skin through the same hole may help minimize the risk of dramatic dimpling, though this also increases the chance that the suture material could be cut by the needle.

This approach may also lead to tearthrough if insufficient dermis is grasped; when working in areas of atrophic skin, it is important to consider this limitation, since the consequences of tearing a wound under tension may make it more difficult to place additional sutures if this approach is ineffective.

Setting back the first throw far from the incised wound edge may result in overeversion; the chief drawback of overeversion is that the dermis may overhang the center of the incised wound edge, barring the epidermal edges from approximating appropriately, leading to a slightly wider final scar. This may be easily solved by carefully beveling the dermis to allow the epidermal edges to meet unimpeded.

References

Marini L. The Haneke-Marini suture: not a "new" technique. *Dermatol Surg.* 1995;21(9):819-820.

Sadick NS, D'Amelio DL, Weinstein C. The modified buried vertical mattress suture. A new technique of buried absorbable wound closure associated with excellent cosmesis for wounds under tension. *J Dermatol Surg Oncol.* 1994;20(11):735-739.

See A, Smith HR. Partially buried horizontal mattress suture: modification of the Haneke-Marini suture. *Dermatol Surg.* 2004;30(12 pt 1):1491-1492.

Vinciullo C, Bekhor P, Sinclair P, Richards S, Rosner L. Credit where credit is due. The Haneke-Marini suture: not a "new" technique. *Dermatol Surg.* 1995;21(9):819.

The Percutaneous Set-Back Dermal Suture

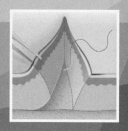

Synonym

Percutaneous Kantor suture

Video 4-10. Percutaneous set-back dermal suture
Access to video can be found via
mhprofessional.com/atlasofsuturingtechniques2e

Application

This technique is designed primarily for the closure of narrow wounds. In anatomic locations such as the scalp and lower leg, there is often insufficient laxity to permit the effective visualization of the undersurface of the undermined wound edge that would be ideal for the placement of set-back dermal sutures.

This technique could theoretically be utilized in other areas, though in practice the standard buried set-back dermal suture should probably be utilized if at all possible to effect better wound-edge approximation.

Suture Material Choice

On the scalp, a 3-0 or 4-0 absorbable suture is probably best, as it allows for robust closure in this area where tension is occasionally moderate to severe. On the lower legs, 3-0 or 4-0 absorbable suture material may be used as well, as this area is sometimes under marked tension. As always, utilizing the smallest gauge suture material that will permit adequate closure under tension is best.

Technique

1. If possible, the wound edge is reflected back using surgical forceps or hooks. Adequate visualization of the underside of the dermis is not required.
2. While gently grasping the skin edge, the suture needle is inserted at 90 degrees into the underside of the dermis 2-4 mm distant from the incised wound edge.
3. The first bite is executed by traversing the dermis and piercing directly up through the epidermis, with the needle exiting the epidermis 2-4 mm from the incised wound edge.
4. The needle is then reloaded on the needle driver in a backhand fashion and inserted at 90 degrees just medial to the exit point. The needle exits the undermined surface of the dermis into the undermined space between the undersurface of the dermis and the deeper subcutaneous tissue, medial to its entry point.
5. The needle is then reloaded, again in a backhand fashion, and inserted into the undersurface of the dermis on the contralateral wound edge, 2-4 mm distant from the incised wound edge. Depending on needle size and the breadth of the wound, this step may be combined with the prior step, saving the need to reload the needle. The needle should traverse the dermis and exit through the epidermis

2-4 mm distant from the incised wound edge.

6. The needle is then reloaded in a standard fashion and inserted in the epidermis just lateral to the exit point at 90 degrees, exiting the undersurface of the dermis in the undermined space.

7. The suture material is then tied utilizing an instrument tie (Figures 4-10A through 4-10K).

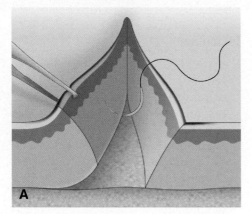

Figure 4-10A. The needle is inserted from the underside of the dermis in the undermined space directly upward through the skin.

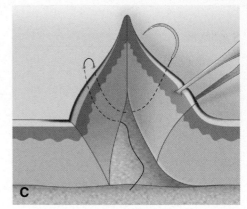

Figure 4-10C. The needle is then inserted on the contralateral side, again from the underside of the dermis, exiting through the skin.

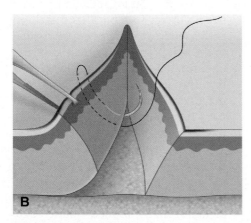

Figure 4-10B. The needle is then reinserted in a backhand fashion just medial to its exit point, exiting through the undersurface of the dermis in the undermined space.

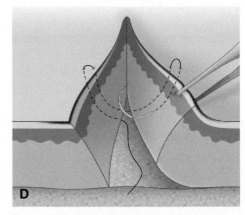

Figure 4-10D. The needle is then reinserted just lateral to its exit point, exiting in the undermined space.

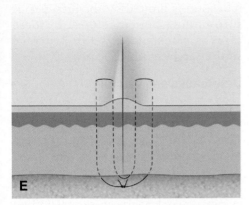

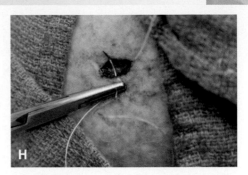

Figure 4-10E. Cross-sectional view of the percutaneous set-back dermal suture.

Figure 4-10H. The needle exits through the undersurface of the dermis in the undermined space, now visible as it arcs toward the center of the wound.

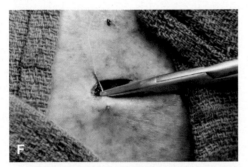

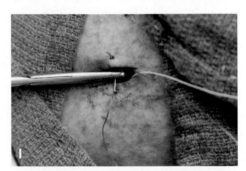

Figure 4-10F. The needle is inserted from the underside of the dermis in the undermined space directly upward through the skin.

Figure 4-10I. The needle is then inserted on the contralateral side, again from the underside of the dermis, exiting through the skin.

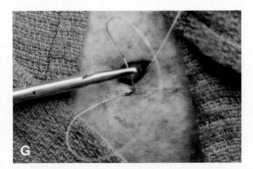

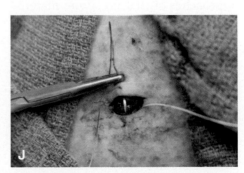

Figure 4-10G. The needle is then reinserted in a backhand fashion just medial to its exit point.

Figure 4-10J. The needle is then reinserted just lateral to its exit point, exiting in the undermined space.

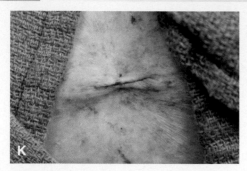

Figure 4-10K. Immediate postoperative appearance. Note the marked wound eversion.

Tips and Pearls

A central advantage of this approach is its ease of execution; since the suture pierces the epidermis and dermis at a 90-degree angle, there is no need to change planes, effect a heart-shaped suture placement, or guarantee that the suture exit point is precisely at the inside edge of the lower dermis, as may be needed with other techniques.

This technique is also appropriate in areas where extensive undermining is not possible; since the undersurface of the dermis does not need to be visualized to effectively place the sutures, the throws can be essentially placed blindly.

An important theoretical advantage of this approach over other percutaneous approaches is that no suture material is left between the wound edges. Since even absorbable suture material may represent a physical impediment to wound healing, this is an important benefit that this approach shares with the standard set-back dermal suture technique.

This technique may also be useful when adding additional sutures to an already largely closed wound. In these cases, there may not be sufficient room to insert a traditional vertically oriented buried suture, both as the space available to insert the needle driver is limited and the degree of possible wound-edge

reflection is limited by the presence of surrounding buried sutures. In these cases, a percutaneous set-back dermal suture can be easily executed.

Drawbacks and Cautions

The percutaneous set-back dermal approach creates significant wound eversion, and the degree of eversion elicited by this approach may be more marked than that seen with the standard set-back dermal suture approach. This pronounced eversion may lead the epidermal portion of the wound edges to separate as the dermis is brought together, as the epidermal edges fail to drape together as they would normally do with the standard set-back dermal technique.

There are two possible approaches to this situation: (1) superficial running or interrupted sutures may be placed to better approximate the epidermal edges, and (2) the defect could be removed with an inward bevel (as is done with the butterfly suture technique), or the dermis may be incised at an inward bevel after the original defect is created, permitting the epidermal edges to come together gently even in the face of the marked eversion seen with this approach. Many clinicians favor a bilayered approach in general, and therefore, placing the epidermal sutures is an easy solution and does not require the degree of preplanning associated with the bevel approach, though a combination of the two solutions may be utilized as well.

Patients should be cautioned that they might develop a significant ridge in the immediate postoperative period. Depending on the suture material used and the density of the sutures, this ridge may last from weeks to months. Explaining that the technique is akin to placing a subcutaneous splint may help the patient develop reasonable and realistic expectations and reduce anxiety regarding the immediate postoperative appearance of the wound.

Epidermal dimpling will often occur with this approach, since the suture material traverses the epidermis. A small degree of dimpling will resolve with time as the absorbable sutures are gradually resorbed, and patients should be warned that this is a likely occurrence and that it is of no long-term clinical consequence.

As with other percutaneous approaches, there is a risk that the suture material may tear through the dermis, particularly if there is significant background atrophy.

Since suture material traverses the epidermis, there is a theoretically greater risk of infection with this technique than with approaches that remain entirely buried on the undersurface of the dermis. Meticulous attention to sterile technique may help mitigate this theoretical risk, and anecdotally, infection is seen no more frequently with this approach than with any other closure technique.

Reference

Kantor J. The percutaneous set-back dermal suture. *J Am Acad Dermatol*. 2015;72(2):e61-62.

The Percutaneous Horizontal Mattress Suture

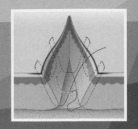

Synonym

Buried horizontal mattress suture

Video 4-11. Percutaneous horizontal mattress suture
Access to video can be found via
mhprofessional.com/atlasofsuturingtechniques2e

Application

As with other percutaneous approaches, this technique is designed to allow for excellent tension relief while concomitantly permitting easy suture placement in relatively tight spaces. It is best suited to areas with thicker dermis, though it may also be utilized in any body area when tension-relieving sutures must be placed and where insertion of the full needle is challenging.

Suture Material Choice

Suture choice is dependent in large part on location. Though suture material travels percutaneously, exiting the epidermis and then reentering, the smallest gauge suture material appropriate for the anatomic location should be utilized. On the back and shoulders, 2-0 or 3-0 suture material is effective, though theoretically the risk of suture spitting or suture abscess formation is greater with the thicker 2-0 suture material, particularly where the material has exited the epidermis entirely. On the extremities, a 3-0 or 4-0 absorbable suture material may be used, and on the face and areas under minimal tension, a 5-0 absorbable suture is adequate.

Technique

1. The wound edge is reflected back using surgical forceps or hooks. In areas under marked tension or where full visualization is not possible, the needle may be blindly inserted from the undermined space.
2. The suture needle is inserted perpendicular to the incision line at a 90-degree angle into the underside of the dermis 4 mm distant from the incised wound edge.
3. The first bite is started by following the needle and traversing from the underside of the dermis in the undermined space and passing entirely through the dermis and exiting the skin.
4. The needle is then reloaded onto the needle driver and inserted through the epidermis either directly through the same hole as the suture followed during exit, or just distal to it, with the needle-oriented parallel to the incision line. A shallow bite is taken, staying in the superficial dermis, exiting on the same side of the incision line distal to the entry point.
5. The needle is then reloaded and inserted into the same hole or just medial to it, while being held perpendicular to the incision line. The needle should travel through the full thickness of the skin, exiting on the undersurface of the undermined dermis.

6. The needle is then reloaded and enters the undersurface of the undermined dermis on the contralateral wound edge, exiting through the surface of the epidermis. This step may be combined with the prior step, and the needle can be inserted into the contralateral wound edge while it is still loaded from the initial pass.

7. The needle is then loaded and inserted either through the same hole or just proximal to it, oriented parallel to the incision line but in the opposite direction as in step (4), following a superficial course and exiting on the same side of the incision line proximal to the incision entry point.

8. The needle is then reloaded in a standard fashion and inserted either through the same hole or just medial to it perpendicular to the incision line, exiting on the undersurface of the undermined dermis.

9. The suture material is then tied utilizing an instrument tie (Figures 4-11A through 4-11J).

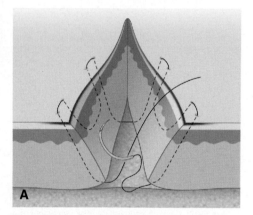

Figure 4-11A. Overview of the percutaneous horizontal mattress suture technique.

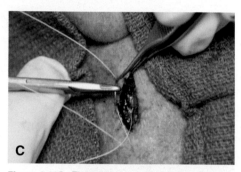

Figure 4-11C. The needle is reinserted directly adjacent to its exit point (or even through the same hole as it exited), now parallel to the incised wound edge.

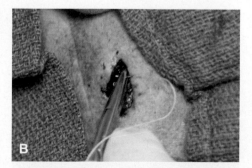

Figure 4-11B. First step of the percutaneous horizontal mattress suture technique. Note that the needle is inserted through the undersurface of the undermined dermis directly upward, exiting the skin set back from the wound edge.

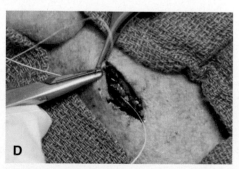

Figure 4-11D. The needle passes superficially through the dermis, exiting at a point equidistant from the incised wound edge.

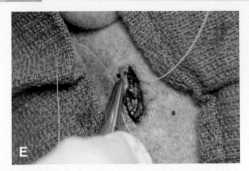

Figure 4-11E. The needle is then reinserted directly adjacent to its exit point (or even through the same hole), now oriented perpendicular to the wound edge to permit it to traverse the wound.

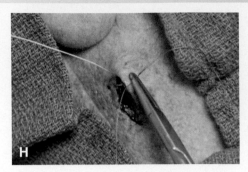

Figure 4-11H. The needle is then reinserted directly adjacent to its exit point (or through the same hole), now oriented perpendicular to the wound edge, exiting in the open wound space.

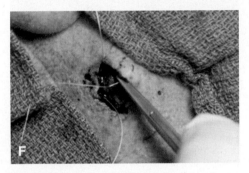

Figure 4-11F. The needle is inserted on the contra-lateral wound edge through the undersurface of the undermined dermis, directly upward, again exiting the skin set back from the wound edge.

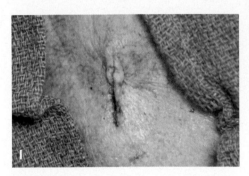

Figure 4-11I. Wound appearance after placement of a single percutaneous horizontal mattress suture.

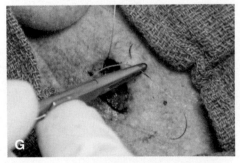

Figure 4-11G. The needle is reinserted directly adjacent to its exit point (or even through the same hole as it exited), now parallel to the incised wound edge, in the direction of the initial entry point.

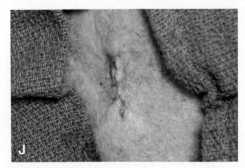

Figure 4-11J. Final wound appearance. Note the marked wound-edge eversion.

Tips and Pearls

This technique is best for use in areas where placement of a traditional buried suture is challenging due to limited space, such as the scalp and lower leg. Even after using small semicircular needles and with extensive undermining, it may be difficult to insert the body of needle into the undersurface of the dermis in these anatomic locations.

This approach may also be used when it is difficult to visualize the undersurface of the dermis, since the needle throws may be placed in an almost blind fashion. The skin is grasped gently to make it taught, and the needle is inserted through the undermined space, exiting on the outside of the skin. This may be executed by feel, an approach well suited to the scalp where minimal dermal elasticity precludes full exposure of the undersurface of the undermined dermis. The ear is another area where this approach may be very useful, since the limited elasticity of the thin dermis on the helix may make placement of traditional vertically oriented buried sutures challenging.

Drawbacks and Cautions

Since suture material exits the skin and then reenters, dimpling may occur. Patients should be warned that this is expected and will resolve with time, though residual dyspigmentation is certainly possible. Reentering the skin through the same hole may help minimize the risk of dramatic dimpling.

Setting back the first throw far from the incised wound edge may result in overeversion; the chief drawback of overeversion is that the dermis may overhand in the center of the incised wound edge, barring the epidermal edges from approximating appropriately, leading to a slightly wider final scar. This may be easily solved by carefully beveling the dermis to allow the epidermal edges to meet unimpeded.

As with other percutaneous approaches, there is a risk that the suture material may tear through the dermis, particularly if there is significant background atrophy. The horizontal orientation may help limit some of this risk, however, since a wider area of dermis is generally grasped.

Theoretically, horizontally oriented sutures may confer a slightly increased risk of epidermal-edge necrosis, since suture material has the potential to constrict the small vessels supplying the wound margin. That said, this complication is rarely seen in practice as long as the bite size is not overly large and suture material is not tied with excessive tension.

References

Epstein E. The buried horizontal mattress suture. *Cutis*. 1979;24(1):104-106.

See A, Smith HR. Partially buried horizontal mattress suture: modification of the Haneke-Marini suture. *Dermatol Surg*. 2004;30(12 pt 1):1491-1492.

CHAPTER 4.12

The Running Buried Dermal Suture

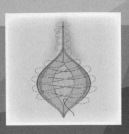

Video 4-12. Running buried dermal suture
Access to video can be found via
mhprofessional.com/atlasofsuturingtechniques2e

Application

This is a hybrid technique, combining the tension relief and lack of transepidermal suture placement of a classic buried suture with the rapidity of placement and lack of resilience of a superficial running technique. This is a niche approach, since the running nature of the technique means that compromise at any point in the course of suture placement may result in wound dehiscence. Therefore, unless absolutely necessary, this approach should not be utilized as a solitary technique for the closure of most wounds.

Suture Material Choice

Suture choice is dependent in large part on location, though as always, the smallest gauge suture material appropriate for the anatomic location should be utilized. On the back and shoulders, 3-0 suture material is effective, though if there is marked tension across the wound, this approach would not be appropriate as the primary closure and would be used best for its pulley benefits. On the extremities, a 3-0 or 4-0 absorbable suture material may be used, and on the face and areas under minimal tension, a 5-0 absorbable suture is adequate.

Technique

1. The wound edge is reflected back using surgical forceps or hooks.
2. While reflecting back the dermis, the suture needle is inserted at 90 degrees into the underside of the dermis 2 mm distant from the incised wound edge.
3. The first bite is executed by following the curvature of the needle and allowing the needle to exit in the incised wound edge. The size of this bite is based on the size of the needle, the thickness of the dermis, and the need for and tolerance of eversion. The needle's zenith with respect to the wound surface should be between the entry and exit points.
4. Keeping the loose end of the suture between the surgeon and the patient, the dermis on the side of the first bite is released. The tissue on the opposite edge is then gently grasped with the forceps.
5. The second bite is executed by inserting the needle into the incised wound edge at the level of the superficial papillary dermis. This bite should be completed by following the curvature of the needle and avoiding catching the undersurface of the epidermis that could result in epidermal dimpling. It then exits approximately 2 mm distal to the wound edge on the undersurface of the dermis. This

should mirror the first bite taken on the contralateral side of the wound.

6. This first anchoring suture is then tied with an instrument tie.

7. The procedure is then repeated sequentially, repeating steps (2) through (5) in sets while moving proximally toward the surgeon for as many throws as are desired, without placing any additional knots until the desired number of loops have been placed.

8. The suture material is then tied utilizing an instrument tie (Figures 4-12A through 4-12F). The final anchoring knot is tied by leaving a loop on the penultimate throw and tying the free end of suture material from the final

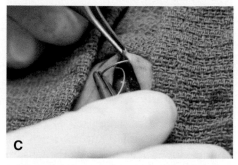

C

Figure 4-12C. The needle is then reinserted at the incised edge on the contralateral wound edge and again follows its curvature, exiting the deep dermis. The suture is then tied off.

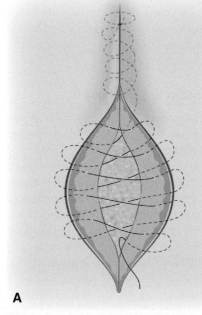

A

Figure 4-12A. Overview of the running buried dermal suture.

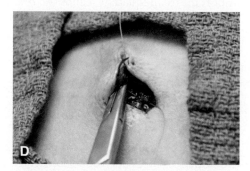

D

Figure 4-12D. First running step of the technique, again following the curvature of the needle.

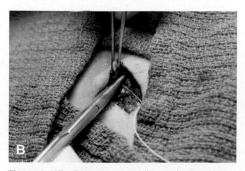

B

Figure 4-12B. Beginning of the first anchoring throw of the buried running dermal suture. The needle entered the deep dermis and followed its curvature, exiting at the incised wound edge.

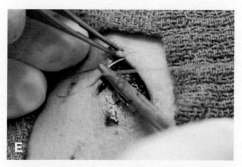

E

Figure 4-12E. The running throw is completed. These continue successively along the course of the wound.

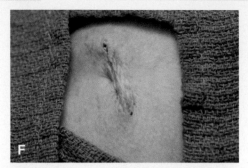

Figure 4-12F. Immediate postoperative appearance.

throw to this loop. The ends of the suture are then trimmed.

Tips and Pearls

This technique may be used as a modified winch or pulley suture, since the multiple loops help minimize the tension across any one loop and permit closure of wounds under marked tension. Because each throw is not tied off, however, it is important to adequately secure the first and final throws with a well-locked knot.

Given the theoretical susceptibility to suture material breakage or compromise, this is a technique that is probably best used in a layered fashion, either superficial to previously placed deep interrupted buried sutures or deep to a set of more superficially placed buried sutures.

If braided absorbable suture is used, the added friction between loops may help lock the suture material in place with each throw, but caution should be taken to pull sufficient suture material with each throw, as this friction may impede the surgeon's ability to pull suture material through the course of multiple loops. Similarly, if monofilament suture is used, it may be easier to pull the additional suture material through, but it may make it more difficult to lock the suture in place before tying.

It may be beneficial to place the running sutures closer together toward the center of the wound than at the poles of

the incision, as this may foster a more pronounced pulley effect at the center of the wound where the tensile forces are greatest.

Given the concern regarding knot breakage, it may be helpful to attempt to better secure the first and final knots at the ends of the running series of loops. This may be done by paying particularly close attention to knot tying, tying an extra full knot, adding extra throws, or leaving a longer tail than would traditionally be executed. An additional approach is to secure the final knot with the aid of a tacking knot, which may similarly provide extra security.

Drawbacks and Cautions

As noted previously, this approach should usually not be used as a solitary closure technique, since there is no redundancy in the closure. It may be useful as an adjunct when there is either minimal tension across a wound (and therefore interrupted buried sutures may be unnecessary) or as a pulley approach to bring recalcitrant wound edges together. It can also be used when deeper layers have been closed whether with a fascial plication suture or with other individual buried sutures.

Like the standard buried dermal suture, this approach provides less wound eversion than other approaches such as the set-back dermal or buried vertical mattress; therefore, a running variation of the latter two techniques may often be preferred to a buried running dermal approach, since wound eversion may be associated with improved cosmesis over the long term.

References

Ftaiha Z, Snow SN. The buried running dermal subcutaneous suture technique. *J Dermatol Surg Oncol.* 1989;15(3):264-266.

Skaria AM. The buried running dermal subcutaneous suture with a tacking knot. *Dermatol Surg.* 2002;28(8):739-741.

The Running Set-Back Dermal Suture

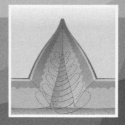

Synonyms

Running Kantor suture, running set-back suture

Video 4-13. Running set-back dermal suture

Access to video can be found via mhprofessional.com/atlasofsuturingtechniques2e

Application

This approach is best used in areas under mild to moderate tension, as it is a running technique that allows rapid placement of multiple buried suture throws. It may be utilized in a variety of anatomic locations, including the face, neck, and extremities. While it may be utilized on the trunk, interrupted set-back sutures are generally more appropriate in this location.

Since it is a running technique, it may be associated with a higher risk of dehiscence, as interruption of the suture material at any point in its course would lead to loss of effectiveness of the entire suture line. Therefore, it is often used in concert with other sutures techniques rather than as a sole closure approach.

Suture Material Choice

Suture choice is dependent in large part on location. Though this technique is designed to bite the deep dermis and remain buried well below the wound surface, the surgeon may choose to utilize a larger gauge suture than would be used for an equivalently placed running simple or running buried vertical mattress suture.

On the extremities, a 3-0 or 4-0 absorbable suture material may be used, and on the face and areas under minimal tension, a 5-0 absorbable suture is adequate. While this approach should probably not be routinely utilized on the back, using a 2-0 absorbable suture on the back with this technique results in only vanishingly rare complications, since the thicker suture remains largely on the underside of the dermis, and suture spitting is an uncommon occurrence.

Braided suture material will allow for better locking of the suture in place, though it will also impede the surgeon's ability to pull suture material through multiple loops, and therefore, adequate suture material should be pulled through with each loop. Monofilament absorbable suture material will pull through more easily, though the lower coefficient of friction means that it will easily slide back through the wound and will therefore not lock in place until tied.

Technique

1. The wound edge is reflected back using surgical forceps or hooks. Adequate visualization of the underside of the dermis is required.
2. While reflecting back the dermis, the suture needle is inserted at 90 degrees into the underside of the dermis 2-6 mm distant from the incised wound edge.
3. The first bite is executed by traversing the dermis following the curvature of the needle and allowing the

needle to exit closer to the incised wound edge. Care should be taken to remain in the dermis to minimize the risk of epidermal dimpling. The needle does not, however, exit through the incised wound edge, but rather 1-4 mm distant from the incised edge. The size of this first bite is based on the size of the needle, the thickness of the dermis, and the need for and tolerance of eversion.

4. Keeping the loose end of the suture between the surgeon and the patient, the dermis on the side of the first bite is released. The tissue on the opposite edge is then reflected back in a similar fashion as on the first side, assuring complete visualization of the underside of the dermis.

5. The second bite is executed by inserting the needle into the underside of the dermis 1-6 mm distant from the incised wound edge. Again, this bite should be executed by following the curvature of the needle and avoiding catching the undersurface of the epidermis that could result in epidermal dimpling. It then exits further distal to the wound edge, approximately 2-6 mm distant from the wound edge. This should mirror the first bite taken on the contralateral side of the wound.

6. A knot is tied using an instrument tie to secure the suture in place. The tail end of the suture is cut with minimal to no tail, and the needle, now attached to suture material that is securely anchored in the dermis, is reloaded.

7. Steps (1) through (5) may then be repeated in pairs, moving toward the surgeon, but without tying additional knots with each throw.

8. Once the end of the wound is reached, the suture material is tied utilizing an instrument or hand tie

(Figures 4-13A through 4-13G). The final anchoring knot is tied by leaving a loop on the penultimate throw and tying the free end of suture material from the final throw to this loop. The ends of the suture are then trimmed.

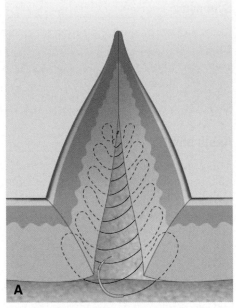

Figure 4-13A. Overview of the running set-back dermal suture.

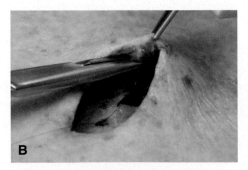

Figure 4-13B. The anchoring suture: a set-back dermal suture is started at the wound apex, and the needle is inserted into the underside of the dermis set back from the wound edge.

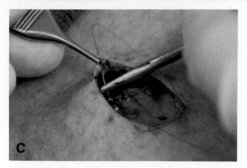

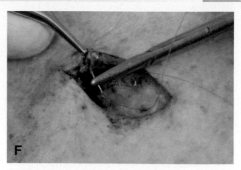

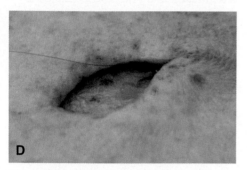

Figure 4-13C. The needle is then inserted at the contralateral side in a similar fashion.

Figure 4-13F. The needle is then inserted on the contralateral wound edge. This alternating pattern is continued along the length of the wound.

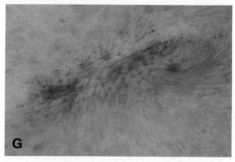

Figure 4-13D. The suture material is tied off, completing the anchoring set-back dermal suture, and the short end of the suture material is trimmed.

Figure 4-13G. Immediate postoperative appearance. Note the pronounced eversion and excellent wound-edge approximation.

Tips and Pearls

As with any running buried technique, this approach provides the benefit of permitting rapid placement of a long string of tension-relieving sutures. The pulley effect of the multiple throws also permits effective closure of wounds under even marked tension.

That said, it is critical to focus on outstanding knot security, since the entire suture line is held in place by the knots at the beginning and end of the set of suture throws.

Adding an additional tacking knot when utilizing this approach is an option

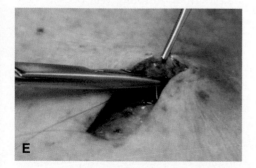

Figure 4-13E. The needle is then inserted into the dermis, exiting set back from the wound edge, moving along the wound edge.

as well. It may provide additional knot security. Alternatively, one could consider placing an additional knot or leaving a longer suture tail when utilizing this approach.

A theoretical benefit of the running approach is that there is less suture material left in situ, since the bulk of retained absorbable suture material is in the knots; as there are knots only at the beginning and end of the row of sutures, this technique theoretically decreases the risk of suture spitting and suture abscess formation. Still, the set-back approach leaves suture material deep to the undersurface of the dermis, and therefore, the risk of suture spitting and suture abscess formation is negligible.

This is an easy to execute running buried suture approach; since the suture follows the arc of the needle on the undersurface of the dermis, there is no need to change planes, effect a heart-shaped suture placement, or guarantee that the suture exit point is precisely at the inside edge of the lower dermis, as may be needed with the running buried vertical mattress suture.

Accurate suture placement is predicated on having a sufficiently undermined plane, since the entire suture loop lays on the undersurface of the dermis. Therefore, broad undermining is a prerequisite for utilizing this technique, since each throw of the needle begins 2-6 mm distant from the incised wound edge on the undermined undersurface of the dermis.

Suture throws may be placed closer together toward the higher-tension areas at the center of the wound to permit greater mechanical advantage and to allow the pulley effect to have a more profound impact at the center of the wound. The throws may then be spaced farther apart toward the apices where the pulley effect is neither needed nor desired, allowing minimization of the quantity of retained buried absorbable suture material left in the wound.

Drawbacks and Cautions

The main drawback of this approach is the same as with any running buried suture. The integrity of the entire suture line rests on the quality of the knots at each end of the row of sutures. Therefore, attention to detail when tying these knots is of paramount importance.

This approach should therefore not be used as a solitary closure technique, but rather may be used deep to interrupted transepidermal sutures or superficial to fascial plication sutures, to afford greater redundancy and add to the resilience of the closure.

The running set-back dermal approach creates significant wound eversion, and the degree of eversion elicited by this approach may, depending on how far set back the dermal bite is taken, elicit significantly more wound eversion than even the running buried vertical mattress technique.

Patients should be cautioned that they might develop a significant ridge in the immediate postoperative period. Depending on the suture material used and the density of the sutures, this ridge may last from weeks to months.

Epidermal dimpling will occasionally occur where the arc of the suture reaches its apex at the dermal-epidermal junction; on the face and areas with thin dermis, this should be assiduously avoided. In truncal areas or those with thick dermis, however, a small degree of dimpling will resolve with time as the absorbable sutures are gradually resorbed. Since tension is distributed broadly across multiple suture loops, the dimpling is not usually overly pronounced, as the tension averages across multiple throws, and therefore, it is less likely that any one area will yield marked dimpling.

Reference

Kantor J. The running set-back dermal suture. *J Am Acad Dermatol.* 2015;72:e163-164.

The Running Buried Vertical Mattress Suture

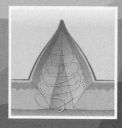

Synonym

Zipper stitch

Video 4-14. Running buried vertical mattress suture

Access to video can be found via mhprofessional.com/atlasofsuturingtechniques2e

Application

This approach is best used in areas under mild to moderate tension, as it is a running technique that allows rapid placement of multiple buried suture throws. It may be utilized in a variety of anatomic locations, including the face, neck, and extremities. While it may be utilized on the trunk, interrupted buried vertical mattress sutures are generally more appropriate in this location.

Since it is a running technique, it may be associated with a higher risk of dehiscence, as interruption of the suture material at any point in its course would lead to loss of effectiveness of the entire suture line. Therefore, it is often used in concert with other sutures techniques rather than as a sole closure approach.

Suture Material Choice

Suture choice is dependent in large part on location. On the extremities, a 3-0 or 4-0 absorbable suture material may be used, and on the face and areas under minimal tension, a 5-0 absorbable suture is adequate. While this approach should probably not be routinely utilized on the back, using a 2-0 or 3-0 absorbable suture in this area would be appropriate.

Braided suture material will allow for better locking of the suture in place, though it will also impede the surgeon's ability to pull suture material through multiple loops, and therefore, adequate suture material should be pulled through with each loop. Monofilament absorbable suture material will pull through more easily, though the lower coefficient of friction means that it will easily slide back through the wound and will therefore not lock in place until tied.

Technique

1. The wound edge is reflected back using surgical forceps or hooks. Adequate visualization of the underside of the dermis is required.
2. While reflecting back the dermis, the suture needle is inserted at 90 degrees into the underside of the dermis 4 mm distant from the incised wound edge.
3. The first bite is executed by following the needle initially at 90 degrees to the underside of the dermis and then, critically, changing direction by twisting the needle driver so that the needle exits in the incised wound edge. This allows the apex of the bite to remain in the papillary dermis while the needle exits in the incised wound edge at the level of the reticular dermis.
4. Keeping the loose end of the suture between the surgeon and the patient, the dermis on the side of the first bite

is released. The tissue on the opposite edge is then reflected back in a similar fashion as on the first side.

5. The second bite is executed by inserting the needle into the incised wound edge at the level of the reticular dermis. It then angles upward and laterally so that the apex of the needle is at the level of the papillary dermis. This should mirror the first bite taken on the contralateral side of the wound.

6. A knot is tied using an instrument tie to secure the suture in place. The tail end of the suture is cut with minimal to no tail, and the needle, now attached to suture material that is securely anchored in the dermis, is reloaded.

7. Steps (1) through (5) may then be repeated, moving in pairs toward the surgeon with each set of throws, but without tying additional knots with each throw.

8. Once the end of the wound is reached, the suture material is tied utilizing an instrument or hand tie (Figures 4-14A through 4-14F). This final anchoring knot is tied by leaving a loop on the penultimate throw

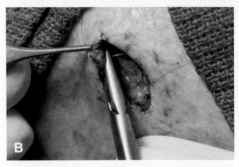

Figure 4-14B. Beginning of the first anchoring throw of the running buried vertical mattress suture. Note that the needle has moved outward and upward before exiting at the incised wound edge.

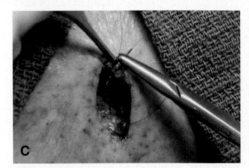

Figure 4-14C. Completion of the first anchoring throw. The needle entered at the incised wound edge. The suture material is then tied off.

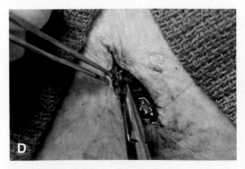

Figure 4-14D. Initiation of the running component of the technique performed in the same fashion as the initial anchoring suture.

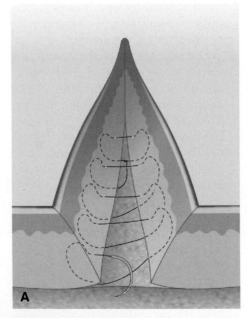

Figure 4-14A. Overview of the running buried vertical mattress suture technique.

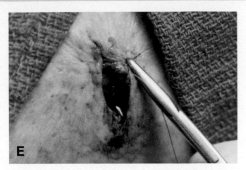

Figure 4-14E. Continuation of the running row of sutures.

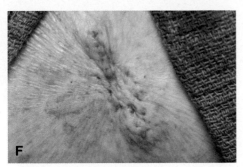

Figure 4-14F. Immediate postoperative appearance. Note the wound eversion.

and tying the free end of suture material from the final throw to this loop. The ends of the suture are then trimmed.

Tips and Pearls

As with any running buried technique, this approach provides the benefit of permitting rapid placement of a long string of tension-relieving sutures. The pulley effect of the multiple throws also permits effective closure of wounds under even marked tension.

That said, it is critical to focus on outstanding knot security, since the entire suture line is held in place by the knots at the beginning and end of the set of suture throws.

Adding an additional tacking knot when utilizing this approach is an option as well, as it may provide additional knot security. Alternatively, one could consider placing an additional knot or leaving a longer suture tail when utilizing this approach.

A theoretical benefit of the running approach is that there is less suture material left in situ, since the bulk of retained absorbable suture material is in the knots; as there are knots only at the beginning and end of the row of sutures, this technique theoretically decreases the risk of suture spitting and suture abscess formation.

Suture throws may be placed closer together toward the higher-tension areas at the center of the wound to permit greater mechanical advantage and to allow the pulley effect to have a more profound impact at the center of the wound. The throws may then be spaced farther apart toward the apices where the pulley effect is neither needed nor desired, allowing minimization of the quantity of retained buried absorbable suture material left in the wound.

Drawbacks and Cautions

The main drawback of this approach is the same as with any running buried suture. The integrity of the entire suture line rests on the quality of the knots at each end of the row of sutures. Therefore, attention to detail when tying these knots is of paramount importance.

This approach should therefore probably not be used as a solitary closure technique, but rather may be used deep to interrupted transepidermal sutures or superficial to fascial plication or deeper buried dermal sutures, to afford greater redundancy and add to the resilience of the closure.

Patients should be cautioned that they may develop a significant ridge in the immediate postoperative period. Depending on the suture material used and the density of the sutures, this ridge may last from weeks to months.

Epidermal dimpling will occasionally occur where the arc of the suture reaches its apex at the dermal-epidermal junction; on the face and areas with thin dermis, this should be assiduously avoided. In truncal areas or those with thick dermis, however, a small degree of dimpling will resolve with time as the absorbable sutures are gradually resorbed. Since tension is distributed broadly across multiple suture loops, the dimpling is not usually overly pronounced, as the tension averages across multiple throws, and therefore, it is less likely that any one area will yield marked dimpling.

References

Ftaiha Z, Snow SN. The buried running dermal subcutaneous suture technique. *J Dermatol Surg Oncol.* 1989;15(3):264-266.

Skaria AM. The buried running dermal subcutaneous suture technique with a tacking knot. *Dermatol Surg.* 2002;28(8):739-741.

Yag-Howard C. Zipper stitch: a novel aesthetic subcutaneous closure. *Dermatol Surg.* 2013;39(9): 1400-1402.

The Running Percutaneous Set-Back Dermal Suture

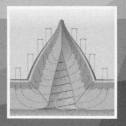

Synonym

Running percutaneous Kantor suture

Video 4-15. Running percutaneous set-back dermal suture

Access to video can be found via mhprofessional.com/atlasofsuturingtechniques2e

Application

This is a niche technique appropriate for the closure of narrow wounds under modest tension. In anatomic locations such as the scalp and lower leg, there is often insufficient laxity to permit effective visualization of the undersurface of the undermined wound edge that would be ideal for the placement of running set-back dermal sutures.

Since this is a running technique, it may be associated with a higher risk of dehiscence, as interruption of the suture material at any point in its course or of one of the knots would lead to loss of effectiveness of the entire suture line.

Suture Material Choice

On the scalp, a 3-0 or 4-0 absorbable suture is probably best, as it allows for robust closure in this area where tension is occasionally moderate to severe. On the lower legs, 3-0 or 4-0 absorbable suture material may be used as well, as this area is sometimes under marked tension. As always, utilizing the smallest gauge suture material that will permit adequate closure under tension is best.

Technique

1. If possible, the wound edge is reflected back using surgical forceps or hooks. Adequate visualization of the underside of the dermis is not required.
2. While gently grasping the skin edge, the suture needle is inserted at 90 degrees into the underside of the dermis 2-4 mm distant from the incised wound edge.
3. The first bite is executed by traversing the dermis and piercing directly up through the epidermis, with the needle exiting the epidermis 2-4 mm from the incised wound edge.
4. The needle is then reloaded on the needle driver in a backhand fashion and inserted at 90 degrees just medial to the exit point. The needle exits the undermined surface of the dermis into the undermined space between the undersurface of the dermis and the deeper subcutaneous tissue.
5. The needle is then reloaded, again in a backhand fashion, and inserted into the undersurface of the dermis on the contralateral wound edge, 2-4 mm distant from the incised wound edge. Depending on needle size and the breadth of the wound, this step may be combined with the prior step, saving the need to reload the needle. The needle should traverse the dermis and exit through the epidermis 2-4 mm distant from the incised wound edge.

6. The needle is then reloaded in a standard fashion and inserted in the epidermis just lateral to the exit point at 90 degrees, exiting the undersurface of the dermis in the undermined space.

7. The suture material is then tied utilizing an instrument tie, and the trailing end of the suture is trimmed.

8. Moving proximally toward the surgeon, steps (1) through (6) are then repeated in pairs; once the desired number of throws are placed, the suture material is then tied off in a secure fashion utilizing an instrument tie (Figures 4-15A through 4-15J). The final anchoring knot is tied by leaving a loop on the penultimate throw and tying the free end of suture material from the final throw to this loop. The ends of the suture are then trimmed.

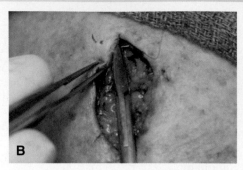

Figure 4-15B. The needle is inserted from the undermined underside of the dermis directly up and through the skin.

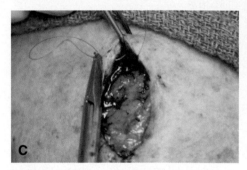

Figure 4-15C. The needle is then reinserted just medial to its exit point, again penetrating directly through the skin and exiting in the undermined space.

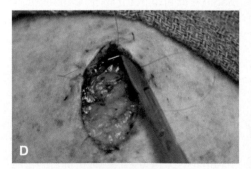

Figure 4-15D. The needle is reinserted on the contralateral side, through the undermined dermis and directly up and through the skin.

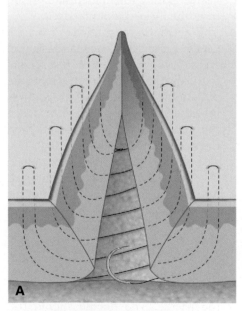

Figure 4-15A. Overview of the running percutaneous set-back dermal suture.

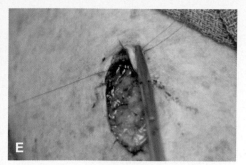

Figure 4-15E. The needle is then reinserted just lateral to its exit point, again penetrating directly through the skin and exiting in the undermined space. The suture material is then tied, and the short end is trimmed.

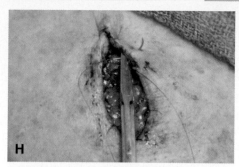

Figure 4-15H. The needle is then inserted on the contralateral wound edge from the underside of the dermis and up through the skin.

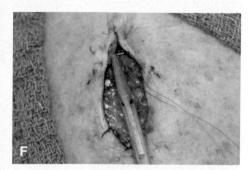

Figure 4-15F. After tying, the needle is inserted further along the wound edge from the underside of the dermis and up through the skin.

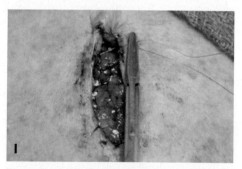

Figure 4-15I. The needle is then reinserted just lateral to its exit point, exiting the underside of the dermis. This pattern continues along the length of the wound until the apex is reached. At that point, the suture material is tied and the knot is buried.

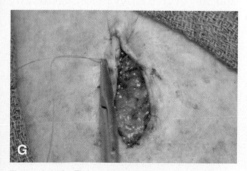

Figure 4-15G. The needle is then reinserted just medial to its exit point, exiting the underside of the dermis.

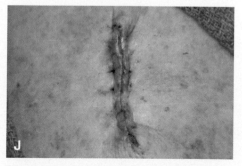

Figure 4-15J. Immediate postoperative appearance.

Tips and Pearls

As noted previously, this is an infrequently utilized approach and is best for closing areas under mild to moderate tension when other running approaches are not feasible. Since knots are tied only at the beginning and the end of the entire line of sutures, this technique is faster than utilizing standard interrupted percutaneous set-back dermal sutures, though this benefit must be weighed against the increased risk of suture line compromise with this approach.

It is critical to focus on outstanding knot security, since the entire suture line is held in place by the knots at the beginning and end of the set of suture throws. Adding an additional tacking knot when utilizing this approach is an option as well. It may provide additional knot security. Alternatively, one could consider placing an additional knot or leaving a longer suture tail.

Although it requires intermittently utilizing a backhand technique, this approach may be easier than other running buried techniques; since the suture pierces the epidermis and dermis at a 90-degree angle, there is no need to change planes or guarantee that the suture exit point is precisely at the inside edge of the lower dermis.

This approach may also be used in wounds under modest tension where extensive undermining is not possible; since the undersurface of the dermis does not need to be visualized to effectively place the sutures, the throws can be essentially placed blindly.

This technique may be conceptualized as a largely buried alternative to the simple running closure, since both approaches do not require wide undermining or an easily reflected wound edge and both approaches may be utilized in areas under modest tension.

An important theoretical advantage of this approach over other running percutaneous approaches is that no suture material is left between the wound edges. Since even absorbable suture material may represent a physical impediment to wound healing, this is an important benefit that this approach shares with the percutaneous and standard set-back dermal suture techniques.

Another theoretical benefit of the running approach is that there is less suture material left in situ, since the bulk of retained absorbable suture material is in the knots; as there are knots only at the beginning and end of the row of sutures, this technique theoretically decreases the risk of suture spitting and suture abscess formation. Still, the standard running set-back approach leaves suture material deep to the undersurface of the dermis, and therefore, the risk of suture spitting and suture abscess formation is negligible.

Drawbacks and Cautions

Like the interrupted percutaneous set-back dermal suture, the running percutaneous set-back dermal approach may result in very dramatic wound eversion, and the degree of eversion elicited by this approach may be more marked than that seen with the standard set-back dermal suture approach. This pronounced eversion may lead the epidermal portion of the wound edges to separate as the dermis is brought together, because the epidermal edges fail to drape together as they would normally do with the standard set-back dermal technique.

There are two possible approaches to this situation: (1) superficial running or interrupted sutures may be placed to better approximate the epidermal edges; and (2) the defect could be initially excised with an inward bevel (as is done with the butterfly suture technique), or the dermis may be incised at an inward bevel after the original defect is created, permitting the epidermal edges to come together gently even in the face of the marked eversion seen with this approach. Many clinicians favor a bilayered approach in general, and therefore, placing the epidermal sutures is an easy approach and does not require the degree of preplanning associated with the bevel approach, though a combination of the two solutions may be utilized as well. Since the running percutaneous set-back dermal approach relies on the security of only two knots to stabilize the entire length of the wound, placing simple interrupted epidermal sutures may be worthwhile.

Patients should be cautioned that they might develop a significant ridge in the immediate postoperative period. Depending on the suture material used and the density of the sutures, this ridge may last from weeks to months.

As with any percutaneous approach, there is a possibility of tear-through, and the consequences of even minimally exposed suture material remaining present at the surface of the wound should be considered.

Epidermal dimpling will often occur with this approach, since the suture material traverses the epidermis. A small degree of dimpling will resolve with time as the absorbable sutures are gradually resorbed, and patients should be warned that this is a likely occurrence and that it is of no long-term clinical consequence.

Since suture material traverses the epidermis, there is a theoretically greater risk of infection with this technique than with approaches that remain entirely buried on the undersurface of the dermis. Meticulous attention to sterile technique may help mitigate this theoretical risk, and anecdotally, infection is seen no more frequently with this approach than with any other closure technique.

Reference

Kantor J. The running percutaneous set-back dermal suture. *J Am Acad Dermatol.* 2015;73:e57-58.

The Running Percutaneous Buried Vertical Mattress Suture

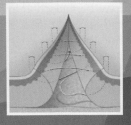

Video 4-16. Running percutaneous buried vertical mattress suture

Access to video can be found via mhprofessional.com/atlasofsuturingtechniques2e

Application

This running technique is designed to allow for moderate tension relief while concomitantly permitting easy suture placement in relatively tight spaces. It is best suited to areas with thicker dermis, though it may also be utilized in any body area when deep sutures are placed and where insertion of the full needle is challenging.

Some authors have advocated this technique as a replacement for standard running buried suture approaches, while others prefer to treat it as a niche approach exclusively for areas where other running fully buried approaches are more challenging to execute.

Suture Material Choice

Suture choice is dependent in large part on location. Though suture material travels percutaneously, exiting the epidermis and then reentering, the smallest gauge suture material appropriate for the anatomic location should be utilized. Often absorbable suture material is used to allow for an entirely buried suture line. If reentry is to be attempted through the same hole as suture exit, monofilament suture material may be preferred over the braided alternatives. On the back and shoulders, 2-0 or 3-0 suture material

is effective, though theoretically, the risk of suture spitting or suture abscess formation is greater with the thicker 2-0 suture material, particularly where the material has exited the epidermis entirely. On the extremities, a 3-0 or 4-0 absorbable suture material may be used, and on the face and areas under minimal tension, a 5-0 absorbable suture is adequate.

In addition to utilizing absorbable suture material, nonabsorbable suture material may also be utilized with this technique. In that event, the knots at the beginning and end of the suture line are tied externally, permitting easy suture removal. In such cases, a monofilament would be preferable to permit easy pull through at suture removal, reinsertion of the needle through the same hole, and a more pronounced pulley effect.

Technique

1. If possible, the wound edge is reflected back using surgical forceps or hooks. In areas under marked tension or where full visualization is not possible, the needle may be blindly inserted from the undermined space.
2. The suture needle is inserted at a 90-degree angle into the underside of the dermis 4 mm distant from the incised wound edge.
3. The first bite is started by following the needle and traversing from the underside of the dermis in the undermined space and passing entirely

through the dermis and exiting the skin.

4. The needle is then reloaded onto the needle driver with a backhanded technique and inserted through the epidermis either directly through the same hole as the suture followed during exit or just medial to it. A shallow bite is taken, and the needle exits on the margin of the incised wound edge.

5. The needle is then reloaded, again in a backhanded fashion, and it is inserted into the contralateral incised wound edge at the same depth as it exited on the first side. The needle again follows a mirror-image superficial course through the dermis, exiting through the epidermis again approximately 4 mm from the wound edge. Alternatively, this step may be combined with the prior step and the needle can be inserted into the contralateral edge while it is still loaded from the initial pass exiting the incised wound edge.

6. The needle is then loaded in a standard fashion and inserted either through the same hole or just lateral to it, following a deeper course and exiting the undersurface of the dermis into the undermined space.

7. The suture material is then tied, securing the anchoring stitch, and the trailing end is trimmed.

8. Steps (1) through (6) are then repeated sequentially for the desired number of throws, moving proximally toward the surgeon after each set of two sutures.

9. The suture material is then tied utilizing an instrument tie (Figures 4-16A through 4-16J). The final anchoring knot is tied by leaving a loop on the penultimate throw and tying the free end of suture material from the final throw to this loop. The ends of the suture are then trimmed.

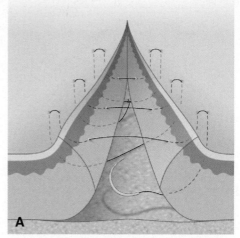

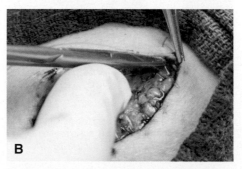

Figure 4-16A. Overview of the running percutaneous buried vertical mattress technique.

Figure 4-16B. Beginning of the initial anchoring percutaneous buried vertical mattress suture. Note that the needle enters the undersurface of the dermis, exiting directly upward through the skin.

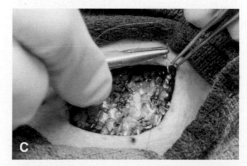

Figure 4-16C. The needle is then inserted with a backhand technique, running more superficially through the dermis, exiting in the incised wound edge.

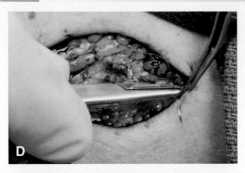

Figure 4-16D. The needle is inserted on the contralateral wound edge, again from the underside of the undermined dermis.

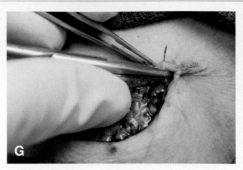

Figure 4-16G. The running technique continues in a similar fashion to the placement of the anchoring suture. Note that each time the suture enters a wound edge, it enters from the deep undermined space through the dermis.

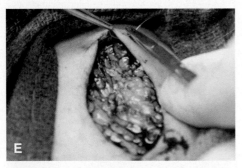

Figure 4-16E. The needle is then reinserted through the same hole or just lateral to it, again running superficially through the dermis and exiting in the incised wound edge.

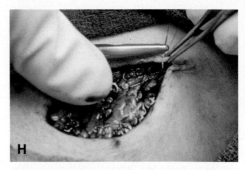

Figure 4-16H. As the percutaneous technique continues, each pass that moves inward toward the wound center is placed superficially, exiting through the incised wound edge.

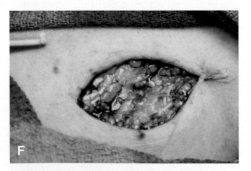

Figure 4-16F. Completed anchoring suture.

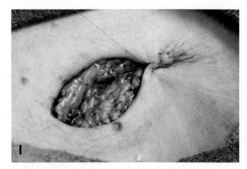

Figure 4-16I. Appearance of the incision as the suture is pulled tight. When using a braided absorbable suture, the suture material should be pulled through with each pass to ensure appropriate locking. With monofilament suture, as is used here, the suture material may be pulled tight intermittently to ensure appropriate wound-edge apposition.

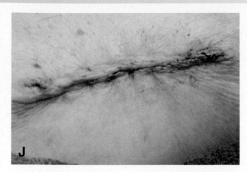

Figure 4-16J. Wound appearance after placement of a full series of running percutaneous buried vertical mattress sutures.

Tips and Pearls

This technique is best for areas where placement of a traditional running buried suture is challenging due to limited space, such as the scalp and lower leg, though it has been advocated as an approach with broader application.

This approach may also be used when it is difficult to visualize the undersurface of the dermis, since the needle throws may be placed in an almost blind fashion. The skin is grasped gently to make it taut, and the needle is inserted through the undermined space, exiting on the outside of the skin. This may be executed by feel, an approach well suited to the scalp where minimal dermal elasticity precludes full exposure of the undersurface of the undermined dermis.

It is critical to focus on outstanding knot security, since the entire suture line is held in place by the knots at the beginning and end of the set of suture throws. Adding an additional tacking knot when utilizing this approach is an option as well and may provide additional knot security. Alternatively, one could consider placing an additional knot throw or leaving a longer suture tail when utilizing this approach.

Like the running percutaneous set-back dermal suture, this technique may be conceptualized as a largely buried alternative to the simple running closure, since both approaches do not require wide undermining or an easily reflected wound edge and both approaches may be utilized in areas under modest tension.

As with any percutaneous approach, there is a possibility of tear-through, and the consequences of even minimally exposed suture material remaining present at the surface of the wound should be considered.

A theoretical benefit of the running approach is that there is less suture material left in situ, since the bulk of retained absorbable suture material is in the knots; as there are knots only at the beginning and end of the row of sutures, this technique theoretically decreases the risk of suture spitting and suture abscess formation.

Drawbacks and Cautions

Since suture material exits the skin and then reenters, dimpling may occur. Patients should be warned that this is expected and will resolve with time. Reentering the skin through the same hole may help minimize the risk of dramatic dimpling, though it carries the attendant risk of damaging the suture material with the needle, potentially leading to suture breakage.

Setting back the first throw far from the incised wound edge may result in overeversion; the chief drawback of overeversion is that the dermis may overhang in the center of the incised wound edge, barring the epidermal edges from approximating appropriately, leading to a slightly wider final scar. This may be easily solved by carefully beveling the dermis to allow the epidermal edges to meet unimpeded.

Patients should be cautioned that they might develop a significant ridge in the immediate postoperative period.

Depending on the suture material used and the density of the sutures, this ridge may last from weeks to months.

Since suture material traverses the epidermis, there is a theoretically greater risk of infection with this technique than with approaches that remain entirely buried on the undersurface of the dermis. Meticulous attention to sterile technique may help mitigate this theoretical risk, and anecdotally, infection is seen no more frequently with this approach than with any other closure technique.

Reference

Justan I. New type of skin suture—fully buried running mattress suture. *J Plast Reconstr Aesthet Surg.* 2010;63(3):e338-339.

The Pulley Buried Dermal Suture

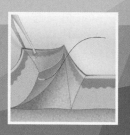

Synonym

Double buried dermal suture

Video 4-17. Pulley buried dermal suture
Access to video can be found via
mhprofessional.com/atlasofsuturingtechniques2e

Application

Wounds under marked tension may be challenging to close even with well-placed buried sutures. The pulley buried dermal suture technique relies on the pulley effect of multiple loops of suture to permit the closure of wounds under even significant tension. In addition, the locking effect of placing a double loop of suture leads the suture material to lock in place after the first throw of the surgical knot, obviating the need for an assistant maintaining the alignment of the wound edges.

Suture Material Choice

Suture choice is dependent in large part on location. Because this technique leaves significant residual suture material both between the incised wound edges and in the superficial dermis from both loops, care should be taken to minimize the liberal use of larger-gauge suture material. On the face, while this approach is only infrequently utilized, a 5-0 absorbable suture is appropriate, and on the distal extremities, a 4-0 suture is generally adequate. Using this technique, a 3-0 absorbable suture works well on the back, though when the area is under marked tension, a 2-0 suture may be needed as well. Braided suture tends to lock more definitively than monofilament, though monofilament suture allows for easy pull through when taking advantage of the pulley effect.

Technique

1. The wound edge is reflected back using surgical forceps or hooks.
2. While reflecting back the dermis, the suture needle is inserted at 90 degrees into the underside of the dermis 2 mm distant from the incised wound edge.
3. The first bite is executed by following the curvature of the needle and allowing the needle to exit in the incised wound edge. The size of this bite is based on the size of the needle, the thickness of the dermis, and the need for and tolerance of eversion. The needle's zenith with respect to the wound surface should be between the entry and exit points.
4. Keeping the loose end of the suture between the surgeon and the patient, the dermis on the side of the first bite is released. The tissue on the opposite edge is then gently grasped with the forceps.
5. The second bite is executed by inserting the needle into the incised

wound edge at the level of the superficial papillary dermis. This bite should be completed by following the curvature of the needle and avoiding catching the undersurface of the epidermis that could result in epidermal dimpling. It then exits approximately 2 mm distal to the wound edge on the undersurface of the dermis. This should mirror the first bite taken on the contralateral side of the wound.

6. Steps (1) through (5) are then repeated, after moving proximally toward the surgeon, with the tail of the suture material resting deep to the loops of suture.

7. The suture material is then tied utilizing an instrument tie (Figures 4-17A through 4-17J).

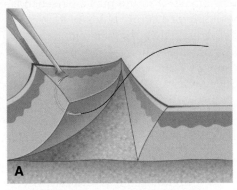

Figure 4-17A. The needle is inserted through the underside of the dermis, following the curvature of the needle and exiting at the incised wound edge.

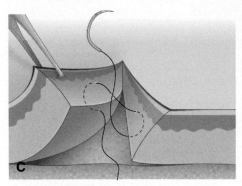

Figure 4-17C. Moving proximally toward the surgeon, with the suture material deep to the sutures and the tail toward the surgeon, the needle is again inserted through the dermis, exiting at the incised wound edge.

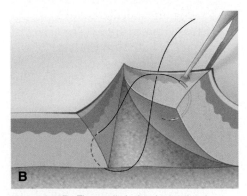

Figure 4-17B. The needle is then inserted at the incised wound edge on the contralateral side, exiting in the deep dermis.

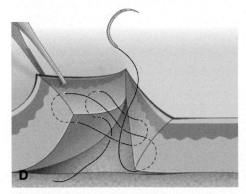

Figure 4-17D. The needle is then reinserted at the incised wound edge on the contralateral side.

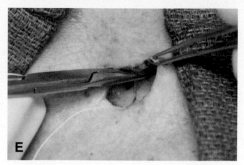

Figure 4-17E. The needle is inserted through the underside of the dermis, following the curvature of the needle and exiting at the incised wound edge.

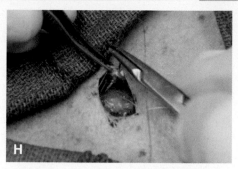

Figure 4-17H. The needle is then reinserted at the incised wound edge on the contralateral side.

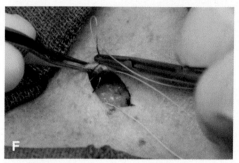

Figure 4-17F. The needle is then inserted at the incised wound edge on the contralateral side, exiting in the deep dermis.

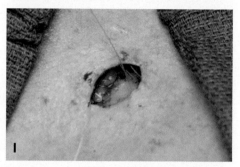

Figure 4-17I. The double loop of suture material with the tail deep to the loops is now visible.

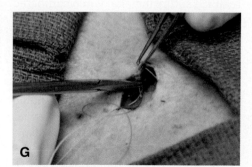

Figure 4-17G. Moving proximally toward the surgeon, with the suture material deep to the sutures and the tail toward the surgeon, the needle is again inserted through the dermis, exiting at the incised wound edge.

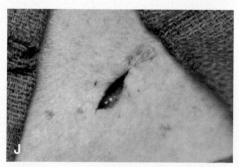

Figure 4-17J. Appearance immediately after tying the suture.

Tips and Pearls

This technique is useful when there is significant tension across the wound and, therefore, a single buried dermal suture may not hold the edges together. As long as undermining has been carried out effectively, utilizing a pulley technique with a thicker gauge suture material should allow for effective closure of all but the tightest wounds.

This technique is also very useful when the surgeon needs the first throw of the knot to securely hold the wound edges together, as this technique is able to effectively lock the suture in position after only a single throw. This obviates the need for an assistant's constant presence in these instances and permits precise placement of the suture and knot to allow for precise epidermal approximation.

It is critical to keep the suture material deep to the loops of suture when using this technique, as this is the mechanism by which the suture locks in place after the first throw. As long as the surgeon conceptualizes this approach as placing a standard buried dermal suture followed by a second standard buried dermal suture closer to the surgeon, this technique can be very simple to learn and is easily reproducible.

As always, the choice of suture material is largely based on the individual surgeon's preference. Braided absorbable suture material has the advantage of locking more reliably than monofilament, though monofilament suture allows for easier pull through and therefore may facilitate the pulley effect of the double loop of suture material.

In areas under extreme tension, a three-loop variation of this approach is possible as well, allowing for an even more dramatic pulley effect. This benefit must be weighed against the added retained suture material that would be associated with the additional loop.

Drawbacks and Cautions

The pulley buried dermal suture, while seemingly a simple approach, can sometimes be difficult to execute properly. Care should be taken to remain at the correct depth when utilizing this technique, as taking overly superficial bites and not following the course of the needle increases the risk of marked wound inversion.

Since pulley sutures leave two loops of suture material in the skin in lieu of one, this may result in an increased risk of foreign-body reaction, suture spitting, or suture abscess formation. Still, since the bulk of retained suture material is in the knots, rather than in the thrown loops of suture, this theoretical risk may not translate into a real-world problem in most cases.

Unlike the pulley set-back dermal suture, the pulley buried dermal suture leaves suture material traversing the incised wound edge, which may similarly increase the theoretical risk of suture spitting or suture abscess formation, especially since the pulley approach may effectively double the volume of non-knot retained suture material when compared to a standard dermal suture.

As with many buried techniques, epidermal dimpling may occur where the arc of the suture reaches its apex at the dermal-epidermal junction; on the face and areas with thin dermis, this should be assiduously avoided. Similarly, areas with sebaceous skin, such as the nose, require meticulous avoidance of dimpling, which has the potential to persist. In truncal areas or those with thick dermis, however, a small degree of dimpling will resolve with time as the absorbable sutures are gradually resorbed.

The tendency toward wound inversion with this approach means that superficial sutures are needed more frequently with this technique than with many others, since the transepidermal sutures are utilized in order to effect eversion of the wound edges. Since obviating the need for superficial sutures may be desirable both in terms of patient comfort and convenience and ultimate cosmetic and functional outcome, this should be considered before broadly applying this technique, and often pulley variations of the buried vertical mattress suture of set-back suture are preferred.

The Pulley Set-Back Dermal Suture

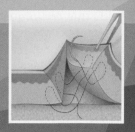

Synonyms

Pulley Kantor suture, double set-back suture, double set-back dermal suture

Video 4-18. Pulley set-back dermal suture

Access to video can be found via mhprofessional.com/atlasofsuturingtechniques2e

Application

This technique is best used in areas under very significant tension. In addition to high-tension wounds in general, areas under marked tension that are prone to wound inversion, such as the back and chest, may be well-served utilizing this technique.

Wounds under marked tension may be challenging to close even with well-placed buried sutures. The pulley set-back dermal suture technique relies on the pulley effect of multiple loops of suture to permit the closure of wounds under even significant tension. In addition, the locking effect of placing a double loop of suture leads the suture material to lock in place after the first throw of the surgical knot, obviating the need for an assistant maintaining the alignment of the wound edges.

Suture Material Choice

Suture choice is dependent in large part on location. Though this technique is designed to bite the deep dermis and remain buried well below the wound surface, the surgeon may choose to utilize a larger gauge suture than would be used for an equivalently placed pulley buried

dermal suture. Using a 2-0 absorbable suture on the back with this technique results in only vanishingly rare complications, since the thicker suture remains largely on the underside of the dermis, and suture spitting is an uncommon occurrence. On the extremities, a 3-0 or 4-0 absorbable suture material may be used, and on the face, if this pulley approach is needed at all, a 5-0 absorbable suture is adequate. Braided suture tends to lock more definitively than monofilament, though monofilament suture allows for easy pull through when taking advantage of the pulley effect.

Technique

1. The wound edge is reflected back using surgical forceps or hooks. Adequate visualization of the underside of the dermis is required.
2. While reflecting back the dermis, the suture needle is inserted at 90 degrees into the underside of the dermis 2-6 mm distant from the incised wound edge.
3. The first bite is executed by traversing the dermis following the curvature of the needle and allowing the needle to exit closer to the incised wound edge. Care should be taken to remain in the dermis to minimize the risk of epidermal dimpling. The needle does not, however, exit through the incised wound edge, but rather 1-4 mm distant from the incised

edge. The size of this first bite is based on the size of the needle, the thickness of the dermis, and the need for and tolerance of eversion.

4. Keeping the loose end of suture between the surgeon and the patient, the dermis on the side of the first bite is released. The tissue on the opposite edge is then reflected back in a similar fashion as on the first side, assuring complete visualization of the underside of the dermis.

5. The second bite is executed by inserting the needle into the underside of the dermis 1-6 mm distant from the incised wound edge. Again, this bite should be executed by following the curvature of the needle and avoiding catching the undersurface of the epidermis that could result in epidermal dimpling. It then exits further distal to the wound edge, approximately 2-6 mm distant from the wound edge. This should mirror the first bite taken on the contralateral side of the wound.

6. Steps (1) through (5) are then repeated after moving proximally toward the surgeon and taking care to leave the tail of the suture material deep to the loops of suture.

7. The suture material is then tied utilizing an instrument tie.

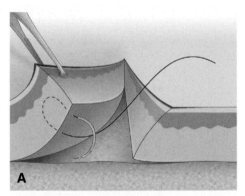

Figure 4-18A. The needle is inserted through the underside of the dermis, exiting the underside of the dermis closer to the incised wound edge but still set back from the incised wound edge.

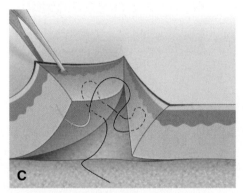

Figure 4-18C. With the loose end of the suture material deep to the active sutures and resting between the surgeon and the needle driver, the needle is then reinserted through the undersurface of the dermis.

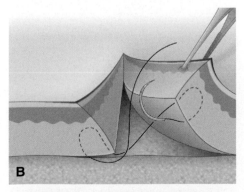

Figure 4-18B. The needle is then inserted through the underside of the dermis on the contralateral wound edge, exiting further away from the incised wound edge on the undersurface of the dermis.

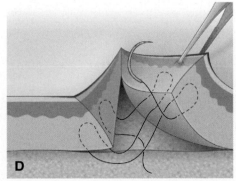

Figure 4-18D. The procedure is again repeated on the contralateral wound edge.

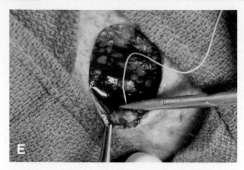

Figure 4-18E. The needle is inserted through the underside of the dermis, exiting the underside of the dermis closer to the incised wound edge but still set back from the incised wound edge.

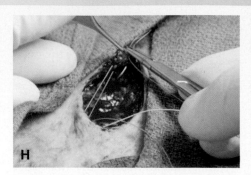

Figure 4-18H. The procedure is again repeated on the contralateral wound edge.

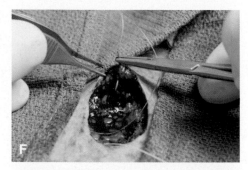

Figure 4-18F. The needle is then inserted through the underside of the dermis on the contralateral wound edge, exiting further away from the incised wound edge on the undersurface of the dermis.

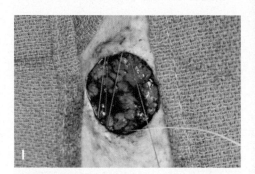

Figure 4-18I. Note the appearance of the suture material prior to pulling it taut.

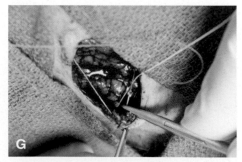

Figure 4-18G. With the loose end of the suture material deep to the active sutures and resting between the surgeon and the needle driver, the needle is then reinserted through the undersurface of the dermis.

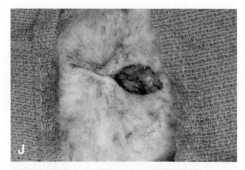

Figure 4-18J. Immediate postoperative appearance. Note the marked wound eversion and the presence of dimpling lateral to the incision line.

Tips and Pearls

One of the chief advantages of this technique is its ease of execution; since the suture follows the arc of the needle on the undersurface of the dermis, there is no need to change planes, effect a heart-shaped suture placement, or guarantee that the suture exit point is precisely at the inside edge of the lower dermis, as may be needed with the pulley buried vertical mattress suture.

Accurate suture placement is predicated on having a sufficiently undermined plane, since the entire suture loop lays on the undersurface of the dermis. Therefore, broad undermining is a prerequisite for utilizing this technique, since the first throw of the needle begins 2-6 mm distant from the incised wound edge.

This technique is useful when there is significant tension across the wound, and a single set-back dermal suture may not hold the edges together. As long as undermining has been carried out effectively, utilizing a pulley technique with a thicker gauge suture material should allow for effective closure of all but the tightest wounds.

This technique is also very useful when the surgeon needs the first throw of the knot to securely hold the wound edges together, as this technique is able to effectively lock the suture in position after only a single throw. This obviates the need for an assistant's constant presence in these instances and permits precise placement of the suture and knot to allow for precise epidermal approximation.

It is critical to keep the suture material deep to the loops of suture when using this technique, as this is the mechanism by which the suture locks in place after the first throw. As long as the surgeon conceptualizes this approach as placing a standard set-back dermal suture followed by a second standard set-back dermal suture closer to the surgeon, this technique can be very simple to learn and is easily reproducible.

As always, the choice of suture material is largely based on the individual surgeon's preference. Braided absorbable suture material has the advantage of locking more reliably than monofilament, though monofilament suture allows for easier pull through and therefore may better facilitate the pulley effect of the double loop of suture material.

In areas under extreme tension, a three-loop variation of this approach is possible as well, allowing for an even more dramatic pulley effect. This benefit must be weighed against the added retained suture material that would be associated with the additional loop. It may instead be preferable to increase the distance between the loops if there is concern for the suture material tearing through the dermis when under tension.

Drawbacks and Cautions

The pulley set-back dermal approach creates significant wound eversion, and the degree of eversion elicited by this approach may, depending on how far set back the dermal bite is taken, elicit significantly more wound eversion than even the pulley buried vertical mattress technique.

Patients should be cautioned that they might develop a significant ridge in the immediate postoperative period. Depending on the suture material used and the density of the sutures, this ridge may last from weeks to months. Explaining that the technique is akin to placing a subcutaneous splint may help the patient develop reasonable and realistic expectations and reduce anxiety regarding the immediate postoperative appearance of the wound.

Epidermal dimpling will occasionally occur where the arc of the suture reaches its apex at the dermal-epidermal junction; on the face and areas with thin dermis, this should be assiduously avoided. Similarly, areas with sebaceous skin, such as the nose, require meticulous avoidance of dimpling, which has the potential to persist. In truncal areas or those with thick dermis, however, a small degree of dimpling will resolve with time as the absorbable sutures are gradually resorbed.

Since pulley sutures leave two loops of suture material in the skin in lieu of one, this may result in an increased risk of foreign-body reaction, suture spitting, or suture-abscess formation. Still, since the bulk of retained suture material is in the knots, rather than in the thrown loops of suture, this theoretical risk may not translate into a real-world problem in most cases.

Reference

Kantor J. The pulley set-back dermal suture: an easy to implement everting suture technique for wounds under tension. *J Am Acad Dermatol.* 2015;72(1):e29-30.

The Pulley Buried Vertical Mattress Suture

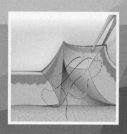

Synonyms

Double buried vertical mattress, dermal buried pulley suture, SICM, modified buried dermal suture

 Video 4-19. Pulley buried vertical mattress suture
Access to video can be found via mhprofessional.com/atlasofsuturingtechniques2e

Application

This technique is best used in areas under very significant tension. Wounds under marked tension may be challenging to close even with well-placed buried sutures. The pulley buried vertical mattress suture technique relies on the pulley effect of multiple loops of suture to permit the closure of wounds under even significant tension. In addition, the locking effect of placing a double loop of suture leads the suture material to lock in place after the first throw of the surgical knot, obviating the need for an assistant maintaining the alignment of the wound edges.

Suture Material Choice

Suture choice is dependent in large part on location. Though suture material traverses the papillary dermis and the incised wound edge, as always, the smallest gauge suture material appropriate for the anatomic location should be utilized. On the back and shoulders, 2-0 or 3-0 suture material is effective, though

theoretically, the risk of suture spitting or suture abscess formation is greater with the thicker 2-0 suture material. This needs to be weighed against the benefit of utilizing a larger CP-2 needle, which will almost never bend even in the thickest dermis, and the benefit of adopting the 2-0 suture material, which is less likely to snap under tension or fail during tension-bearing activities, leading to attendant dehiscence. On the extremities, a 3-0 or 4-0 absorbable suture material may be used, and on the face and areas under minimal tension, a 5-0 absorbable suture is adequate.

Braided suture tends to lock more definitively than monofilament, though monofilament suture allows for easy pull through when taking advantage of the pulley effect.

Technique

1. The wound edge is reflected back using surgical forceps or hooks. Adequate visualization of the underside of the dermis is desirable.
2. While reflecting back the dermis, the suture needle is inserted at 90 degrees into the underside of the dermis, 4 mm distant from the incised wound edge.
3. The first bite is executed by following the needle initially at 90 degrees to the underside of the dermis and then, critically, changing direction by twisting the needle driver so that the needle exits in the incised wound

edge. This allows the apex of the bite to remain in the papillary dermis while the needle exits in the incised wound edge at the level of the reticular dermis.

4. Keeping the loose end of the suture between the surgeon and the patient, the dermis on the side of the first bite is released. The tissue on the opposite edge is then reflected back in a similar fashion as on the first side.

5. The second bite is executed by inserting the needle into the incised wound edge at the level of the reticular dermis. It then angles upward and laterally so that the apex of the needle is at the level of the papillary

dermis. This should mirror the first bite taken on the contralateral side of the wound.

6. Keeping the tail of the suture material between the surgeon and the first set of loops, steps (1) through (5) are then repeated, after moving proximally toward the surgeon. The second set of loops may be placed 2-6 mm apart depending on the size of the defect, the thickness of the dermis, and the degree of tension on the wound.

7. The suture material is then tied utilizing an instrument tie (Figures 4-19A through 4-19I).

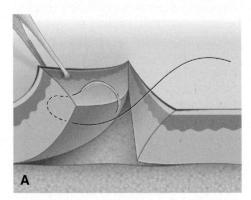

Figure 4-19A. The needle is inserted through the dermis, angling upward and outward before exiting at the incised wound edge.

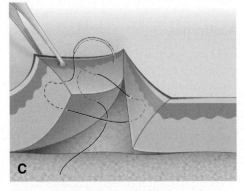

Figure 4-19C. Keeping the tail of the suture deep to the suture throws and toward the surgeon, the first step is then repeated, with the needle entering deep and exiting at the incised wound edge.

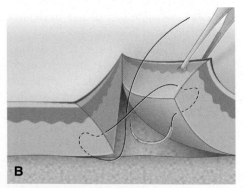

Figure 4-19B. The needle is then inserted through the incised wound edge on the contralateral side, again moving superolaterally before exiting deep.

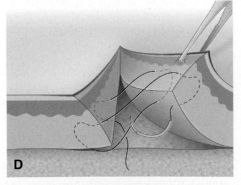

Figure 4-19D. Again with the tail deep, the needle is inserted through the incised wound edge on the contralateral side.

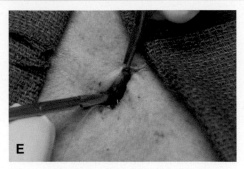

Figure 4-19E. The needle is inserted through the dermis, angling upward and outward before exiting at the incised wound edge.

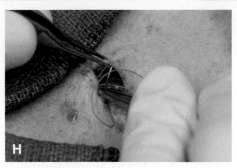

Figure 4-19H. Again with the tail of the suture deep, the needle is inserted through the incised wound edge on the contralateral side.

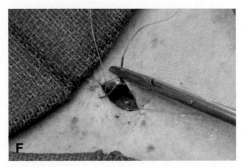

Figure 4-19F. The needle is then inserted through the incised wound edge on the contralateral side, again moving superolaterally before exiting deep.

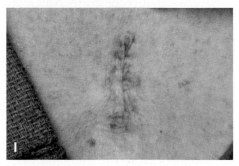

Figure 4-19I. Immediate postoperative appearance. Note the wound-edge eversion.

Tips and Pearls

This technique requires some practice to master, though once mastered, it is straightforward to execute. The first bite may be finessed by first reflecting the wound edge back sharply during needle insertion and then returning the edge medially after the apex has been reached. This approach helps lead the needle in the correct course without an exaggerated change in direction with the needle driver.

A similar approach may be utilized by surgeons who favor skin hooks over surgical forceps; here again, the hook may be used to hyper-reflect the skin edge back during the first portion of the first

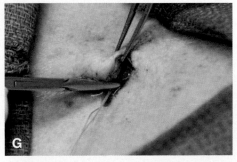

Figure 4-19G. Keeping the tail of the suture deep to the suture throws and toward the surgeon, the first step is then repeated, with the needle entering deep and exiting at the incised wound edge.

bite and then similarly pull the incised wound edge toward the center of the wound during the second portion of the first bite. This will encourage the needle to follow the desired heart-shaped path without necessitating a dramatic twist of the needle driver as the needle changes course.

The apex of the needle should be in the papillary dermis; if the needle courses too superficially, dimpling may occur. While such dimpling is sometimes almost unavoidable, it remains best to avoid it if possible since: (1) patients may sometimes have some concern regarding the immediate postoperative appearance, and (2) dimpling signifies that the suture material traverses very superficially, raising concern that it could be associated with an increased risk of suture spitting.

This technique is useful when there is significant tension across the wound and a single buried vertical mattress suture may not hold the edges together. As long as undermining has been carried out effectively, utilizing a pulley technique with a thicker gauge suture material should allow for effective closure of all but the tightest wounds.

This technique is also very useful when the surgeon needs the first throw of the knot to securely hold the wound edges together, as this technique is able to effectively lock the suture in position after only a single throw. This obviates the need for an assistant's constant presence in these instances and permits precise placement of the suture and knot to allow for precise epidermal approximation.

It is critical to keep the suture material deep to the loops of suture when using this technique, as this is the mechanism by which the suture locks in place after the first throw. As long as the surgeon conceptualizes this approach as placing a standard buried vertical mattress suture followed by a second buried vertical mattress suture closer to the surgeon, this technique can be very simple to learn and is easily reproducible.

As always, the choice of suture material is largely based on the individual surgeon's preference. Braided absorbable suture material has the advantage of locking more reliably than monofilament, though monofilament suture allows for easier pull through and therefore may facilitate the pulley effect of the double loop of suture material.

In areas under extreme tension, a three-loop variation of this approach is possible as well, allowing for an even more dramatic pulley effect. This benefit must be weighed against the added retained suture material that would be associated with the additional loop. It may be preferable to increase the distance between the loops if there is concern for the suture material tearing through the dermis when under tension.

Drawbacks and Cautions

While the eversion is less pronounced than that seen in other techniques, such as the pulley set-back dermal suture, patients may still be left with a small ridge in the immediate postoperative period.

Epidermal dimpling will occasionally occur where the arc of the suture reaches its apex at the dermal-epidermal junction; on the face and areas with thin dermis, this should be assiduously avoided. Similarly, areas with sebaceous skin, such as the nose, require meticulous avoidance of dimpling, which has the potential to persist. In truncal areas or those with thick dermis, however, a small degree of dimpling will resolve with time as the absorbable sutures are gradually resorbed.

Since pulley sutures leave two loops of suture material in the skin in lieu of one, this may result in an increased risk of foreign-body reaction, suture spitting, or suture abscess formation. Still, since the bulk of retained suture material is in the knots, rather than in the thrown loops of suture, this theoretical risk may not translate into a real-world problem in most cases.

References

Giandoni MB, Grabski WJ. Surgical pearl: the dermal buried pulley suture. *J Am Acad Dermatol.* 1994;30(6):1012-1013.

Jeon IK, Kim JH, Roh MR, Chung KY. The subcutaneous inverted cross mattress stitch (SICM stitch) in our experience. *Dermatol Surg.* 2013;39(5):794-795.

Whalen JD, Dufresne RG, Collins SC. Surgical pearl: the modified buried dermal suture. *J Am Acad Dermatol.* 1999;40(1):103-104.

Yag-Howard C. Novel surgical approach to subcutaneous closure: the subcutaneous inverted cross mattress stitch (SICM stitch). *Dermatol Surg.* 2011;37(10):1503-1505.

The Half Pulley Buried Vertical Mattress Suture

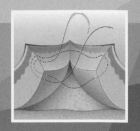

Synonyms

Dermal buried pulley suture, modified buried dermal suture

Video 4-20. Half pulley buried vertical mattress suture

Access to video can be found via mhprofessional.com/atlasofsuturingtechniques2e

Application

This technique is best used in areas under very significant tension and can be conceptualized as existing on the spectrum between single and double buried vertical mattress sutures. Wounds under marked tension may be challenging to close even with well-placed buried sutures. The half pulley buried dermal suture technique relies on the pulley effect of an additional single loop of suture to permit the closure of wounds under even significant tension. In addition, the effect of placing an extra bite of suture leads the suture material to lock in place after the first throw of the surgical knot, obviating the need for an assistant maintaining the alignment of the wound edges.

Suture Material Choice

Suture choice is dependent in large part on location. Since some suture material traverses the papillary dermis and the incised wound edge, as always, the smallest gauge suture material appropriate for the anatomic location should be utilized. On the back and shoulders, 2-0 or 3-0 suture material is effective, though theoretically, the risk of suture spitting or suture abscess formation is greater with the thicker 2-0 suture material. This needs to be weighed against the benefit of utilizing a larger CP-2 needle, which will almost never bend even in the thickest dermis, and the benefit of adopting the 2-0 suture material, which is less likely to snap under tension or fail during tension-bearing activities, leading to attendant dehiscence. On the extremities, 3-0 or 4-0 absorbable suture material may be used, and on the face and areas under minimal tension, though this technique would only rarely be used, a 5-0 absorbable suture is adequate.

Braided suture tends to lock more definitively than monofilament, though monofilament suture allows for easy pull through when taking advantage of the pulley effect.

Technique

1. The wound edge is reflected back using surgical forceps or hooks. Adequate visualization of the underside of the dermis is desirable.
2. While reflecting back the dermis, the suture needle is inserted at 90 degrees into the underside of the dermis 4 mm distant from the incised wound edge.
3. The first bite is executed by following the needle initially at 90 degrees to the underside of the dermis and then changing direction by twisting

the needle driver so that the needle exits in the incised wound edge. This allows the apex of the bite to remain in the papillary dermis while the needle exits in the incised wound edge at the level of the reticular dermis.

4. Keeping the loose end of the suture between the surgeon and the patient, the dermis on the side of the first bite is released. The tissue on the opposite edge is then reflected back in a similar fashion as on the first side.

5. The second bite is executed by inserting the needle into the incised wound edge at the level of the reticular dermis. It then angles upward and laterally so that the apex of the needle is at the level of the papillary

dermis. This should mirror the first bite taken on the contralateral side of the wound.

6. Keeping the tail of the suture material between the surgeon and the first set of loops, the needle is then inserted into the undersurface of the dermis slightly further set back from the wound edge than the first throw.

7. The needle then exits in the deep reticular dermis, just deep to the exit point of the first loop of suture.

8. With both ends of the suture material now exiting from the same side of the wound (generally the surgeon's left), the suture material is then tied utilizing an instrument tie (Figures 4-20A through 4-20F).

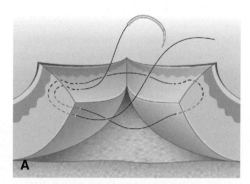

Figure 4-20A. Overview of the half pulley buried vertical mattress suture.

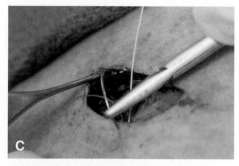

Figure 4-20C. The needle is then inserted at the incised wound edge on the contralateral side.

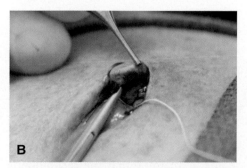

Figure 4-20B. The needle is inserted through the deep dermis and exits at the incised wound edge, as with a buried vertical mattress suture.

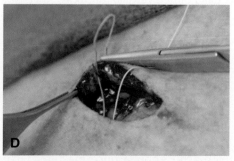

Figure 4-20D. After moving slightly upward and outward, the needle exits the dermis.

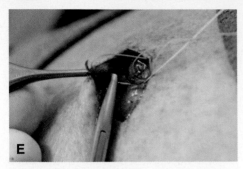

Figure 4-20E. The needle is then reinserted on the contralateral side through the dermis and exits near the incised wound edge, forming a pulley system of a one-and-one-half buried vertical mattress suture.

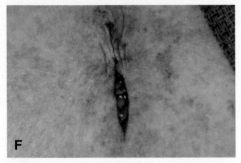

Figure 4-20F. Immediate postoperative appearance after placing a single half pulley buried vertical mattress suture.

Tips and Pearls

This technique may be conceptualized as a buried vertical mattress suture with an additional bite or as a 1½ loop buried vertical mattress pulley suture. It is therefore slightly faster to execute than the pulley buried vertical mattress, since this technique saves one needle throw. That said, since there is one less loop of suture, the pulley effect may similarly be less pronounced, though this needs to be weighed against the theoretical benefit of less retained suture material in this technique than in a double buried vertical mattress suture.

This technique requires some practice to master, though once mastered, it is straightforward to execute. The first bite may be finessed by first reflecting the

wound edge back sharply during needle insertion and then returning the edge medially after the apex has been reached. This approach helps lead the needle in the correct course without an exaggerated change in direction with the needle driver.

The apex of the needle should be in the papillary dermis; if the needle courses too superficially, dimpling may occur. This technique is useful when there is significant tension across the wound and a single buried vertical mattress suture may not hold the edges together.

This technique is also very useful when the surgeon needs the first throw of the knot to securely hold the wound edges together, as this technique is able to effectively lock the suture in position after only a single throw. This obviates the need for an assistant's constant presence in these instances and permits precise placement of the suture and knot to allow for precise epidermal approximation.

The extra throw may also be completed with an oblique or near-horizontal orientation, since it is very important that this extra throw bite sufficient dermis to support the tension of the wound. The extra throw may also be executed as a single set-back dermal suture, though doing so may lead to some discrepancy in the depth of the wound edges, necessitating the placement of depth-correcting epidermal sutures.

Drawbacks and Cautions

While the eversion is less pronounced than that seen with other techniques, such as the pulley set-back dermal suture, patients may still be left with a small ridge in the immediate postoperative period. While this is desirable, it is also important to warn patients of this outcome; explaining that the technique is akin to placing a subcutaneous splint may help the patient develop reasonable and realistic expectations and reduce anxiety regarding the immediate postoperative appearance of the wound.

Epidermal dimpling will occasionally occur where the arc of the suture reaches its apex at the dermal-epidermal junction; on the face and areas with thin dermis, this should be assiduously avoided. Similarly, areas with sebaceous skin, such as the nose, require meticulous avoidance of dimpling, which has the potential to persist. In truncal areas or those with thick dermis, however, a small degree of dimpling will resolve with time as the absorbable sutures are gradually resorbed.

Since this pulley approach leaves an extra single loop of suture material in the skin, this may result in an increased risk of foreign-body reaction, suture spitting, or suture abscess formation. Still, since the bulk of retained suture material is in the knots, rather than in the thrown loops of suture, this theoretical risk may not translate into a real-world problem in most cases.

There is also a theoretical concern that the extra loop of suture could lead to some wound-edge necrosis, particularly if it is oriented in a horizontal fashion, though this is not usually seen in practice. Finally, since the suture material is tied together on one side of the wound, there may be less precise epidermal approximation than is seen with other techniques, such as the pulley set-back dermal suture and the pulley buried vertical mattress.

References

Giandoni MB, Grabski WJ. Surgical pearl: the dermal buried pulley suture. *J Am Acad Dermatol.* 1994;30(6):1012-1013.

Whalen JD, Dufresne RG, Collins SC. Surgical pearl: the modified buried dermal suture. *J Am Acad Dermatol.* 1999;40(1):103-104.

CHAPTER 4.21

The Double Butterfly Suture

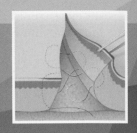

Video 4-21. Double butterfly suture

Access to video can be found via mhprofessional.com/atlasofsuturingtechniques2e

Application

This technique is best used in areas under very significant tension. Wounds under marked tension may be challenging to close even with well-placed buried sutures. The double butterfly suture technique relies on the pulley effect of multiple horizontally oriented diagonal loops of suture to permit the closure of wounds under even significant tension. Since the loops are horizontally oriented, a broader bite of dermis is included with each throw, adding to the theoretical robustness of this closure technique.

Suture Material Choice

As always, suture material choice depends on preference and location. Though this technique is designed for wounds under significant tension on the trunk, it is commonly utilized with a 3-0 suture. While adopting a 2-0 gauge suture material is sometimes useful, especially to avoid bending smaller needles, the knot for this suture is buried in line with the incision and at the base of the dermis, and therefore, suture material spitting is a risk. Use of an absorbable monofilament (polydioxanone) has been proposed as providing superior outcomes over a braided absorbable suture.

Technique

1. This technique ideally requires that the wound edges be incised with a reverse bevel, allowing the epidermis to overhang the dermis in the center of the wound.

2. The wound edge is reflected back using surgical forceps or hooks. Adequate full visualization of the underside of the dermis is very helpful.

3. While reflecting back the dermis, the suture needle is inserted into the undersurface of the dermis approximately 3 mm set back from the medial edge of the dermis at the base of the bevel. The needle driver is held like a pencil at 90 degrees to the incised wound edge, and the needle may be held on the needle driver at an oblique angle to facilitate suture placement.

4. The first bite is executed by placing gentle pressure on the needle so that it moves laterally and upward, forming a horizontal loop that on cross section resembles the wing of a butterfly. The needle then exits the undersurface of the dermis after following its curvature, similarly set back from the incised wound edge.

5. Keeping the loose end of the suture between the surgeon and the patient, the dermis on the side of the first bite is released. The tissue on the opposite edge is then reflected back in a similar fashion as on the first side.

6. The second bite is executed by inserting the needle into the undersurface

of the dermis on the contralateral side distal to the exit point, with a backhand technique if desired and the needle still pointing in the same direction as the first throw, and completing a loop that forms an S when viewed along with the first loop.

7. The needle is then reinserted into the contralateral wound edge in line with its exit point, now heading toward the surgeon, in a mirror image of step (6).

8. Finally, the needle is then reinserted into the contralateral side in a mirror image of the first throw (step 4). Thus, the entry point of the first suture loop and the exit point of the last suture loop are directly across from each other on the undersurface of the dermis.

9. The suture material is then tied utilizing an instrument tie (Figures 4-21A through 4-21J).

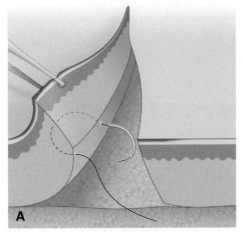

Figure 4-21A. First bite of the double butterfly suture. Note that the needle courses parallel to the incised wound edge, taking a more superficial portion of dermis in the center of its trajectory.

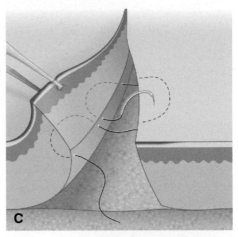

Figure 4-21C. The needle is then reloaded so that it points in the opposite direction of the first two bites and enters on the contralateral side of the wound at approximately the level of its exit point.

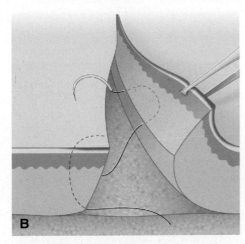

Figure 4-21B. The needle then enters the contralateral wound edge approximately level with its exit point, still on the same trajectory as the first bite.

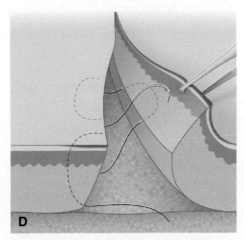

Figure 4-21D. Preparing for the final bite of the double butterfly suture, again with the needle entering at the same level as its exit point so that the final exit point of the needle will be directly across from the initial entry point placed at the start of this technique.

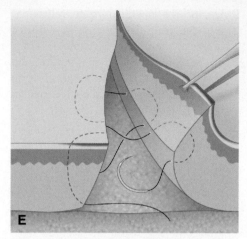

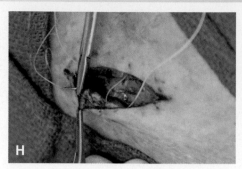

Figure 4-21H. The needle is then reloaded so that it points in the opposite direction of the first two bites and enters on the contralateral side of the wound at approximately the level of its exit point.

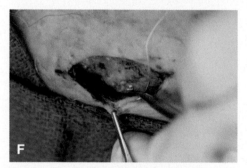

Figure 4-21E. Overview of the double butterfly suture technique.

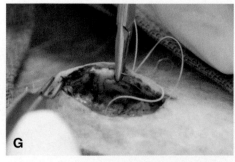

Figure 4-21F. First bite of the double butterfly suture. Note that the needle courses parallel to the incised wound edge, taking a more superficial portion of dermis in the center of its trajectory.

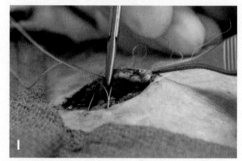

Figure 4-21I. Final bite of the double butterfly suture, again with the needle entering at the same level as its exit point so that the final exit point of the needle is now directly across from the initial entry point placed at the start of this technique.

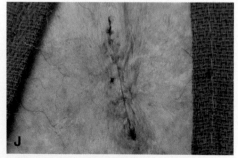

Figure 4-21G. The needle then enters the contralateral wound edge approximately level with its exit point, still on the same trajectory as the first bite.

Figure 4-21J. Immediate postoperative appearance after placement of a central double butterfly suture and multiple set-back dermal sutures at the apices. Note the wound eversion.

Tips and Pearls

This technique is designed for areas under marked tension, though it may be used in any anatomic location. As such, utilizing a sufficiently robust needle may be very helpful in mitigating the risk of needle bending that can be seen when attempting to place the needle in the thick dermis of the back.

It is helpful to conceptualize this technique as forming an S, which is then turned into a figure 8. Importantly, the double butterfly technique is *not* executed by performing two sets of butterfly sutures sequentially.

As with the pulley buried vertical mattress approach, the first bite may be finessed by first reflecting the wound edge back sharply during needle insertion and then returning the edge medially after the apex has been reached. This approach helps lead the needle in the correct course without an exaggerated change in direction with the needle driver, though the needle is oriented parallel to the incised wound edge, as opposed to the perpendicular approach utilized with the buried vertical mattress.

The apex of the needle should be in the papillary dermis; if the needle courses too superficially, dimpling may occur. In particularly high-tension areas, the suture loops may be placed close together in order to mitigate the risk of an accordion effect. The horizontal orientation of the suture loops means that a relatively significant amount of dermis is included within each suture loop. Particularly in areas under marked tension where there is concern regarding the ability of the dermis to withstand tensile forces, this represents an advantage over other double or pulley approaches.

Drawbacks and Cautions

The need to bevel the wound edges means that this technique requires a small degree of preplanning. The bevel may, however, be useful for other techniques as well (such as the modified buried horizontal mattress suture), and it may help with wound-edge apposition in general, though there is also the theoretical risk of contracture leading to a small separation between the wound edges. If the butterfly suture is utilized without beveling the wound edges, a small amount of dermis may overhang in the incised wound edges, preventing wound-edge apposition. In this event, surgical scissors or a blade may be used to trim back the overhanging dermis to permit the epidermal wound edges to come together unimpeded.

Some authors have raised concerns regarding possible wound-edge necrosis associated with any horizontally oriented suture placement. Advocates of this approach report that wound-edge necrosis has not been seen as a complication, and indeed, the only time that necrosis seems to be an issue is with superficially placed horizontal mattress sutures, rather than with their buried counterparts. This is likely due to a constrictive effect on the incised wound edge, which is not typically seen with buried sutures.

While the suture loops may be relatively close together, especially under areas of marked tension, the loops themselves should not overlap, as this has the potential to compress the wound edges together, leading to central bunching of the wound edges.

Given the marked eversion associated with this technique, patients may be left with a small ridge in the immediate postoperative period. While this is desirable, it is also important to warn patients of this outcome; explaining that the technique is akin to placing a subcutaneous splint may help the patient develop reasonable and realistic expectations and reduce anxiety regarding the immediate postoperative appearance of the wound.

References

Breuninger H. Double butterfly suture for high tension: a broadly anchored, horizontal, buried interrupted suture. *Dermatol Surg.* 2000;26(3):215-218.

Breuninger H, Keilbach J, Haaf U. Intracutaneous butterfly suture with absorbable synthetic suture material. Technique, tissue reactions, and results. *J Dermatol Surg Oncol.* 1993;19(7):607-610.

The Half Pulley Buried Dermal Suture

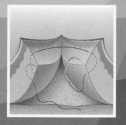

Synonyms

Lateral pulley buried dermal suture, set back pulley dermal suture

 Video 4-22. Half pulley buried dermal suture
Access to video can be found via mhprofessional.com/atlasofsuturingtechniques2e

Application

This technique is best used in areas under very significant tension and can be conceptualized as existing on the spectrum between single and double buried vertical mattress sutures. It is similar to the half pulley buried vertical mattress suture, but with the extra loop placed at the beginning, rather than the end, of the technique.

Wounds under marked tension may be challenging to close even with well-placed buried sutures. The half pulley buried dermal suture technique relies on the pulley effect of multiple loops of suture to permit the closure of wounds under even significant tension. In addition, the locking effect of placing a double loop of suture leads the suture material to lock in place after the first throw of the surgical knot, obviating the need for an assistant maintaining the alignment of the wound edges.

Suture Material Choice

Suture choice is dependent in large part on location. Though suture material traverses the papillary dermis and the incised wound edge, as always, the smallest gauge suture material appropriate for the anatomic location should be utilized. On the back and shoulders, 2-0 or 3-0 suture material is effective, though theoretically, the risk of suture spitting or suture abscess formation is greater with the thicker 2-0 suture material. This needs to be weighed against the benefit of utilizing a larger CP-2 needle, which will almost never bend even in the thickest dermis, and the benefit of adopting the 2-0 suture material, which is less likely to snap under tension or fail during tension-bearing activities, leading to attendant dehiscence. On the extremities, a 3-0 or 4-0 absorbable suture material may be used. Braided suture tends to lock more definitively than monofilament, though monofilament suture allows for easy pull through when taking advantage of the pulley effect.

Technique

1. The wound edge is reflected back using surgical forceps or hooks. Adequate visualization of the underside of the dermis is required.
2. While reflecting back the dermis, the suture needle is inserted at 90 degrees into the underside of the dermis 4-8 mm distant from the incised wound edge.
3. The first bite, which represents the extra pulley loop, is executed by traversing the dermis following the curvature of the needle and allowing the needle to exit closer to the

115

incised wound edge. Care should be taken to remain in the dermis to minimize the risk of epidermal dimpling. The needle does not, however, exit through the incised wound edge, but rather 3-4 mm distant from the incised edge, as would be done with a set-back dermal suture. The size of this first loop is based on the size of the needle and the thickness of the dermis and should be designed as a modestly sized extra loop, which will allow for a pulley effect.

4. Keeping the loose end of the suture between the surgeon and the patient, the needle is then reinserted again on the same side of the dermis as the first loop, just distal to the entry and exit points of the first loop of the suture, but again through the undermined undersurface of the dermis. It should

enter approximately 3-8 mm set back from the incised wound edge. The needle then exits at the wound margin as in a simple buried dermal suture.

5. The tissue on the opposite side of the wound is then reflected back in a similar fashion as on the first side, and the third bite is executed by inserting the needle into the dermis at the wound edge. This bite should be executed by following the curvature of the needle and avoiding catching the undersurface of the epidermis. It then exits the undersurface of the dermis approximately 3-8 mm lateral to the incised wound margin. This should mirror the second bite taken on the contralateral side of the wound.

6. The suture material is then tied utilizing an instrument tie (Figures 4-22A through 4-22E).

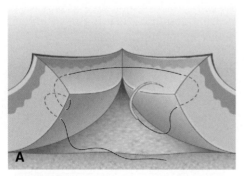

Figure 4-22A. Overview of the half pulley buried dermal suture.

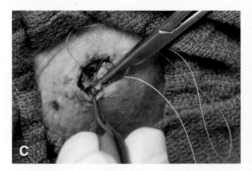

Figure 4-22C. The needle is then inserted through the dermis, exiting at the incised wound edge.

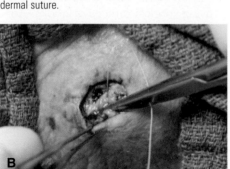

Figure 4-22B. The suture is started by placing the needle through the dermis, markedly set back from the wound edge.

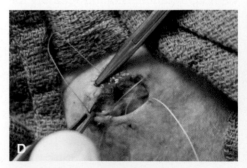

Figure 4-22D. The needle is then reinserted on the contralateral side through the incised wound edge, exiting in the dermis.

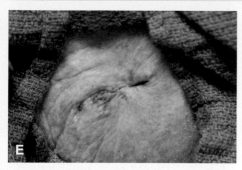

Figure 4-22E. Immediate postoperative appearance after placing a single half pulley buried dermal suture.

Tips and Pearls

Like the half pulley buried vertical mattress suture, this technique may be conceptualized as a simple buried dermal suture with an additional loop or as a 1½ loop simple buried dermal pulley suture, though with the extra loop taken at the beginning, rather than at the end, of the technique. In this way, it is also similar to a half version of the modified buried horizontal mattress suture (Chapter 4.23), though with the two loops separated vertically rather than horizontally. It is slightly faster to execute than other pulley sutures, since this technique saves one needle throw. That said, since there is one less loop of suture, the pulley effect may similarly be less pronounced, though this needs to be weighed against the theoretical benefit of less retained suture material in this technique than in a pulley buried dermal suture.

This technique is useful when there is significant tension across the wound and a single buried suture may not hold the edges together.

As always, the choice of suture material is largely based on the individual surgeon's preference. Braided absorbable suture material has the advantage of locking more reliably than monofilament, though monofilament suture allows for easier pull through and therefore may facilitate the pulley effect of the extra loop of suture material.

Drawbacks and Cautions

Epidermal dimpling will occasionally occur where the arc of the suture reaches its apex at the dermal-epidermal junction; on the face and areas with thin dermis, this should be assiduously avoided. Similarly, areas with sebaceous skin, such as the nose, require meticulous avoidance of dimpling, which has the potential to persist. In truncal areas or those with thick dermis, however, a small degree of dimpling will resolve with time as the absorbable sutures are gradually resorbed.

Since this pulley approach leaves an extra single loop of suture material in the skin, this may result in an increased risk of foreign-body reaction, suture spitting, or suture-abscess formation. Still, since the bulk of retained suture material is in the knots, rather than in the thrown loops of suture, this theoretical risk may not translate into a real-world problem in most cases.

There is also a theoretical concern that the extra loop of suture could lead to some wound-edge necrosis, particularly if it is oriented in an oblique fashion, though this is not usually seen in practice. Finally, since the additional loop of suture material is located on the side of the first bite, the pulley effect may not be as pronounced as in other pulley techniques, since there is no back-and-forth pulley effect between the two sides of the wound.

References

Huang L. The lateral pulley buried dermal suture. *Australas J Dermatol.* 2011;52(3):207-208.

Huang L. The setback pulley dermal suture for skin defects. *Am Surg.* 2011;77(5):647-648.

The Modified Buried Horizontal Mattress Suture

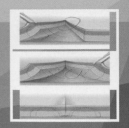

Synonyms

Modified subcutaneous buried horizontal mattress suture, four-throw buried horizontal mattress suture

 Video 4-23. Modified buried horizontal mattress suture
Access to video can be found via mhprofessional.com/atlasofsuturingtechniques2e

Application

This is a niche technique, useful occasionally when closing wounds under significant tension. It may be employed in a variety of locations, including the scalp, trunk, and lower leg. It requires four separate throws but leads to only a minimal pulley effect, reducing its usefulness in many situations. It was originally described when used in concert with a reverse beveled excision, as with a butterfly suture approach.

Suture Material Choice

As always, suture material choice depends on preference and location; while the suture material remains on the undersurface of the dermis, it does traverse the midpapillary dermis, and therefore, care should be taken to utilize the smallest caliber of suture that provides adequate tensile strength. Similarly, the knot remains relatively superficial at the level of the reticular dermis, particularly when performing this technique as described in the literature, suggesting the need to utilize the finest suture available.

On the extremities, a 4-0 absorbable suture material may be used, and on the face and areas under minimal tension, a 5-0 absorbable suture is adequate, though this technique would rarely be used. Using this technique, a 3-0 absorbable suture works well on the back, though when the area is under marked tension, a 2-0 suture may be needed as well.

Technique

1. The wound edge is reflected back using surgical forceps or hooks. The needle enters along the underside of the dermis adjacent to the incised wound edge, exiting set back at the undersurface of the undermined wound.
2. The needle is then reloaded, the skin is reflected back, and the needle is inserted through the undersurface of the undermined dermis adjacent to its exit point, exiting at the underside of the dermis adjacent to the wound.
3. The needle is reloaded and enters the dermal-epidermal junction directly across from its exit point, and a bite is taken following the curvature of the needle and exiting at the undersurface of the undermined dermis.
4. The needle is then reloaded, and the final bite is taken by entering at the undermined undersurface of the dermis and exiting in the underside of the dermis adjacent to the incised wound edge.

5. The suture material is then tied utilizing an instrument tie (Figures 4-23A through 4-23K).

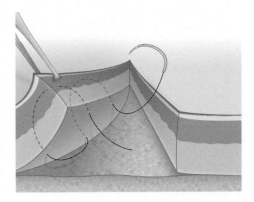

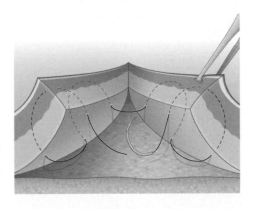

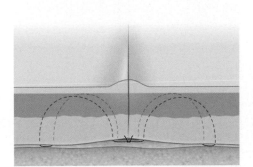

Figure 4-23A. Overview of the modified buried horizontal mattress suture.

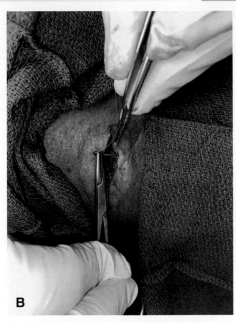

Figure 4-23B. The wound edge is reflected back using surgical forceps or hooks. The needle enters along the underside of the incised wound edge.

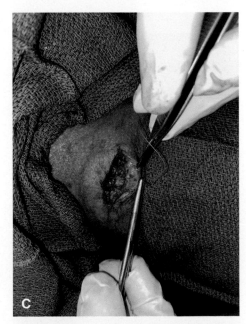

Figure 4-23C. The needle exits further set back along the undersurface of the undermined wound.

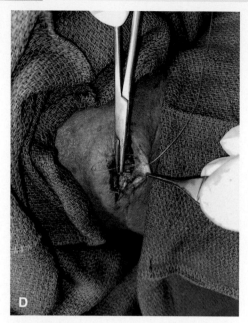

Figure 4-23D. The needle is then reloaded, the skin is reflected back, and the needle is inserted through the undersurface of the undermined dermis adjacent to its exit point.

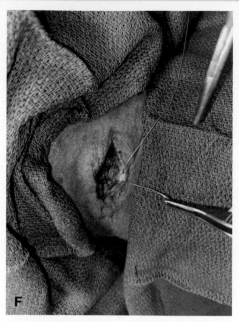

Figure 4-23F. Appearance after the first set of sutures is placed.

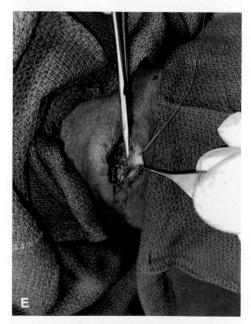

Figure 4-23E. The needle exits closer to the wound edge on the undersurface of the wound.

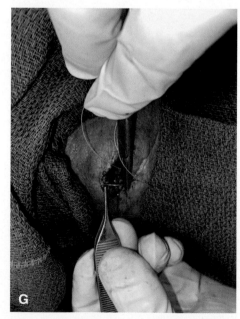

Figure 4-23G. The needle is reloaded and enters the dermal-epidermal junction directly across from its exit point.

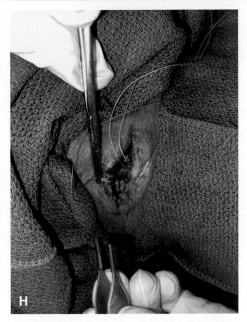

Figure 4-23H. A bite is taken following the curvature of the needle and exiting at the undersurface of the undermined dermis.

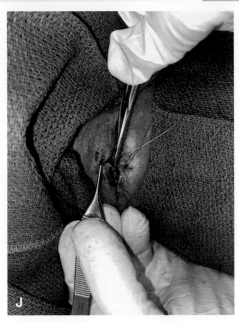

Figure 4-23J. The needle exits at the undersurface of the dermis adjacent to the incised wound edge.

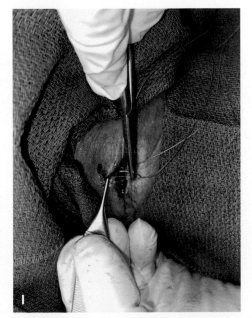

Figure 4-23I. The needle is then reloaded, and the final bite is taken by entering at the undermined undersurface of the dermis.

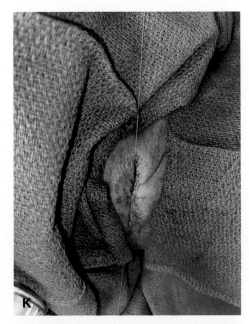

Figure 4-23K. The suture material is then tied utilizing an instrument tie.

Tips and Pearls

This can be conceptualized as a horizontal mattress suture where each throw of the suture material is vertically oriented. Therefore, it is in some ways more similar to the traditional horizontal mattress suture than the originally described buried horizontal mattress suture, though it requires additional throws.

It can also be thought of as a double set-back suture (since, in the images in the article describing the technique, each throw enters and exits on the underside of the undermined dermis), but one lacking a true pulley effect.

As with any buried technique, the apex of the needle should be in or deep to the papillary dermis; if the needle courses too superficially, dimpling may occur.

The chief advantage of this technique is the greater tensile strength that this suture can carry when compared with other techniques. This advantage, however, must be weighed against the additional effort required (since there are four distinct vertically oriented throws involved) and the larger amount of suture material that remains to be absorbed.

Drawbacks and Cautions

While some have suggested this as a standard technique for excisional surgery, in general, this technique should not be adopted in all areas, and there are better options for use in areas with a robust dermis under moderate to marked tension, such as the back and shoulders, including the set-back suture or buried vertical mattress suture, particularly when combined with a fascial plication suture.

Patients may still be left with a small ridge in the immediate postoperative period. While this is desirable, it is also important to warn patients of this outcome.

Reference

Meng F, Andrea S, Cheng S, Wang Q, Huo R. Modified subcutaneous buried horizontal mattress suture compared with vertical buried mattress suture. *Ann Plast Surg.* 2017;79(2):197-202.

The Suspension Suture

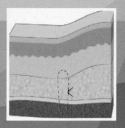

Synonyms

Pexing suture, ImPli, tacking suture, buried basting suture

 Video 4-24. Suspension suture
Access to video can be found via
mhprofessional.com/atlasofsuturingtechniques2e

Application

This is a niche technique designed to fix a defect to a deeper structure. This approach has also been referred to as a pexing suture or tacking suture and is utilized typically in several situations. First, when repairing a defect that crosses a natural sulcus, it is important to tack down the skin overlying the sulcus so that the natural depression is not blunted, or bridged, by the repair. Second, it is used when working near cosmetic subunit boundaries and free margins to avoid functional challenges such as ectropion and eclabium, as well as cosmetic distortion of sensitive areas such as the lip and eyebrows. It is also useful in order to fix a flap in place and minimize tension on the distal portion of the flap. It can also be used to fix the base of a graft to underlying structures, minimizing the risk of dead space formation and graft failure. Finally, this approach may also be used to prevent nasal valve collapse in the appropriate setting.

Suture Material Choice

Suture choice is dependent in large part on location, though this technique is usually utilized on the face. While some authors have advocated for nonabsorbable clear monofilament suture to provide a lasting suspension effect, in general, absorbable suture material is adequate and may mitigate some of the concerns related to leaving a nonabsorbable foreign body in place for an extended period of time. A 4-0 absorbable suture may often be utilized for this approach on the face. While utilizing smaller gauge absorbable suture material is reasonable, it may not provide sufficient tensile strength to adequately and reliably fix the tissue to the periosteum.

Technique

1. The wound edge is reflected back using surgical forceps or hooks, and adequate visualization of the underside of the dermis is desirable.
2. While reflecting back the dermis, the suture needle is inserted at 90 degrees into the underside of the dermis 2-6 mm distant from the incised wound edge.
3. The first bite is executed by traversing the dermis following the curvature of the needle and allowing the needle to exit closer to the incised wound edge. This will minimize the risk of vascular compromise. Care should be taken to remain in the dermis to minimize the risk of epidermal dimpling. The needle does not, however, exit through the incised wound edge, but rather 1-4 mm distant from the incised edge or, in

select cases, potentially further back from the wound edge.

4. The flap of skin may be gently pulled by the suture material so that the location of the first bite directly overlies the planned fixation point. This permits the surgeon to double-check the final position of the suspension suture. The needle is then blindly inserted through the fat and deeper structures until the bone is reached. A 3-mm bite of the periosteum is then taken, and the needle is brought back up through the soft tissues into the open center of the wound.

5. The suture material is then tied utilizing an instrument tie. Hand tying may be utilized as well, which may be useful if the depth of the defect is significant (Figures 4-24A through 4-24F).

Tips and Pearls

This technique is very useful when working around the eyelids and lips, though its use demands familiarity with the underling anatomy so that no sensitive deeper structures are injured or entrapped during

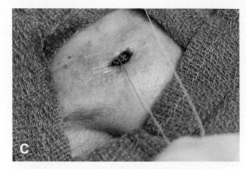

Figure 4-24C. The suture material is gently pulled to determine the location of the desired anchoring point.

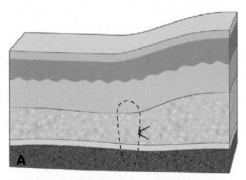

Figure 4-24A. Overview of the suspension suture technique.

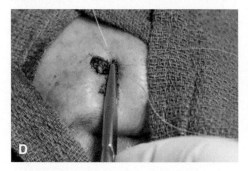

Figure 4-24D. A bite of periosteum is taken over the desired suspension point. Note that the needle is inserted blindly through the subcutaneous fat until the periosteum is reached.

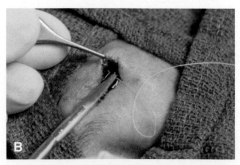

Figure 4-24B. A set-back suture bite is taken from the dermis overlying the anticipated anchoring point on the lower forehead.

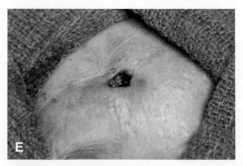

Figure 4-24E. The suture has now been tied, tacking the dermis to a fixed point, leading to subtle dimpling.

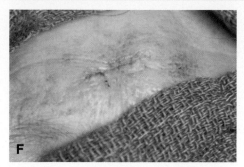

Figure 4-24F. Immediate postoperative appearance.

the blind placement of the deep anchoring suture. The deep suture should also be placed parallel to the underlying vascular plexus to similarly mitigate this risk.

Placement is based on several considerations, including the degree of tension across the advanced tissue, the presence of a bony prominence, which can be used easily for suspension purposes, and the absence of underlying nerves, which could inadvertently become strangulated by the anchoring suture.

The first half of this suture technique, where the suture material is fixed to the underside of the dermis, may be conceptualized as a single throw of a set-back dermal suture. Depending on the location of the repair and the degree of suspension necessary, a single throw of this technique may be adequate. When reconstructing longer sulci, such as the mental sulcus, a series of spaced suspension sutures can be placed to assure that the natural crease is not bridged by the repair.

Pulling on the suture once it is anchored to the periosteum may help assure the surgeon that the suture is indeed tacked down to an immobile surface.

A central advantage of this technique is that it may permit the use of linear closures in areas where otherwise a flap would have been advisable to minimize free-margin distortion. Thus, for example, closures on the lower forehead or upper malar area may be closed in a linear fashion if the advancing skin (the superior and inferior portions of the repairs, respectively) is effectively tacked down.

A three-point variation of this approach is possible as well, which allows wound-edge approximation and a tacking effect to occur all with one suture placement. This is accomplished by first placing either a buried vertical mattress or set-back dermal suture at the two wound edges and then taking a bite of the underlying periosteum prior to tying the knot. The suture material thus fixes the wound edges together as well as to the underlying anchoring point. This approach, however, may result in sub-optimal wound-edge eversion and places additional stress on the suture material, increasing the risk of scar spread. Moreover, it is only appropriate if the anchor target lies in the approximate midpoint of the defect, since it recreates a natural sulcus but does not permit differential pull from one side of the defect; therefore, this approach is of little utility when attempting to avoid cosmetic distortion of sensitive areas.

This technique may also be used as an alternative to cartilage grafting when reconstructing the nose. Loss of alar cartilage may lead to nasal valve collapse, which traditionally was addressed by placing an auricular cartilage graft along the reconstructed alar rim in order to maintain valve patency. A simple and elegant alternative is placing a suture in the ala and fixing it to a point superolaterally in the maxillary periosteum, permitting the nasal valve to remain open and obviating the need for a cartilage graft in many cases.

In select cases, a suspension suture may be used to fix a flap or graft to fascia or other soft tissue structures, rather than periosteum, in order to secure its position or decrease the tension across superficial sutures at the time of final closure.

Drawbacks and Cautions

Since the underside of the dermis is often tacked to the periosteum, this technique may result in an area of depression at the site of suspension suture placement. It is therefore important to utilize this approach exclusively in areas with adequate laxity, as poorly placed suspension sutures could theoretically result in an aggravated degree of distortion in cosmetically sensitive areas. Moreover, the presence of only minimal laxity increases the risk of subsequent dehiscence and ischemia.

The anchoring portion of this suture technique carries the risk of damage to an underlying vascular or neural plexus. Familiarity with the underlying bony anatomy is therefore of paramount importance, as it also permits the surgeon to select the best location for suspension suture placement. Such areas include the mental crease, zygomatic arch, malar eminence, and supraorbital and infraorbital ridges. As suture material is tacked to the periosteum—and traverses muscle and fascia—patients should be warned that they may experience more pain with this approach than would be experienced with a typical bilayered closure.

References

Robinson JK. Suspension sutures aid facial reconstruction. *Dermatol Surg.* 1999;25(3):189-194.

Robinson JK. Suspension sutures in facial reconstruction. *Dermatol Surg.* 2003;29(4):386-393.

Salasche SJ, Jarchow R, Feldman BD, Devine-Rust MJ, Adnot J. The suspension suture. *J Dermatol Surg Oncol.* 1987;13(9):973-978.

Wang JH, Finn D, Cummins DL. Suspension suture technique to prevent nasal valve collapse after Mohs micrographic surgery. *Dermatol Surg.* 2014;40(3):345-347.

Webster RC, Davidson TM, Reardon EJ, Smith RC. Suspending sutures in blepharoplasty. *Arch Otolaryngol.* 1979;105(10):601-604.

Yag-Howard C. Novel approach to decreasing tension when approximating wound edges in advancement flaps: the ImPli stitch. *Dermatol Surg.* 2012;38:661-663.

The Percutaneous Suspension Suture

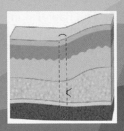

 Video 4-25. Percutaneous suspension suture
Access to video can be found via
mhprofessional.com/atlasofsuturingtechniques2e

Application

Like the traditional suspension suture, this is a niche technique designed to fix the edge of a defect to a deeper structure and may also be utilized typically in four situations: (1) when repairing a defect that crosses a natural sulcus, (2) when working near cosmetic subunit boundaries and free margins, to avoid functional challenges such as ectropion and eclabium, as well as cosmetic distortion of sensitive areas such as the lip and eyebrows, (3) when fixing a flap in place to minimize tension on the distal portion of the flap, and (4) when fixing a graft to underlying structures to minimize the risk of dead space/hematoma formation and maintain close approximation between the underside of the graft and the underlying vascular bed.

Since the dermal component of the suture is percutaneous, however, it consistently results in immediate postoperative dimpling. The advocates of this technique have suggested that the dimpling resolves spontaneously over time, though unless the technique is truly necessary in order to be able to fix the tissue—which may be the case if it is challenging to insert the needle and needle driver through an undermined tunnel of skin—it would probably be preferable to perform a standard suspension suture in order to minimize the risk of long-term dimpling at the site of percutaneous suture placement.

Suture Material Choice

Suture choice is dependent in large part on location, though this technique is usually utilized on the face. Since the suture is placed percutaneously, absorbable suture is preferred. A 4-0 or 5-0 absorbable suture may be used on the face. While utilizing smaller gauge absorbable suture material is reasonable, it may not provide sufficient tensile strength to adequately and reliably fix the tissue to the periosteum.

Technique

1. Unlike the traditional suspension suture, visualization of the percutaneous tacking site on the mobile flap of skin is not necessary.
2. The suture needle is inserted at 90 degrees into the underside of the dermis at the point in the undermined flap where fixation to the underlying anchoring point is desired. The needle then pierces through the epidermis.
3. The first bite is completed by either reinserting the needle back through the epidermis with the twist of a wrist or by grasping the needle where it exits the epidermis and reintroducing it directly down through the epidermis so that it exits 2-4 mm away from the entry point.

4. The flap of skin may be gently pulled by the suture material so that the location of the first bite directly overlies the planned fixation point. This permits the surgeon to double-check the final position of the suspension suture. The needle is then blindly inserted through the fat and deeper structures until the bone is reached. A 3-mm bite of the periosteum is then taken, and the needle is brought back through the soft tissues into the open center of the wound.

5. The suture material is then tied utilizing an instrument tie. Hand tying may be utilized as well, which may be useful if the depth of the defect is significant (Figures 4-25A through 4-25F).

Tips and Pearls

As with the traditional suspension suture, this technique's use demands familiarity with the underlying anatomy so that no sensitive deeper structures are injured

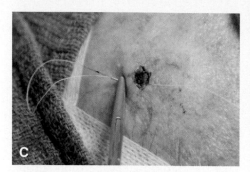

Figure 4-25C. The needle is then inserted just medial to its exit point through the skin, exiting on the underside of the dermis in the undermined space.

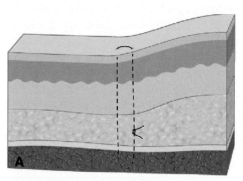

Figure 4-25A. Overview of the percutaneous suspension suture.

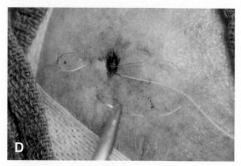

Figure 4-25D. Appearance after placing the percutaneous component of the suture.

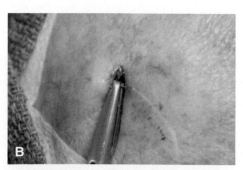

Figure 4-25B. The needle is inserted from the underside of the dermis in the undermined space, up directly through the skin.

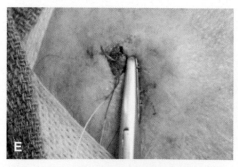

Figure 4-25E. The needle is then inserted blindly through the fat until the periosteum is reached, and a small bite of periosteum is taken. The suture is then tied, suspending the skin over the target point over the periosteum.

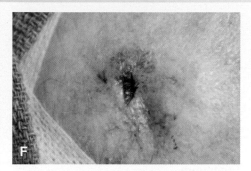

Figure 4-25F. Immediate postoperative appearance.

or strangled during the blind placement of the deep anchoring suture. The deep suture should also be placed parallel to the underlying vascular plexus to similarly mitigate this risk.

Placement is based on several considerations, including the degree of tension across the advanced tissue, the presence of a bony prominence, which can be used easily for suspension purposes, and the absence of underlying nerves, which could inadvertently become entrapped by the anchoring suture.

While a series of spaced percutaneous suspension sutures can be placed to assure that a natural crease is not bridged by a surgical repair, it may be best to minimize the number of sutures placed in order to mitigate the risk of pronounced persistent dimpling of the overlying skin.

Pulling on the suture once it is anchored to the periosteum may help assure the surgeon that the suture is indeed tacked down to an immobile surface in cases where this approach is used for this purpose.

As with the traditional suspension suture, an advantage of this technique is that it may permit the use of linear closures in areas where otherwise a flap would have been advisable to minimize free-margin distortion. Thus, for example, closures on the lower forehead may be closed in a linear fashion if the advancing skin (the superior portion of the repair) is effectively tacked down, thus avoiding raising the ipsilateral eyebrow.

Drawbacks and Cautions

The percutaneous nature of this approach effectively guarantees an area of depression at the site of suspension suture placement. It is therefore important to utilize this approach exclusively in areas with adequate laxity, as poorly placed suspension sutures could theoretically result in an aggravated degree of distortion in cosmetically sensitive areas. Moreover, the presence of only minimal laxity increases the risk of subsequent dehiscence and ischemia. Therefore, this technique is best used in the event that placement of traditional suspension sutures is not feasible. Alternatively, if this approach is used as a percutaneous basting suture for graft placement, fast-absorbing suture could be used to ensure that the dimpling does not persist.

The anchoring portion of this suture technique carries the risk of damage to an underlying vascular or neural plexus. Familiarity with the underlying bony anatomy is therefore of paramount importance, as it also permits the surgeon to select the best location for suspension suture placement. As suture material is tacked to the periosteum—and traverses muscle and fascia—patients should be warned that they may experience more pain with this approach than would be experienced with a typical bilayered closure.

Reference

Cruz A, Wang AR, Campbell R, Chang KH, Dufresne R. The percutaneous suspension suture. *Dermatol Surg.* 2012;38(6):929-931.

The Pinpoint Pexing Suspension Suture

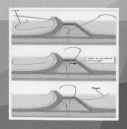

Video 4-26. The pinpoint pexing suspension suture

Access to video can be found via mhprofessional.com/atlasofsuturingtechniques2e

Application

Like the traditional buried suspension suture, this is a niche technique designed to fix the edge of a defect to a deeper structure and may also be utilized typically in four situations: (1) when repairing a defect that crosses a natural sulcus, (2) when working near cosmetic subunit boundaries and free margins, to avoid functional challenges such as ectropion and eclabium, as well as cosmetic distortion of sensitive areas such as the lip and eyebrows, (3) when fixing a flap in place to minimize tension on the distal portion of the flap, and (4) when fixing a graft to underlying structures to minimize the risk of dead space/hematoma formation and maintain close approximation between the underside of the graft and the underlying vascular bed.

The end result of this technique is a buried suspension suture, but it begins with an initial step that is percutaneous in order to better assess the ideal location for suture placement; the percutaneous portion is removed prior to tying, as noted below.

Suture Material Choice

Suture choice is dependent in large part on location, though this technique is usually utilized on the face. A 4-0 or 5-0 absorbable suture may be used.

Technique

1. The suture needle is inserted at 90 degrees from the outside of the skin overlying the desired tacking point directly through the dermis, exiting on the undersurface of the undermined flap at the point where fixation to the underlying anchoring point is desired.
2. The needle is then regrasped and inserted through the fat and deeper structures until the bone is reached (for periosteal suspension) or through more superficial structures (for simple tacking). A bite is then taken, and the needle is brought back through the soft tissues into the open center of the wound. Gentle tension can be used to ensure than an adequate bite was taken.
3. The needle is then reloaded, and a bite of the underside of the undermined dermis directly adjacent to the initial entry point is taken. Again, very gentle tension can be used to ensure that an adequate bite was taken.
4. The tail of the suture that traverses the entire thickness of the flap can then be pulled through so that the only remaining bites are the deep bite and the bite at the underside of the dermis.
5. The suture material is then tied using an instrument tie. Hand tying may be utilized as well, which may be useful if the depth of the defect is significant (Figures 4-26A through 4-26G).

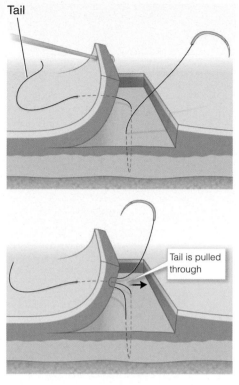

Tail

Tail is pulled through

Tail

Figure 4-26A. Overview of the pinpoint pexing suture.

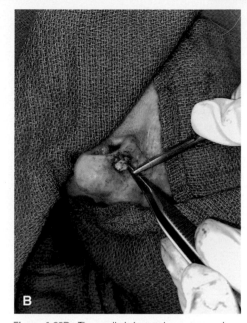

Figure 4-26B. The needle is inserted percutaneously at the desired location, directly through the elevated skin flap.

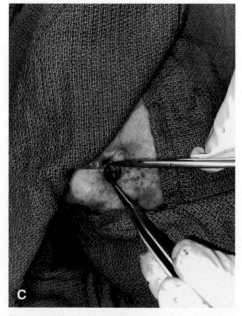

Figure 4-26C. The graft is reflected back, and the needle is gently pulled through. The needle is then reloaded.

Tips and Pearls

The initial transepidermal throw is used with this technique simply for placement purposes; one of the challenges of all suspension sutures is appropriately aligning the superficial and deep bites. By placing a temporary throw through the

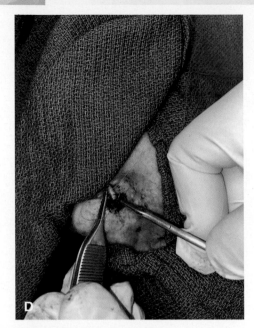

Figure 4-26D. The needle is inserted blindly through the fat until the periosteum is reached, and a small bite of periosteum is taken (or, for graft tacking, this bite would include only more superficial structures).

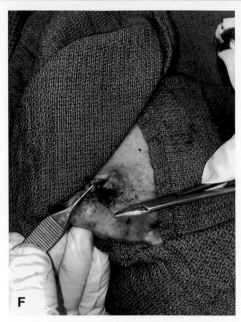

Figure 4-26F. The tail of the suture from the original percutaneous pass is pulled through so that no percutaneous suture remains, and the suture is tied.

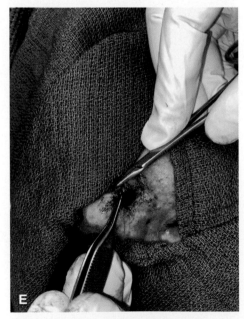

Figure 4-26E. The needle is then reloaded and inserted through the underside of the elevated flap directly adjacent to the percutaneous suture that marks the ideal location. A small bite through the dermis is taken.

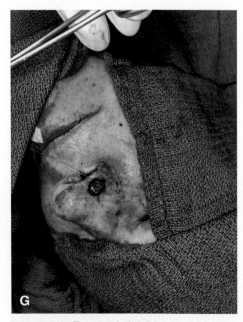

Figure 4-26G. The suture is tied, fixing the graft in place.

outside surface in the desired location, the ideal spot is pinpointed so that it is ideally situated, and after the final throw through the underside of the dermis is placed, the initial bite (now at the tail of the suture) is simply pulled through. As with the traditional suspension suture, this technique's use demands familiarity with the underlying anatomy so that no sensitive deeper structures are injured or strangled during the blind placement of the deep anchoring suture. The deep suture should also be placed parallel to the underlying vascular plexus to similarly mitigate this risk.

Placement is based on several considerations, including the degree of tension across the advanced tissue, the presence of a bony prominence, which can be used easily for suspension purposes, and the absence of underlying nerves, which could inadvertently become entrapped by the anchoring suture.

In addition to tacking to periosteum, this technique can be very useful when fixing a graft in place.

As with the traditional suspension suture, an advantage of this technique is that it may permit the use of linear closures in areas where otherwise a flap would have been advisable to minimize free-margin distortion. Thus, for example, closures on the lower forehead may be closed in a linear fashion if the advancing skin (the superior portion of the repair) is effectively tacked down, thus avoiding raising the ipsilateral eyebrow.

Drawbacks and Cautions

As with any suspension suture, the anchoring portion of this suture technique carries the risk of damage to an underlying vascular or neural plexus. Familiarity with the underlying bony anatomy is therefore of paramount importance, as it also permits the surgeon to select the best location for suture placement if the suture will be tacked to periosteum.

Caution should be exerted in not tying the suture too tightly, as this can lead to permanent dimpling at the site of suture placement.

Reference

Nelson T, Mortimer N, Salmon P. Refining the "pin-point technique" for pexing sutures in facial reconstructive surgery. *Dermatol Surg.* 2020;46(1):135-136.

CHAPTER 4.27

The Tie-Over Suture

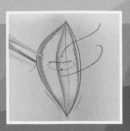

Video 4-27. Tie-over suture
Access to video can be found via
mhprofessional.com/atlasofsuturingtechniques2e

Application

This niche technique is useful when attempting to recreate a natural sulcus when the defect lies parallel to the sulcus. It involves encircling a buried vertical mattress suture with an anchoring suture that attaches to deeper structures such as the periosteum. It is a tissue-to-suture technique, since the anchoring suture is tied not to the overlying dermis but rather to a previously placed buried vertical mattress suture.

Suture Material Choice

This technique is generally utilized on the face, and therefore, the smallest gauge suture material with appropriate tensile strength should be utilized. Generally, a 4-0 or 5-0 absorbable suture material provides adequate security when anchoring to the periosteum. Nonabsorbable material could theoretically be utilized and may provide a longer-lasting depressive effect on the tissue, but this benefit is likely outweighed by the increased risk of foreign-body reaction and suture material extrusion.

Technique

1. The wound edge is reflected back using surgical forceps or hooks. Adequate visualization of the underside of the dermis is desirable.

2. While reflecting back the dermis, the suture needle is inserted at 90 degrees into the underside of the dermis 4 mm distant from the incised wound edge.

3. The first bite is executed by following the needle initially at 90 degrees to the underside of the dermis and then, critically, changing direction by twisting the needle driver so that the needle exits in the incised wound edge. This allows the apex of the bite to remain in the papillary dermis while the needle exits in the incised wound edge at the level of the reticular dermis.

4. Keeping the loose end of the suture between the surgeon and the patient, the dermis on the side of the first bite is released. The tissue on the opposite edge is then reflected back in a similar fashion as on the first side.

5. The second bite is executed by inserting the needle into the incised wound edge at the level of the reticular dermis. It then angles upward and laterally so that the apex of the needle is at the level of the papillary dermis. This should mirror the first bite taken on the contralateral side of the wound.

6. The suture material is then tied utilizing an instrument tie.

7. Once the buried vertical mattress suture has been completed, starting from one side of the tied buried vertical mattress suture, the needle

is blindly inserted through the fat and deeper structures until the bone is reached. A 3-mm bite of the periosteum is then taken, and the needle is brought back up through the soft tissues into the open center of the wound on the contralateral side of the buried vertical mattress suture and lifted above the buried vertical mattress suture.

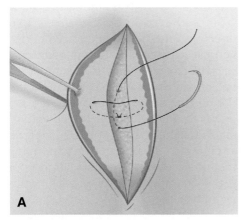

Figure 4-27A. Surgeon's eye view of the tie-over suture. A buried vertical mattress suture has been placed, and a suspension suture is now being secured perpendicular to the buried vertical mattress suture.

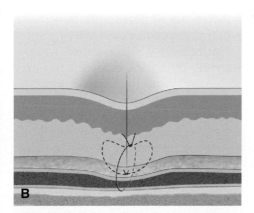

Figure 4-27B. Cross-sectional view of the tie-over suture. Note that the suspension suture connects the deeper tissues to the previously placed buried vertical mattress suture.

8. The suture material is then tied over the buried vertical mattress suture using an instrument tie, anchoring down the buried vertical mattress suture (Figures 4-27A through 4-27G).

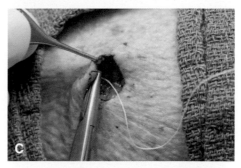

Figure 4-27C. The buried vertical mattress suture is started by inserting the needle into the deep dermis, angling upward, and exiting at the incised wound edge.

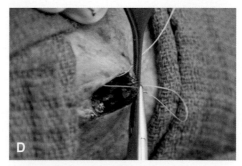

Figure 4-27D. A mirror-image technique is utilized on the contralateral wound edge.

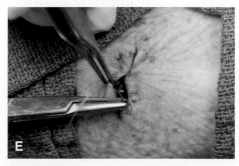

Figure 4-27E. After placing the buried vertical mattress suture, the needle is blindly inserted parallel to the wound axis and perpendicular to the buried vertical mattress suture.

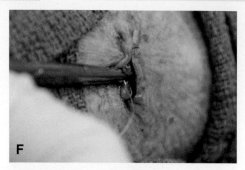

Figure 4-27F. The needle exits on the contralateral side of the buried vertical mattress suture. It is then tied over the buried vertical mattress suture, pulling the suture down and creating a sulcus.

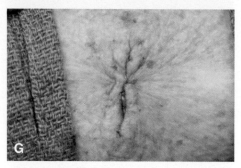

Figure 4-27G. Immediate postoperative appearance.

Tips and Pearls

While originally described for use with the buried vertical mattress suture, this technique may also be used to anchor periosteum to a set-back dermal suture. Since the technique entails the placement of a large amount of suture material (a minimum of six knots) in a single location, a set-back dermal starting suture may be preferable in order to lessen the risk of foreign-body reaction and suture material extrusion.

Since a previously placed buried suture is anchored to underlying periosteum, unlike the traditional suspension suture, this technique can only be used when the buried suture directly overlies a natural sulcus. Therefore, it is most widely used with defects along the nasofacial sulcus, though theoretically it could be utilized over other sulci and creases as well.

Drawbacks and Cautions

The relatively large amount of suture material that is left in situ with this technique means that the chances of foreign-body reaction, suture abscess, or suture spitting are probably higher than with other suspension suture approaches. This should be taken into account before broadly adopting this approach.

Since the anchoring suture is tied directly to the previously placed buried vertical mattress suture, the additional torque placed on the buried suture may translate into a greater risk of suture material rupture or at least of added tension on the dermis where the buried vertical mattress suture is anchored. Therefore, attention to detail in placing and tying the buried vertical mattress suture is of particular importance when utilizing this technique.

As with any suspension suture, there is a risk of damaging underlying structures when placing the anchoring bite of suture material. Comfort with and knowledge of the underlying anatomy, and particularly the location of neural and vascular bundles, are of paramount importance when adopting this approach.

Finally, there is a risk of creating a long-standing depression at the site of suture placement. While the immediate postoperative dimpling generally resolves, this depends largely on the patient's fibrotic response, and an exaggerated fibrotic response may translate into a permanent depression at the site of suture placement.

Reference

Otley CC. The tie-over suture for re-creating the nasofacial sulcus. *Dermatol Surg.* 2000; 26(3):270-272.

The Buried Vertical Mattress Suspension Suture

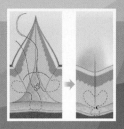

Synonyms

Criss-cross tie-over tacking suture, three-point suspension suture

Video 4-28. Buried vertical mattress suspension suture
Access to video can be found via
mhprofessional.com/atlasofsuturingtechniques2e

Application

Like the tie-over suture, this technique is useful when attempting to recreate a natural sulcus when the defect lies parallel to the sulcus. It may be conceived as a hybrid between the traditional suspension suture and the tie-over suture, as it entails combining a buried vertical mattress suture with an anchoring suture that attaches to deeper structures, but rather than separately executing a buried vertical mattress suture and a tie-over suture, these two steps are combined into one. Since its application is limited to areas where the buried vertical mattress suture directly overlies the natural sulcus, this represents a niche technique.

Suture Material Choice

This technique is generally utilized on the face, and therefore, the smallest gauge suture material with appropriate tensile strength should be utilized. Generally, a 4-0 or 5-0 absorbable suture material provides adequate security when anchoring to the periosteum. Nonabsorbable material could theoretically be utilized and may provide a longer-lasting depressive effect on the tissue, but this benefit is likely outweighed by the increased risk of foreign-body reaction and suture material extrusion.

Technique

1. The wound edge is reflected back using surgical forceps or hooks. Adequate visualization of the underside of the dermis is desirable.
2. While reflecting back the dermis, the suture needle is inserted at 90 degrees into the underside of the dermis 4 mm distant from the incised wound edge.
3. The first bite is executed by following the needle initially at 90 degrees to the underside of the dermis and then, critically, changing direction by twisting the needle driver so that the needle exits in the incised wound edge. This allows the apex of the bite to remain in the papillary dermis while the needle exits in the incised wound edge at the level of the reticular dermis.
4. Keeping the loose end of the suture between the surgeon and the patient, the dermis on the side of the first bite is released. The tissue on the opposite edge is then reflected back in a similar fashion as on the first side.
5. The second bite is executed by inserting the needle into the incised wound edge at the level of the reticular dermis. It then angles upward

and laterally so that the apex of the needle is at the level of the papillary dermis. This should mirror the first bite taken on the contralateral side of the wound.

6. The suture material is then tied utilizing an instrument tie, but importantly, the suture material is not cut, thus leaving a long tail.

7. Once the buried vertical mattress suture has been completed, starting from the side of the tied buried vertical mattress suture where the long tail is present, the needle is blindly inserted through the fat and deeper structures until the bone is reached. A 3-mm bite of the periosteum is then taken, and the needle is brought back up through the soft tissues into the open center of the wound on the contralateral side of the buried vertical mattress suture and lifted above the buried vertical mattress suture.

8. The suture material is then tied to the loose tail over the buried vertical mattress suture using an instrument tie, anchoring down the buried vertical mattress suture (Figures 4-28A through 4-28E).

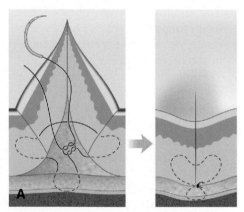

Figure 4-28A. Overview of the buried vertical mattress suspension suture, simplified version.

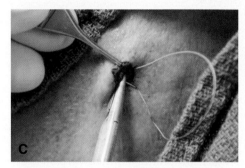

Figure 4-28C. The needle is then inserted through the dermis, moving upward and outward, and exits through the incised wound edge, forming half of a buried vertical mattress suture.

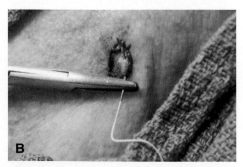

Figure 4-28B. The needle is inserted blindly through the fat, grasping fascia or periosteum, as appropriate, to effect the tacking component of the suture.

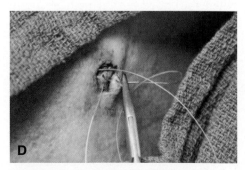

Figure 4-28D. The needle is then inserted on the contralateral wound edge through the wound margin, exiting in the dermis, in a mirror image.

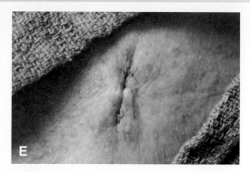

Figure 4-28E. Immediate postoperative appearance. Note the wound inversion.

Tips and Pearls

Since the buried suture is anchored to the underlying periosteum, unlike the traditional suspension suture, this technique can only be used when the buried suture directly overlies a natural sulcus. Therefore, it is most widely used with defects along the nasofacial sulcus, though theoretically, it could be utilized over other sulci and creases as well.

A variation of this technique, the modified crisscross tie-over suture, was designed to assure that the second knot (securing the anchoring suture to the buried vertical mattress) remains buried lateral or deep to the buried vertical mattress, since the original iteration of this technique may result in the second knot riding above the buried vertical mattress suture, increasing the risk of suture abscess formation. In the modified version of this technique, the deep anchoring throw is placed ipsilateral to the loose tail and does not encircle the buried vertical mattress suture. This encourages the second knot to remain firmly buried while resulting in the same degree of tissue suspension.

A simplified version of this technique (as shown in the figures) permits placement of the buried vertical mattress suture and the suspension suture all with a single set of knots; the suspension suture may be placed first, followed by placement of the buried vertical mattress suture, and then the suture can be tied, minimizing the number of knots that will need to be absorbed. This three-point suspension suture, or buried vertical mattress suspension suture, may be preferable to the other variations as less suture material will be left in the dermis to be hydrolyzed.

Drawbacks and Cautions

The relatively large amount of suture material that is left in situ with this technique means that the chances of foreign-body reaction, suture abscess, or suture spitting are probably higher than other suspension suture approaches. This should be taken into account before broadly adopting this approach, and while some proponents have suggested that these complications are rarely, if ever, seen, others have stated that this may be a frequent occurrence.

In the standard version of this approach, since the anchoring suture is tied directly to the loose tail of the buried vertical mattress suture, the additional torque placed on the buried suture may translate into a greater risk of suture material rupture, or at least of added tension on the dermis where the buried vertical mattress suture is anchored. Therefore, attention to detail in placing and tying the buried vertical mattress suture is of particular importance when utilizing this technique.

As with any suspension suture, there is a risk of damaging underlying structures when placing the anchoring bite of suture material. Comfort with and knowledge of the underlying anatomy, and particularly the location of neural and vascular bundles, are of paramount importance when adopting this approach.

Finally, there is a risk of creating a long-standing depression at the site of suture placement. While the immediate postoperative dimpling generally resolves, this depends largely on the patient's fibrotic response, and an exaggerated fibrotic response may translate into a permanent depression at the site of suture placement.

References

Albertini JG. The criss-cross tie-over tacking suture. *Dermatol Surg.* 2002;28(2):188-189.

Finley EM. The crisscross tie-over tacking suture revisited. *Dermatol Surg.* 2003;29(3):281-283.

The Corset Plication Suture

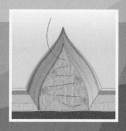

Synonym

Running fascial plication suture

Video 4-29. Corset plication suture
Access to video can be found via mhprofessional.com/atlasofsuturingtechniques2e

Application

This technique is designed for wounds under marked tension, especially those on the back and shoulders, and can be conceptualized as a running variation of a vertically oriented fascial plication suture. Like fascial plication, it is a deep technique, permitting the tension of wound closure to shift from the dermis to the fascia and concomitantly creating a lower-tension closure that is associated with less scar spread. In addition to tension reduction, this approach also leads to a modest increase in the apparent length-to-width ratio of an excised ellipse and improved dead-space minimization.

Suture Material Choice

Suture choice is dependent in large part on location. Since this technique is designed to bite the fascia, generally a larger-gauge suture can be utilized. Therefore, for the back and shoulders, a 2-0 or 3-0 monofilament absorbable suture may be used. As the running technique is predicated on pulling through multiple lengths of suture material, monofilament suture material should be utilized to minimize

the coefficient of friction. Since suture material traverses the fascia, the incidence of suture abscess formation is vanishingly rare.

Technique

1. The wound edges are reflected back to permit visualization of the deep bed of the wound. In deep excisions, such as those performed for melanoma or large cysts, the muscle fascia may be directly visible. Otherwise, visualizing the subcutaneous fat is appropriate as well.
2. Starting at one pole of the ellipse, the suture needle is inserted at 90 degrees through the deep fat 2-4 mm medial to the undermined edge of the wound.
3. The first bite is executed by entering the fascia and following the curvature of the needle, allowing the needle to exit closer to the incised wound edge. The suture material may be gently pulled to test that a successful bite of fascia has been taken.
4. Keeping the loose end of the suture distal to the first bite, attention is then shifted to the opposite side of the wound. The second bite is executed by repeating the procedure on the contralateral side.
5. Steps (2) through (4) are then repeated sequentially in pairs moving toward the contralateral pole of the wound.
6. Once the desired number of paired bites have been taken, the suture is

then pulled tight and tied onto itself using either an instrument or hand tie (Figures 4-29A through 4-29F).

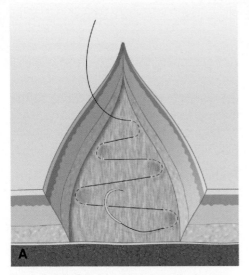

Figure 4-29A. Overview of the corset plication suture.

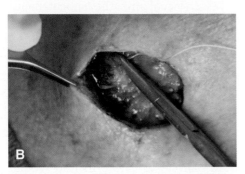

Figure 4-29B. The needle is inserted (here blindly) through the deep fascia on one side of the wound.

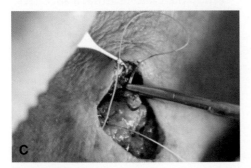

Figure 4-29C. This is then repeated on the contralateral side of the wound.

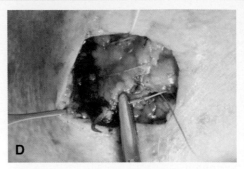

Figure 4-29D. The pattern of alternating fascial bites continues along the course of the wound.

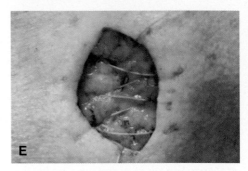

Figure 4-29E. Appearance of the wound with multiple bites of the corset plication suture in place.

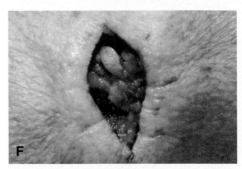

Figure 4-29F. Appearance after tying the corset plication suture. Note that the wound now appears more fusiform.

Tips and Pearls

This technique can be conceptualized as a pulley version of a vertically oriented fascial plication suture. The multiple loops of suture material serve to exert a pulley effect, allowing even the tightest wound to be effectively brought together.

Like the fascial plication approach, this technique is very useful for wounds under marked tension, especially for large defects on the back and shoulders.

As with the fascial plication suture, this approach often leads to a more fusiform defect, even when an oval-shaped excision has been performed. Therefore, it may be useful when attempting to keep a defect as short as possible without dog-ear formation. In cases where this approach is anticipated, it may be worthwhile to create a defect with a length-to-width ratio of less than 3 to 1, as is traditionally employed, as that may be sufficient to lead to a sufficiently tapered ellipse.

As with the fascial plication suture, this technique is also useful when large space-occupying lesions, such as cysts or lipomas, have been extirpated. In these cases, placing dermal sutures alone results in significant residual dead space that may be associated with a higher risk of hematoma or seroma formation, as well as subsequent infection. Corset plication may serve to help minimize this dead space by pulling deeper structures centrally and thereby filling the potential space.

Drawbacks and Cautions

Since this is a running variation of the fascial plication technique, its efficacy is predicated on both suture material integrity and adequate knot security. The value of the entire row of corset sutures would be nullified by either breakage anywhere along the row of suture material or knot failure. Therefore, its proponents have suggested utilizing a 2-0 monofilament suture in order to mitigate the risk of suture breakage, since this material has significant tensile strength. That said, since this technique is exclusively used when wounds are under marked tension, suture material failure remains a

risk. Additionally, adding an extra throw when tying the knots may help mitigate the risk of knot failure.

Another important drawback of this approach is the potential for increased postoperative pain when compared with utilizing dermal sutures alone, or even when compared with placing a single fascial plication suture. Depending on how deep the suture material traverses through fascia and the underlying muscle, pain may sometimes be experienced that is out of proportion to the defect size and depth, particularly since this technique involves the placement of multiple throws of suture material through the fascia.

The lateral bites in the fascia should be taken no closer than 1-2 mm from the undermined edge of the tissue. Taking bites too far laterally, where there is no undermined plane between fascia and dermis, may result in dimpling at the lateral edges. This dimpling occurs when the bites of fascia are directly contiguous with the overlying dermis and epidermis, and the suture's lateral tension on the fascia also pulls on the dermis. While the dimpling may resolve with time, it is best avoided if possible.

While there is a theoretical risk of distortion of the ellipse caused by these running fascial sutures, this is not typically seen in practice. Because this approach entails multiple passes of suture material through the fascia, the risks of pain and infection are theoretically higher than with placing one or two interrupted fascial plication sutures. While this is balanced by the theoretical benefit of the pulley effect of this technique, this pulley effect is almost never needed even in the largest wounds given the ability of a single fascial plication suture to bring together even high-tension wounds. Coupled with the chance that the entire line of sutures can be annulled by breakage anywhere in the suture material or a single knot failure, this approach probably should be used less frequently than the standard fascial plication technique.

References

Dzubow LM. The use of fascial plication to facilitate wound closure following microscopically controlled surgery. *J Dermatol Surg Oncol.* 1989;15(10):1063-1066.

Kantor J. The fascial plication suture: an adjunct to layered wound closure. *Arch Dermatol.* 2009;145(12):1454-1456.

Tierney E, Kouba DJ. A subcutaneous corset plication rapidly and effectively relieves tension on large linear closures. *Dermatol Surg.* 2009;35(11):1806-1808.

The Imbrication Suture

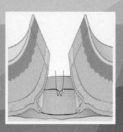

Video 4-30. Imbrication suture
Access to video can be found via
mhprofessional.com/atlasofsuturingtechniques2e

Application

This technique is designed for wounds under marked tension, especially those on the scalp and upper forehead. It is a deep tissue support technique, permitting the tension of wound closure to shift from the dermis to the galea or fascia, thereby creating a lower-tension closure that is associated with less scar spread. Like the fascial plication technique, in addition to tension reduction, this approach also leads to an increase in the apparent length-to-width ratio of an excised ellipse and improved dead-space minimization.

Suture Material Choice

Suture choice is dependent in large part on location. As this technique is designed to bite the galea or the undersurface of the deep fat, generally a 3-0 (on the scalp), 4-0, or even 5-0 absorbable suture may be used. Since suture material is left deep to the subcutaneous fat, the incidence of suture abscess formation is vanishingly rare.

Technique

1. After adequate undermining in the subgaleal (on the scalp and upper forehead) or suprafrontalis (on the lower forehead) plane, and after any lagging fat has been extirpated, the wound edges are reflected back using surgical forceps or hooks.

2. While reflecting back the wound edge, including the galea (or deep fat, as applicable), the suture needle is inserted at 90 degrees into the underside of the deep tissue 4-8 mm distant from the incised wound edge but medial to the edge of the undermined plane.

3. The first bite is executed by entering the deep tissue and following the curvature of the needle parallel to the wound edge. The suture material may be gently pulled to test that a successful bite of deep tissue has been taken.

4. Keeping the loose end of suture between the surgeon and the patient, attention is then shifted to the opposite side of the wound. The second bite is executed by repeating the procedure on the contralateral side.

5. The suture material is then tied utilizing an instrument tie. Hand tying may be utilized as well, particularly if the wound is deep and the instruments cannot be easily inserted to complete the tie (Figures 4-30A through 4-30D).

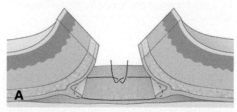

Figure 4-30A. Overview of the imbrication suture.

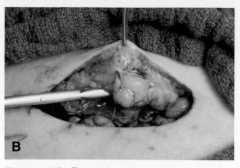

Figure 4-30B. The needle is inserted through the fascia, far lateral to the incised wound edge. Depending on the depth of the defect, this may be performed in muscle or fascia, as long as the depth is kept constant on each side.

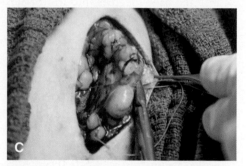

Figure 4-30C. The procedure is repeated in a mirror image on the contralateral wound edge.

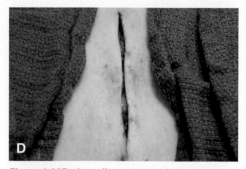

Figure 4-30D. Immediate postoperative appearance. Note that the wound has an exaggerated fusiform appearance.

Tips and Pearls

This technique is useful for wounds under marked tension, especially for larger defects on the scalp and forehead.

If needed, a galeotomy—relaxing incisions through the galea—may be placed parallel to the long axis of the wound to facilitate even greater tissue movement. Like the fascial plication approach, this can therefore be conceptualized as an alternative to pulley sutures that affords both a decrease in tension across the wound surface (by shifting tension from the dermis to the galea) and an increase in the length-to-width ratio of the ellipse.

Like the fascial plication technique, this approach often leads to a more fusiform defect, even when an oval-shaped excision has been performed. Therefore, it may be useful when attempting to keep a defect as short as possible without dog-ear formation. In cases where this approach is anticipated, it may be worthwhile to create a defect with a length-to-width ratio of less than 3 to 1, as is traditionally employed, as that may be sufficient to lead to a tapered ellipse.

If possible, a single galeal imbrication suture may be placed at the center of the wound. This balances the benefit of dead-space minimization and tension relief with the desire to minimize suture material piercing the galea that may be associated with a theoretical increase in infection rate.

In large wounds under marked tension, a series of spaced imbrication sutures may be placed as well. Except for the largest wounds, typically no more than three or four sutures are needed to effectively imbricate the underlying galea.

This technique is also useful when large space-occupying lesions, such as pilar cysts, have been excised from the scalp. In these cases, placing dermal sutures alone results in a significant residual dead space that may be associated with a higher risk of hematoma or seroma formation, as well as subsequent infection. Imbrication may serve to help minimize this dead space by pulling deeper structures centrally and thereby filling the potential space.

A double, or pulley, version of this approach is possible as well, and may be useful when the imbricated tissues are under marked tension. As with any pulley approach, this affords a mechanical advantage and allows the imbricated tissues to be drawn together with greater ease. As an added benefit, this also permits immediate locking of the suture material after the first knot throw, which may obviate the need for an assistant in some cases.

Drawbacks and Cautions

It is important that the surgeon have excellent familiarity with the relevant tissue planes when executing deep-tissue imbrication. Since deep tissues are incised, undermined, extirpated, and then imbricated, there is the theoretical potential for damage to an underlying neural or vascular plexus in the course of wound preparation and suturing. As long as meticulous attention is paid to the depth of undermining and the correct tissue planes (subgaleal generally, or suprafrontalis on the lower central forehead), this is not generally a problem, though certainly this technique should not be applied in any of the "danger zones" of the face where damage to the facial nerve, or other vital structures, is possible.

Another possible drawback of this approach is the potential for increased postoperative pain when compared with utilizing dermal sutures alone. While this is not a typical occurrence, depending on how deep the suture material traverses through frontalis muscle, pain may sometimes be experienced that is out of proportion to the defect size and depth.

Since the integrity of the galea has been compromised, there is similarly a theoretically increased risk of infection with this technique. That said, many closures on the scalp and upper forehead, even when placing only dermal sutures, benefit from subgaleal undermining, and therefore, this risk is not unique to this technique.

The lateral bites in the undersurface of the galea should be taken no closer than 1-2 mm from the lateral undermined edge of the deep tissue. In addition, for horizontally oriented excisions on the forehead, the surgeon may wish to differentially undermine so that a broad area is undermined at the superior portion of the wound but only a relatively narrow area is undermined at its inferior edge. This will aid in avoiding adding a dramatic lift to the lower forehead.

Reference

Radonich MA, Bisaccia E, Scarborough D. Management of large surgical defects of the forehead and scalp by imbrication of deep tissues. *Dermatol Surg.* 2002;28(6):524-526.

The Guitar String Suture

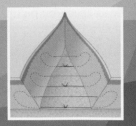

Application

This is a niche technique useful for reducing the size of a defect prior to flap or graft repair in wounds under marked tension. It is most commonly employed on the scalp, trunk, and extremities, though its use has been described elsewhere as well. It should probably be avoided on the face, where possible anatomic distortion and the long-term fibrotic bands from the placement of these sutures are undesirable. Of note, this technique does not entirely close a defect; instead, it serves to pull the wound edges closer together, reducing the size of the defect prior to definitive closure.

Suture Material Choice

Suture choice is dependent in large part on location. Since this technique is designed to hold a fair amount of tension, generally a 3-0 or 2-0 absorbable suture is appropriate. As a large amount of suture material will remain relatively superficially in the bed of the wound, longer-lasting absorbable suture material (such as polydioxanone) should probably be avoided.

Technique

1. The desired axis of partial wound closure is visualized, and the wound edge on one side of the desired axis is reflected back using surgical forceps

   or hooks. Adequate visualization of the underside of the dermis is required.
2. While reflecting back the dermis, the suture needle is inserted at 90 degrees into the underside of the dermis 7-9 mm distant from the incised wound edge.
3. The first bite is executed by traversing the dermis following the curvature of the needle and allowing the needle to exit closer to the incised wound edge. Care should be taken to remain in the dermis to minimize the risk of epidermal dimpling. The needle does not, however, exit through the incised wound edge, but rather 5 mm distant from the incised edge. The size of this first bite is based on the size of the needle and the thickness of the dermis.
4. Keeping the loose end of the suture between the surgeon and the patient, the dermis on the side of the first bite is released. The tissue on the opposite edge is then reflected back in a similar fashion as on the first side, assuring complete visualization of the underside of the dermis.
5. The second bite is executed by inserting the needle into the underside of the dermis 5 mm distant from the incised wound edge. Again, this bite should be performed by following the curvature of the needle and avoiding catching the undersurface of the epidermis that could result

in epidermal dimpling. It then exits further distal to the wound edge, approximately 6-9 mm distant from the wound edge. This should mirror the first bite taken on the contralateral side of the wound.

6. The suture material is then pulled centrally, reducing the size of the open wound, and the suture material is tied utilizing an instrument tie. Hand tying may be utilized as well. The use of an assistant to hold the wound edges in place as far medially as possible may be helpful (Figures 4-31A through 4-31E).

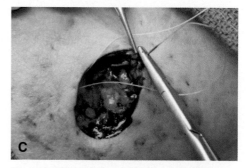

Figure 4-31C. On the contralateral wound edge, the needle is inserted close to the incised wound edge, exiting further set back along the undermined undersurface of the dermis.

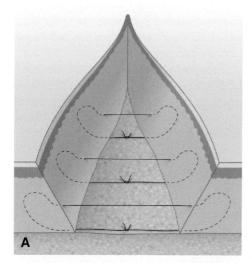

Figure 4-31A. Overview of the guitar string suture technique demonstrating its use with a series of buried vertical mattress sutures.

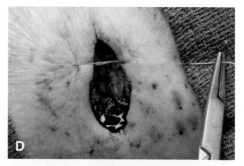

Figure 4-31D. The suture is tied as tightly as possible.

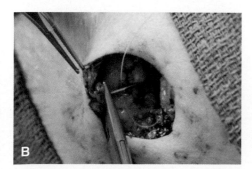

Figure 4-31B. The needle is inserted from the underside of the dermis, exiting set back from the incised wound edge.

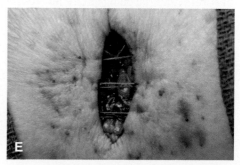

Figure 4-31E. Immediate postoperative appearance after placing a series of guitar string sutures.

Tips and Pearls

Like the purse string suture—when it is used solely for reducing defect size—this technique does not alone result in complete defect closure. It is therefore best suited to areas that are under marked tension, areas where a skin graft will be used, or where even a large flap may have difficulty closing a defect. After placement of the guitar string sutures, a full- or partial-thickness skin graft may be used to cover the residual defect.

A double, or pulley, variation of this approach is possible as well, which may aid in adding additional medial tension on the suture material by taking advantage of the pulley effect. The benefits of the pulley effect, however, should be weighed against both the increase in retained suture material and the possible increased risk of tissue necrosis from the high-tension closure that may be undertaken utilizing this approach.

This technique's name, of course, is derived from the appearance of the residual suture material between the wound edges, as the taut suture material has the appearance of guitar strings as it traverses over the underlying subcutaneous fat or fascia.

Drawbacks and Cautions

This technique results in a large volume of suture material being left in the wound for many months. Even after the suture material is hydrolyzed, it leaves behind palpable fibrotic bands that may take months to absorb entirely, and there is a theoretical risk that these bands will not disappear entirely.

The large volume of foreign-body material that is left in the wound may increase the theoretical risk of infection. Moreover, depending on the depth of these sutures, other complications, such as sinus tract formation, are possible as well. Though these complications have not been described by proponents of this technique, they remain theoretically possible depending on individual patient circumstances and local technique variations.

The tension inherent in this approach also increases the theoretical risk of tissue necrosis and long-term residual dimpling at the lateral borders of the wound. While epidermal dimpling will occasionally occur where the arc of the suture reaches its apex at the dermal-epidermal junction, generally, a small degree of dimpling will resolve with time as the absorbable sutures are gradually resorbed.

Reference

Redondo P. Guitar-string sutures to reduce a large surgical defect prior to skin grafting or flap movement. *Dermatol Surg.* 2014;40(1):69-72.

The Dog-Ear Tacking Suture

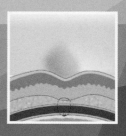

Video 4-32. Dog-ear tacking suture
Access to video can be found via
mhprofessional.com/atlasofsuturingtechniques2e

Application

This is a niche technique used for reducing the appearance of dog ears, or standing cones, at the ends of elliptical excisions or local flaps. While dog-ear minimization is generally accomplished by excising lesions with fusiform incisions, this often extends the length of the wound significantly, which is undesirable. This technique was designed as an approach to mitigate the raised dog-ear appearance of the standing cone while concomitantly avoiding unnecessarily extending the length of the wound.

Suture Material Choice

Suture choice is dependent in large part on location. Since this technique is designed to bite the deep dermis and the underlying fascia or periosteum, the surgeon may choose to utilize a larger gauge suture than would be used for an equivalently placed buried suture. On the back and extremities, a 2-0, 3-0, or 4-0 absorbable suture material may be used, and on the face and other areas under minimal tension, a 4-0 or 5-0 absorbable suture is adequate.

Technique

1. The apex of the wound where the incipient dog ear is anticipated is widely undermined. The wound edge at this apex is reflected back using surgical forceps or hooks, and adequate visualization of the underside of the dermis is required.

2. While reflecting back the dermis, the suture needle is inserted at 90 degrees into the underside of the dermis 4-6 mm distant from the apex.

3. The first bite is executed by traversing the dermis following the curvature of the needle and allowing the needle to exit farther from the incised wound edge. Care should be taken to remain in the dermis to minimize the risk of epidermal dimpling. The needle exits approximately 8 mm distant from the incised edge, though this depends on the size of the standing cone that is being smoothed. Keeping the loose end of suture between the surgeon and the patient, the dermis is released.

4. The standing cone may be gently pulled by the suture material so that the location of the first bite directly overlies the planned fixation point. This permits the surgeon to double-check the final position of the suture. The needle is then blindly inserted through the fat and deeper structures until bone is reached. A 3-mm bite of the periosteum or fascia is then taken, and the needle is brought back up through the soft tissues into the open center of the wound.

5. The suture material is then tied utilizing an instrument tie (Figures 4-32A through 4-32D).

151

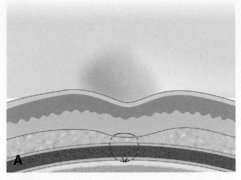

Figure 4-32A. Overview of the dog-ear tacking suture.

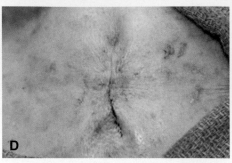

Figure 4-32D. Immediate postoperative appearance demonstrating dimpling at each apex where dog-ear tacking sutures were placed. This dimpling resolves with time, though residual fibrosis helps mitigate the formation of dog ears as the suture material is absorbed.

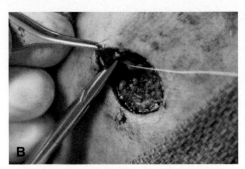

Figure 4-32B. The needle is inserted through the undersurface of the undermined dermis, exiting set back from the wound edge at the apex of the wound.

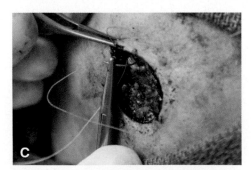

Figure 4-32C. The needle is then passed blindly through the periosteum, anchoring the suture in place.

Tips and Pearls

This technique works best when the standing cone is fixed to a truly immobile tissue, such as the periosteum. Therefore, this approach is of particular utility on the forehead and other areas over bony prominences. On the trunk and extremities, where no truly fixed underlying anchoring point is present, the standing cone can be fixed to the muscle fascia. Though this does not lead to as dramatic a degree of downward pull as when the dog ear is fixed to the periosteum, it does have a positive impact on the height of the standing cone.

In some locations, such as convexities over the forehead, even defects repaired with a 4:1 ellipse may still display residual standing cones at the apices; therefore, this approach may be used as an adjunct in such cases as well.

This technique can be conceptualized as a suspension suture for the standing cone, where the dog ear is anchored downward to prevent the residual focal elevation that will otherwise be seen in such cases. Since no additional tissue is excised, this technique will occasionally lead to a rippling effect in the areas where it is utilized, though this is generally preferable to the dramatic bump that would otherwise be present when dog ears are left behind.

Some experience is helpful in deciding what degree of residual standing cone appearance is acceptable. Wounds on the lower legs, for example, often heal well, and residual standing cones may smooth out spontaneously, likely due to the tension over bony prominences; conversely, standing cones over cheeks and other areas with abundant soft tissue often resolve only minimally over time, and therefore, leaving significant dog ears in these locations should be assiduously avoided if possible.

In some cases, instead of taking a single bite from the undersurface of the dermis, it may be more effective to take two bites, as if a set-back dermal suture were being taken from the imaginary line splitting the standing cone. These two bites are then anchored to a central anchoring point deep to the theoretical midpoint of the standing cone. A percutaneous variation of this approach, with the tacking performed to the lateral surface of the wound rather than its base, has also been described.

This approach, when used in concert with a technique such as the fascial plication suture that leads a round or oval defect to appear more fusiform, may permit closure of wounds with significantly less standing cone removal, leading to shorter—and therefore more cosmetically appealing—scars.

Drawbacks and Cautions

As with any suspension suture, since the underside of the dermis is tacked to periosteum, this technique may result in an area of depression at the site of suture placement.

The anchoring portion of this suture technique carries the risk of damage to an underlying vascular or neural plexus. Familiarity with the underlying bony anatomy is therefore of paramount importance, as it also permits the surgeon to select appropriate locations for dog-ear tacking suture placement.

As suture material is tacked to the periosteum—and traverses muscle and fascia—patients should be warned that they may experience more pain with this approach than would be experienced with a typical bilayered closure.

When tacking to the underlying fascia, since the anchoring point is not entirely immobile, it is possible that the degree of standing cone reduction will be only modest. Therefore, such cases may require a greater degree of standing cone excision than those overlying bony prominences.

The residual focal rippling of the epidermis caused by tissue redundancy will generally resolve with time, though in areas with significant actinic damage and solar elastosis, the lack of underlying elasticity may lead to residual textural changes that do not resolve. In these unusual cases, surgical revision may be useful to excise the residual area, as would be done for a dog-ear removal, thus leading to a more acceptable cosmetic outcome.

References

Cronin MM, Li Y, Cronin TA, Cronin TA. The snug tip stitch: a tissue-sparing technique for the correction of small dog ears. *Dermatol Surg.* November 3, 2020 [epub ahead of print].

Kantor J. The dog ear tacking suture technique. *J Am Acad Dermatol.* 2015;73:e25-26.

The Buried Purse-String Suture

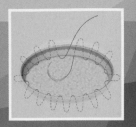

Video 4-33. Buried purse-string suture
Access to video can be found via
mhprofessional.com/atlasofsuturingtechniques2e

Application

This technique is designed to either shrink the size of a defect or obviate it entirely, depending on the degree of tension and the size of the defect. It is a niche technique, since the purse-string effect tends to lead to a slight puckering in the surrounding skin, a feature that may be acceptable (and will likely resolve with time) on areas such as the forearms and back but is less desirable in cosmetically sensitive locations such as the face. The running nature of the technique means that compromise at any point in the course of suture placement may result in wound dehiscence, though for this reason, a larger gauge suture material is generally utilized.

Suture Material Choice

Suture choice is dependent in large part on location, though as always, the smallest gauge suture material appropriate for the anatomic location should be utilized. On the back and shoulders, 2-0 or 3-0 suture material is effective, and on the extremities and scalp, a 3-0 or 4-0 absorbable suture material may be used. When used on the face, a 5-0 absorbable suture is adequate. Since the technique requires easy pull through of suture material, monofilament absorbable suture is generally preferable.

Technique

1. The wound edge at the far end of the round- or oval-shaped wound, parallel to the incision line, is reflected back.

2. With the tail of the suture material resting between the surgeon and the far end of the wound, the needle is inserted into the underside of the dermis on the far edge of the wound with a trajectory running parallel to the incision. Generally, this entry point in the dermis should be approximately 3-6 mm set back from the epidermal edge, depending on the thickness of the dermis and the anticipated degree of tension across the closure. The needle, and therefore the suture, should pass through the deep dermis at a uniform depth. Bite size is dependent on needle size, though in order to minimize the risk of necrosis, it may be prudent to restrict the size of each bite. The needle should exit the dermis at a point equidistant from the cut edge from where it entered.

3. The needle is then grasped with the surgical pickups and simultaneously released by the hand holding the needle driver. As the needle is freed from the tissue with the pickups, the needle is grasped again by the needle driver in an appropriate position to repeat the preceding step to the left of the previously placed suture.

4. A small amount of suture material is pulled through and the needle is inserted into the dermis to the left of the previously placed suture, and the same movement is repeated.
5. The same technique is repeated moving stepwise around the entire wound until the needle exits close to the original entry point at the far end of the wound.
6. Once the desired number of throws have been placed, the suture material is then pulled taut, leading to complete or partial closure of the wound, and tied utilizing an instrument tie (Figures 4-33A through 4-33F).

Tips and Pearls

This technique is designed as an efficient method of wound area reduction. In many cases, placing a purse-string suture can effect complete wound closure, and it therefore represents an alternative to a layered repair of a fusiform incision.

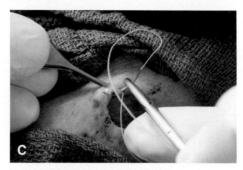

Figure 4-33C. The prior step is repeated sequentially around the periphery of the wound.

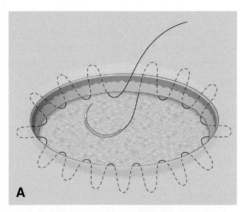

Figure 4-33A. Overview of the buried purse-string suture technique.

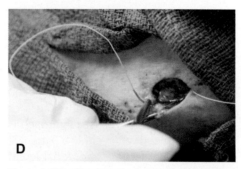

Figure 4-33D. A backhand technique may be used when following the curvature of the wound back to the suture's inception point.

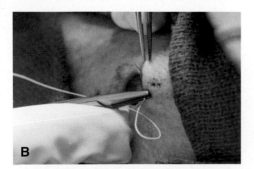

Figure 4-33B. The needle is inserted through the underside of the undermined dermis, set back from the wound edge and with a trajectory paralleling the wound edge.

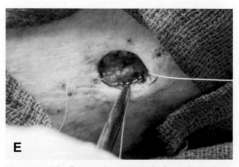

Figure 4-33E. This continues until the inception point is reached. The suture material is then pulled taut and tied.

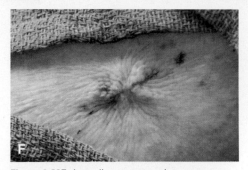

Figure 4-33F. Immediate postoperative appearance after placement of the buried purse-string technique. Note the slight residual pucker, though the wound edges are well approximated overall.

It has been suggested that some defects on the back and extremities, particularly in elderly patients with loose skin, are better closed with a purse-string approach than with a traditional linear closure, since linear closures often heal with a residual scar and require a significantly longer excision line, while the puckering that may be present immediately postoperatively with purse-string closures is likely to resolve with time. That said, in the right hands, linear closures on the trunk and extremities often heal with subtle scarring, even when wounds are closed under tension.

On a pragmatic level, this approach is generally utilized when either a patient is unwilling to undergo a traditional linear closure or when their comorbidities make the additional length of the incision for a linear closure an unrealistic option.

As with linear running dermal techniques, this technique may be used as a modified winch or pulley suture, since the multiple loops help minimize the tension across any one loop and permit closure of wounds under marked tension. Because each throw is not tied off, however, it is important to adequately secure the knot.

Tying a purse-string closure under significant tension may be challenging, as suture material tends to slip after the first knot throw. Utilizing hemostats to secure

the suture ends in position during suture lockdown may help mitigate this problem.

Absorbable purse-string sutures may also be used to reduce the size of a defect prior to graft placement, in a fashion similar to the guitar string suture. Similarly, a modified purse-string closure has been described that involves a buried purse-string closure following by placement of standard percutaneous sutures to yield better wound-edge approximation and decreased bunching.

Drawbacks and Cautions

As with other running dermal techniques, this approach leaves a fair amount of absorbable suture material in the dermis. Therefore, foreign-body reactions, suture abscess formation, and infection are possibilities. The entire suture line is secured with a single knot, and since most of the bulk of any suture line is in the knots, rather than the lengths of suture material between knots, this technique may be less susceptible to suture abscess or suture spitting than others.

The pucker effect of this closure resolves rapidly in atrophic skin, though it can persist in other areas; patients should realize that some degree of residual puckering toward the center of the wound is to be expected. Additionally, this technique may be used to help recreate the nipple-areola complex if full reconstruction is not desired and the nipple is lost to a local tumor.

Since the entire closure is held by a single knot, this approach may be associated with a higher rate of wound dehiscence, as knot failure or failure in the suture material at any point leads to an immediate loss of tension on the closure. Given the concern regarding knot breakage, it may be helpful to attempt to better secure the knot. This may be done by paying particularly close attention to knot tying, tying an extra full knot, adding extra throws, or leaving a longer tail than would traditionally be executed.

A recent study has suggested, however, that the postoperative cosmesis of a purse-string closure is no better than a wound allowed to heal by secondary intention, though wounds closed with purse-string sutures may heal approximately 2 weeks faster than those allowed to heal by secondary intention.

This approach provides less wound eversion than vertically oriented approaches such as the set-back dermal or buried vertical mattress sutures. Therefore, consideration should be given to adding additional superficially placed everting sutures, such as the vertical mattress suture, in order to mitigate this problem. Still, since this approach is generally adopted when the surgeon has accepted that the cosmetic outcome may be less than ideal, it may be reasonable to use this approach as a solitary closure.

References

Cohen PR, Martinelli PT, Schulze KE, Nelson BR. Closure of round cutaneous postoperative wounds with the purse string suture. *South Med J.* 2006;99(12):1401-1402.

Cohen PR, Martinelli PT, Schulze KE, Nelson BR. The cuticular purse string suture: a modified purse string suture for the partial closure of round postoperative wounds. *Int J Dermatol.* 2007;46(7):746-753.

Cohen PR, Martinelli PT, Schulze KE, Nelson BR. The purse-string suture revisited: a useful technique for the closure of cutaneous surgical wounds. *Int J Dermatol.* 2007;46(4):341-347.

Collett T, Smith A, Liu Y, et al. Underappreciated utility of the purse-string suture in head and neck skin cancer defect reconstruction. *Dermatol Surg.* 2019;45(2):216-222.

Field LM. Inadvertent and undesirable sequelae of the stellate purse-string closure. *Dermatol Surg.* 2000;26(10):982.

Greenbaum SS, Radonich M. Closing skin defects with purse-string suture. *Plast Reconstr Surg.* 1998;101(6):1749-1751.

Harrington AC, Montemarano A, Welch M, Farley M. Variations of the pursestring suture in skin cancer reconstruction. *Dermatol Surg.* 1999;25(4):277-281.

Hoffman A, Lander J, Lee PK. Modification of the purse-string closure for large defects of the extremities. *Dermatol Surg.* 2008;34(2):243-245.

Joo J, Custis T, Armstrong AW, et al. Purse-string suture vs second intention healing: results of a randomized, blind clinical trial. *JAMA Dermatol.* 2015;151:265-270.

Kim BY, Chun SH, Kim IH. The modified purse-string suture: a useful technique for the repair of cutaneous surgical wounds. *J Am Acad Dermatol.* 2017;77(5):e131-132.

Ku BS, Kwon OE, Kim DC, et al. A case of erosive adenomatosis of nipple treated with total excision using purse-string suture. *Dermatol Surg.* 2006;32(8):1093-1096.

Lackey J, Mendese G, Grande D. Using an absorbable purse-string suture to reduce surgical defects of the nose before placement of full-thickness skin grafts. *Dermatol Surg.* 2015;41:657-660.

Marquart JD, Lawrence N. The purse-string lock-down. *Dermatol Surg.* 2009;35:853-855.

Nicholas L, Bingham J, Marquart J. Percutaneous buried modification of the purse-string closure. *Dermatol Surg.* 2014;40(9):1052-1054.

Patel KK, Telfer MR, Southee R. A "round block" purse-string suture in facial reconstruction after operations for skin cancer surgery. *Br J Oral Maxillofac Surg.* 2003;41(3):151-156.

Peled IJ, Zagher U, Wexler MR. Purse-string suture for reduction and closure of skin defects. *Ann Plast Surg.* 1985;14(5):465-469.

Randle HW. Modified purse string suture closure. *Dermatol Surg.* 2004;30(2 pt 1):237.

Romiti R, Randle HW. Complete closure by purse-string suture after Mohs micrographic surgery on thin, sun-damaged skin. *Dermatol Surg.* 2002;28(11):1070-1072.

Spencer JM, Malerich SA, Moon SD. A regional survey of purse-string sutures for partial and complete closure of Mohs surgical defects. *Dermatol Surg.* 2014;40(6):679-685.

Teitelbaum S. The purse-string suture. *Plast Reconstr Surg.* 1998;101(6):1748-1749.

Zhu JW, Wu XJ, Lu ZF, Cai SQ, Zheng M. Purse-string suture for round and oval defects: a useful technique in dermatologic surgery. *J Cutan Med Surg.* 2012;16(1):11-17.

The Percutaneous Purse-String Suture

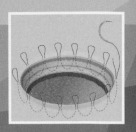

Application

As with the buried purse-string closure, this technique is designed to use circumferential tissue advancement to either shrink the size of a defect or obviate it entirely, depending on the degree of tension and the size of the defect. It is a niche technique, since the purse-string effect tends to lead to a slight puckering in the surrounding skin, a feature that may be acceptable (and will likely resolve with time) on areas such as the forearms and back but is less desirable in cosmetically sensitive locations such as the face. The running nature of the technique means that compromise at any point in the course of suture placement may result in wound dehiscence, though for this reason, a larger gauge suture material is generally utilized. This percutaneous approach is most useful either for relatively narrow wounds or those with marked atrophy of the surrounding skin, such as on the shins and scalp.

Suture Material Choice

Suture choice is dependent in large part on location, though as always, the smallest gauge suture material appropriate for the anatomic location should be utilized. On the extremities and scalp, where this technique is generally used, a 3-0 or 4-0 absorbable suture material may be used. On the back and shoulders, 2-0 or 3-0 suture material is effective. Since the technique requires easy pull through of suture material, monofilament absorbable suture is generally preferable.

Technique

1. At the wound edge at the far end of the round- or oval-shaped wound, the needle is inserted at 90 degrees through the epidermis parallel to the incision line 5-20 mm set back from the wound edge. Alternatively, if absorbable suture material is used, the needle may enter from the underside of the dermis so that the final knot will be buried.

2. The curvature of the needle is followed keeping the same distance from the wound edge so that the needle exits through the epidermis 10-15 mm to the left of the entry point at the same distance set back from the wound edge by following a trajectory running parallel to the incision. Bite size is dependent on needle size. The needle should exit the dermis at a point equidistant from the cut edge from where it entered.

3. The needle is then grasped with the surgical pickups and simultaneously released by the hand holding the needle driver. As the needle is freed from the tissue with the pickups, the needle is grasped again by the needle driver in an appropriate position

to repeat steps (1) through (3). With each throw, however, the needle pierces the epidermis through the exit hole of the prior throw.

4. A small amount of suture material is pulled through with each throw.

5. The same technique is repeated moving stepwise around the entire wound until the needle exits through the original entry point at the far end of the wound.

6. The suture material is then pulled taut, leading to complete or partial closure of the wound, and tied utilizing an instrument tie (Figures 4-34A through 4-34G).

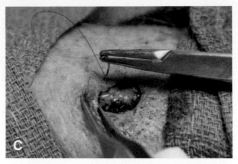

Figure 4-34C. The needle is reinserted directly adjacent to its exit point, or even through the same hole, oriented parallel to the wound edge and set back from the wound edge.

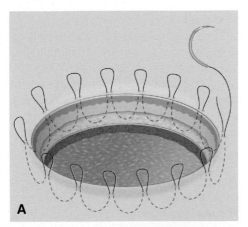

Figure 4-34A. Overview of the percutaneous purse-string technique.

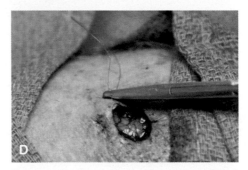

Figure 4-34D. The needle then moves directly through the dermis, exiting the undersurface of the dermis, and then curves back up through the undersurface of the dermis, exiting the skin further along the curvature of the wound.

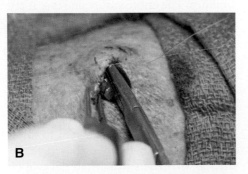

Figure 4-34B. The needle is inserted from the inside of the wound up and directly through the dermis, exiting the epidermis.

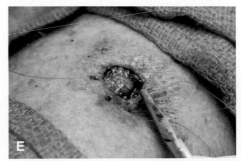

Figure 4-34E. This pattern continues around the perimeter of the wound, where a backhand technique may be used when heading away from the surgeon.

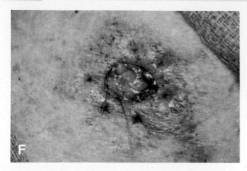

Figure 4-34F. Once all sutures have been placed, the final throw ends with the needle exiting the undersurface of the dermis adjacent to the initial entry point. The suture material is subsequently pulled taut and tied.

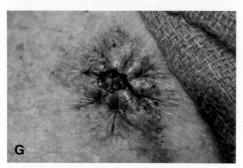

Figure 4-34G. Immediate postoperative appearance. With this technique, wounds are sometimes only partially closed, as seen here. The residual wound may heal via granulation, or a transepidermal suture may be placed.

Tips and Pearls

Unlike the fully buried purse-string approach, this technique allows for additional recruitment of the surrounding tissue by permitting placement of the sutures markedly set back from the wound edge. This may therefore be a technique of choice if maximal tension is expected on the wound.

This variation may also be useful when the wound is relatively narrow, such as on the shin, or when the skin is very atrophic and the full thickness of the dermis needs to be recruited to provide stability and minimize suture tear-through.

This technique is designed as an efficient method of wound-area reduction. In many cases, placing a purse-string suture can effect complete wound closure, and therefore, it represents an alternative to a layered repair of a fusiform incision.

On a pragmatic level, this approach is generally utilized when either a patient is unwilling to undergo a traditional linear closure or their comorbidities make the additional length of the incision for a linear closure an unrealistic option.

The knot may be buried by beginning and ending this technique on the interior of the wound (as opposed to starting outside the skin), although the tension across the knot generally pulls it inward if the standard technique is used and the suture line is started on the exterior of the skin.

Tying a purse-string closure under significant tension may be challenging, as suture material tends to slip after the first knot throw. Utilizing hemostats to secure the suture ends in position during suture lockdown may help mitigate this problem.

Drawbacks and Cautions

As with other running dermal techniques, this approach leaves a fair amount of absorbable suture material in the dermis. Therefore, foreign-body reactions, suture abscess formation, and infection are possibilities. The entire suture line is secured with a single knot, and since most of the bulk of any suture line is in the knots, rather than the lengths of suture material between knots, this technique may be less susceptible to suture abscess or suture spitting than others.

Utilizing the same holes for exit and entry of the needle is designed to minimize residual skin dimpling but increases the risk that the suture material will be cut by the needle as it renters the same hole. Since the entire closure rests on the resiliency of a single strand of suture, this risk should not be overlooked. A simple variation of this technique, where the needle is reinserted through a hole just lateral to the exit point, may help mitigate this potential risk.

Skin dimpling is often seen with this approach, particularly since these wounds are often closed under significant tension. This does generally resolve with time, but patients should be warned to expect these changes in the immediate postoperative period.

As with the buried purse-string closure, the pucker effect of this closure resolves rapidly in atrophic skin, though it can persist in other areas; patients should realize that some degree of residual puckering toward the center of the wound is to be expected.

Since the entire closure is held by a single knot, this approach may be associated with a higher rate of wound dehiscence, as knot failure or failure in the suture material at any point leads to an immediate loss of tension on the closure. Given the concern regarding knot breakage, it may be helpful to attempt to better secure the knot. This may be done by paying particularly close attention to knot tying, tying an extra full knot, adding extra throws, or leaving a longer tail that would traditionally be executed.

While arguable better than the fully buried purse-string closure, this approach provides less wound eversion than vertically oriented approaches such as the set-back dermal or buried vertical mattress sutures. Therefore, consideration should be given to adding additional superficially placed everting sutures, such as the vertical mattress suture, in order to mitigate this problem. Still, since this approach is generally adopted when the surgeon has accepted that the cosmetic outcome may be less than ideal, it may be reasonable to use this approach as a solitary closure.

References

Cohen PR, Martinelli PT, Schulze KE, Nelson BR. Closure of round cutaneous postoperative wounds with the purse string suture. *South Med J.* 2006;99(12):1401-1402.

Cohen PR, Martinelli PT, Schulze KE, Nelson BR. The cuticular purse string suture: a modified purse string suture for the partial closure of round postoperative wounds. *Int J Dermatol.* 2007;46(7):746-753.

Cohen PR, Martinelli PT, Schulze KE, Nelson BR. The purse-string suture revisited: a useful technique for the closure of cutaneous surgical wounds. *Int J Dermatol.* 2007;46(4):341-347.

Field LM. Inadvertent and undesirable sequelae of the stellate purse-string closure. *Dermatol Surg.* 2000;26(10):982.

Greenbaum SS, Radonich M. Closing skin defects with purse-string suture. *Plast Reconstr Surg.* 1998;101(6):1749-1751.

Harrington AC, Montemarano A, Welch M, Farley M. Variations of the pursestring suture in skin cancer reconstruction. *Dermatol Surg.* 1999;25(4):277-281.

Hoffman A, Lander J, Lee PK. Modification of the purse-string closure for large defects of the extremities. *Dermatol Surg.* 2008;34(2):243-245.

Ku BS, Kwon OE, Kim DC, et al. A case of erosive adenomatosis of nipple treated with total excision using purse-string suture. *Dermatol Surg.* 2006;32(8):1093-1096.

Marquart JD, Lawrence N. The purse-string lockdown. *Dermatol Surg.* 2009;35:853-855.

Nicholas L, Bingham J, Marquart J. Percutaneous buried modification of the purse-string closure. *Dermatol Surg.* 2014;40(9):1052-1054.

Patel KK, Telfer MR, Southee R. A "round block" purse-string suture in facial reconstruction after operations for skin cancer surgery. *Br J Oral Maxillofac Surg.* 2003;41(3):151-156.

Randle HW. Modified purse string suture closure. *Dermatol Surg.* 2004;30(2 pt 1):237.

Romiti R, Randle HW. Complete closure by purse-string suture after Mohs micrographic surgery on thin, sun-damaged skin. *Dermatol Surg.* 2002;28(11):1070-1072.

Spencer JM, Malerich SA, Moon SD. A regional survey of purse-string sutures for partial and complete closure of Mohs surgical defects. *Dermatol Surg.* 2014;40(6):679-685.

Teitelbaum S. The purse-string suture. *Plast Reconstr Surg.* 1998;101(6):1748-1749.

Zhu JW, Wu XJ, Lu ZF, Cai SQ, Zheng M. Purse-string suture for round and oval defects: a useful technique in dermatologic surgery. *J Cutan Med Surg.* 2012;16(1):11-17.

The Figure 8 Double Purse-String Suture

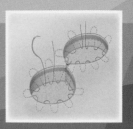

Application

This is a variation of the purse-string approach for larger defects. Like the standard purse-string technique, it is designed to either shrink the size of a defect or obviate it entirely, depending on the degree of tension and the size of the defect. It is a niche technique, as it leads to a slight puckering in the surrounding skin, a feature that may be acceptable (and will likely resolve with time) on areas such as the forearms and back but is less desirable in cosmetically sensitive locations such as the face.

Suture Material Choice

Suture choice is dependent in large part on location, though as always, the smallest gauge suture material appropriate for the anatomic location should be utilized. On the back and shoulders, 2-0 or 3-0 suture material is effective, and on the extremities and scalp, a 3-0 or 4-0 absorbable suture material may be used. In the unlikely event this technique is used on the face, a 4-0 or 5-0 absorbable suture is adequate. Since the technique requires easy pull through of suture material, monofilament absorbable suture is generally preferable. If suture removal is planned, a monofilament nonabsorbable suture is also an option.

Technique

1. After extensive undermining is performed, a single buried vertically oriented suture is placed at the center of the wound; a set-back dermal suture may be utilized.

2. Once the wound has been bisected, the wound edge at the far end of one of the nascent round- or oval-shaped wounds, parallel to the incision line, is reflected back.

3. With the tail of the suture material resting between the surgeon and the far end of the wound, the needle is inserted into the underside of the dermis on the far edge of the wound with a trajectory running parallel to the incision. Generally, this entry point in the dermis should be approximately 3-6 mm set back from the epidermal edge, depending on the thickness of the dermis and the anticipated degree of tension across the closure. The needle, and therefore the suture, should pass through the deep dermis at a uniform depth. Bite size is dependent on needle size, though in order to minimize the risk of necrosis, it may be prudent to restrict the size of each bite. The needle should exit the dermis at a point equidistant from the cut edge from where it entered.

4. The needle is then grasped with the surgical pickups and simultaneously released by the hand holding the

needle driver. As the needle is freed from the tissue with the pickups, the needle is grasped again by the needle driver in an appropriate position to repeat the preceding step to the left of the previously placed suture.

5. A small amount of suture material is pulled through, and the needle is inserted into the dermis to the left of the previously placed suture, and the same movement is repeated.

6. The same technique is repeated moving stepwise around the entire wound until the needle exits close to the original entry point at the far end of the wound.

7. Once the desired number of throws have been placed, the suture material

is then pulled taut, leading to complete or partial closure of the wound, and tied utilizing an instrument tie.

8. The same procedure (steps 2 through 7) is then repeated on the adjacent open wound (Figures 4-35A through 4-35H).

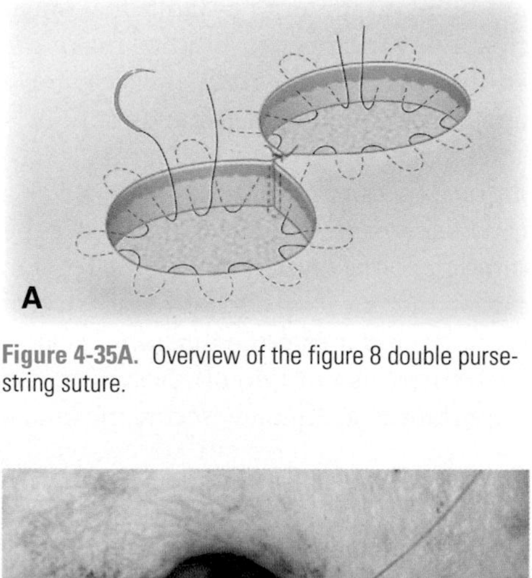

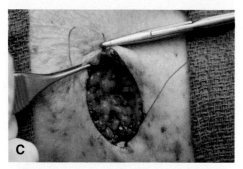

Figure 4-35C. On the contralateral wound edge, the needle is inserted set back from the wound edge, exiting in the undermined undersurface of the dermis.

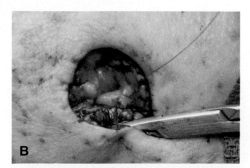

Figure 4-35A. Overview of the figure 8 double purse-string suture.

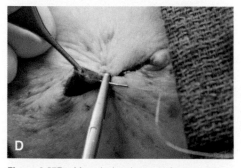

Figure 4-35D. After placing the central suture, the purse-string suture is started by inserting the suture in the dermis, parallel to the wound edge.

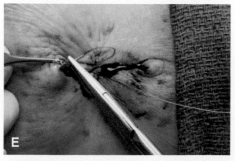

Figure 4-35B. The central suture is placed; this may be a nonabsorbable simple interrupted suture or (as shown here) a buried suture. The needle is inserted from the underside of the dermis, exiting set back from the incised wound edge.

Figure 4-35E. This is continued along the edge of the wound.

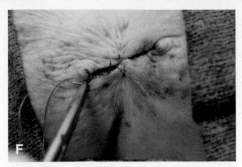

Figure 4-35F. Once the end is reached, this may be continued with a backhand technique.

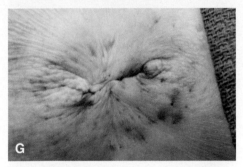

Figure 4-35G. Appearance after placing the purse-string sutures along one side.

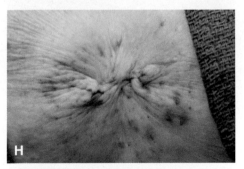

Figure 4-35H. This procedure is then repeated on the contralateral side of the central suture. Immediate postoperative appearance.

Tips and Pearls

Bisecting the original defect permits even large areas to be closed with a purse-string technique.

It has been suggested that some defects on the back and extremities, particularly in elderly patients with loose skin, are better closed with a purse-string approach than with a traditional linear closure, since linear closures often heal with a residual scar and require a significantly longer excision line, while the puckering that may be present immediately postoperatively with purse-string closures is likely to resolve with time. That said, in the right hands, linear closures on the trunk and extremities often heal with subtle scarring, even when wounds are closed under tension. Moreover, a recent randomized controlled trial demonstrated that the cosmetic outcome of a purse-string closure is comparable to secondary intention healing.

On a pragmatic level, like the standard purse-string closure, this approach is generally utilized when either a patient is unwilling to undergo a traditional linear closure or their comorbidities make the additional length of the incision for a linear closure an unrealistic option.

As with linear running dermal techniques, this technique may be used as a modified winch or pulley suture, since the multiple loops help minimize the tension across any one loop and permit closure of wounds under marked tension. Because each throw is not tied off, however, it is important to adequately secure the knots.

Drawbacks and Cautions

As with other running dermal techniques, this approach leaves a fair amount of absorbable suture material in the dermis. Therefore, foreign-body reactions, suture abscess formation, and infection are possibilities. That said, since the entire suture line is secured with a single knot, and since most of the bulk of any suture line is in the knots, rather than the lengths of suture material between knots, this technique may be less susceptible to suture abscess or suture spitting than others.

Nonabsorbable monofilament suture may also be used, in which case, suture removal may be performed approximately 2 weeks postoperatively.

The pucker effect of this closure resolves rapidly in atrophic skin, though it can persist in other areas; patients should realize that some degree of residual puckering toward the center of the wound is to be expected.

This approach provides less wound eversion than vertically oriented approaches such as the set-back dermal or buried vertical mattress sutures. Therefore, consideration should be given to adding additional superficially placed everting sutures, such as the vertical mattress suture, in order to mitigate this problem. Still, since this approach is generally adopted when the surgeon has accepted that the cosmetic outcome may be less than ideal, it may be reasonable to use this approach as a solitary closure.

References

Cohen PR, Martinelli PT, Schulze KE, Nelson BR. Closure of round cutaneous postoperative wounds with the purse string suture. *South Med J.* 2006;99(12):1401-1402.

Cohen PR, Martinelli PT, Schulze KE, Nelson BR. The cuticular purse string suture: a modified purse string suture for the partial closure of round postoperative wounds. *Int J Dermatol.* 2007;46(7):746-753.

Cohen PR, Martinelli PT, Schulze KE, Nelson BR. The purse-string suture revisited: a useful technique for the closure of cutaneous surgical wounds. *Int J Dermatol.* 2007;46(4):341-347.

Field LM. Inadvertent and undesirable sequelae of the stellate purse-string closure. *Dermatol Surg.* 2000;26(10):982.

Greenbaum SS, Radonich M. Closing skin defects with purse-string suture. *Plast Reconstr Surg.* 1998;101(6):1749-1751.

Harrington AC, Montemarano A, Welch M, Farley M. Variations of the pursestring suture in skin cancer reconstruction. *Dermatol Surg.* 1999;25(4):277-281.

Hoffman A, Lander J, Lee PK. Modification of the purse-string closure for large defects of the extremities. *Dermatol Surg.* 2008;34(2):243-245.

Joo J, Custis T, Armstrong AW, et al. Purse-string suture vs second intention healing: results of a randomized, blind clinical trial. *JAMA Dermatol.* 2015;151:265-270.

Ku BS, Kwon OE, Kim DC, et al. A case of erosive adenomatosis of nipple treated with total excision using purse-string suture. *Dermatol Surg.* 2006;32(8):1093-1096.

Lin H, Li W. Complete closure using a double purse-string closure for skin defects. *Dermatol Surg.* 2009;35(9):1406-1409.

Nicholas L, Bingham J, Marquart J. Percutaneous buried modification of the purse-string closure. *Dermatol Surg.* 2014;40(9):1052-1054.

Patel KK, Telfer MR, Southee R. A "round block" purse-string suture in facial reconstruction after operations for skin cancer surgery. *Br J Oral Maxillofac Surg.* 2003;41(3):151-156.

Peled IJ, Zagher U, Wexler MR. Purse-string suture for reduction and closure of skin defects. *Ann Plast Surg.* 1985;14(5):465-469.

Randle HW. Modified purse string suture closure. *Dermatol Surg.* 2004;30(2 pt 1):237.

Romiti R, Randle HW. Complete closure by purse-string suture after Mohs micrographic surgery on thin, sun-damaged skin. *Dermatol Surg.* 2002;28(11):1070-1072.

Spencer JM, Malerich SA, Moon SD. A regional survey of purse-string sutures for partial and complete closure of Mohs surgical defects. *Dermatol Surg.* 2014;40(6):679-685.

Teitelbaum S. The purse-string suture. *Plast Reconstr Surg.* 1998;101(6):1748-1749.

Zhu JW, Wu XJ, Lu ZF, Cai SQ, Zheng M. Purse-string suture for round and oval defects: a useful technique in dermatologic surgery. *J Cutan Med Surg.* 2012;16(1):11-17.

The Stacked Double Purse-String Suture

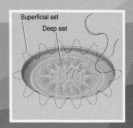

Superficial set
Deep set

Video 4-36. Stacked double purse-string suture
Access to video can be found via mhprofessional.com/ atlasofsuturingtechniques2e

Application

Like all purse-string approaches, this technique is designed to either shrink the size of a defect or obviate it entirely, depending on the degree of tension and the size of the defect. It is a niche technique, since the purse-string effect tends to lead to a slight puckering in the surrounding skin, a feature that may be acceptable (and will likely resolve with time) on areas such as the forearms and back but is less desirable in cosmetically sensitive locations such as the face. This technique relies on first performing a purse-string closure of the fascia or deeper structures followed by a second purse-string layer through the dermis.

Suture Material Choice

Suture choice is dependent in large part on location, though as always, the smallest gauge suture material appropriate for the anatomic location should be utilized. On the back and shoulders, 2-0 or 3-0 suture material is effective, and on the extremities and scalp, a 3-0 or 4-0 absorbable suture material may be used. In the unlikely event this technique is used on the face, a 4-0 or 5-0 absorbable suture is adequate. Since the technique requires easy pull through of suture material, monofilament absorbable suture is generally preferable.

Technique

1. Wide and deep undermining is performed around the defect.
2. The wound edge at the far end of the round- or oval-shaped wound, parallel to the incision line, is reflected back.
3. With the tail of the suture material resting between the surgeon and the far end of the wound, the needle is inserted into the deep dermis or superficial fascia on the far edge of the wound with a trajectory running parallel to the incision. The needle, and therefore the suture, should pass through the deep dermis or fascia at a uniform depth. Bite size is dependent on needle size, though in order to minimize the risk of necrosis, it may be prudent to restrict the size of each bite. The needle should exit at a point equidistant from the cut edge from where it entered.
4. The needle is then grasped with the surgical pickups and simultaneously released by the hand holding the needle driver. As the needle is freed from the tissue with the pickups, the needle is grasped again by the needle driver in an appropriate position to repeat the preceding step to the left of the previously placed suture.
5. A small amount of suture material is pulled through, and the needle is inserted into the deep dermis or superficial fascia to the left of the

previously placed suture, and the same movement is repeated.

6. The same technique is repeated moving stepwise around the entire wound until the needle exits close to the original entry point at the far end of the wound.

7. Once the desired number of throws have been placed, the suture material is then pulled taut, leading to a partial closure of the wound, and tied utilizing an instrument tie.

8. Steps (2) through (7) are then repeated, but now in the mid-dermis, closer to the incised wound edge, so that two sets of nested circumferentially oriented sutures are ultimately placed (Figures 4-36A through 4-36I).

Tips and Pearls

This technique may be thought of as a hybrid between corset plication and a traditional purse-string closure and is designed as an efficient method of wound area reduction. In many cases, placing a stacked double purse-string suture can

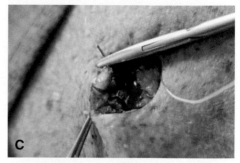

Figure 4-36C. This is repeated moving around the wound edge.

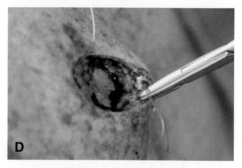

Figure 4-36D. When the contralateral side of the wound is reached, a backhand technique may be used for loading the needle.

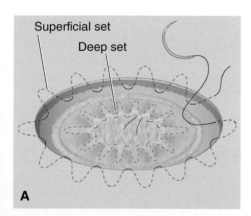

Figure 4-36A. Overview of the stacked purse-string technique.

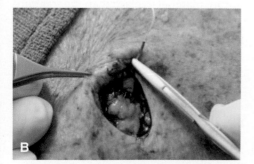

Figure 4-36B. The needle is inserted parallel to the defect in the deep dermis.

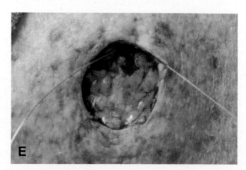

Figure 4-36E. Appearance after placement of the deep set of purse-string sutures.

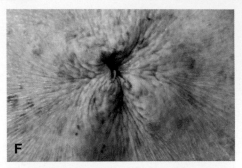

Figure 4-36F. Appearance after tying the deep set of purse-string sutures.

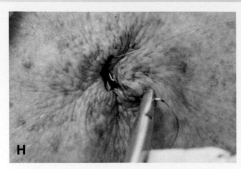

Figure 4-36H. This is repeated moving around the wound.

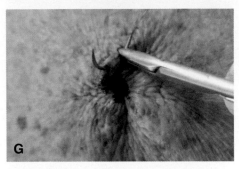

Figure 4-36G. The needle is then inserted parallel to the wound edge through the superficial dermis.

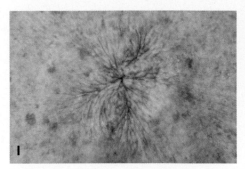

Figure 4-36I. Immediate postoperative appearance after placement of both sets of purse-string sutures. Note the stellate appearance.

effect complete wound closure, and therefore, it represents an alternative to a layered repair.

On a pragmatic level, this approach is generally utilized when either a patient is unwilling to undergo a traditional linear closure or their comorbidities make the additional length of the incision for a linear closure an unrealistic option.

As with linear running dermal techniques, this technique may be used as a modified winch or pulley suture, since the multiple loops help minimize the tension across any one loop and permit closure of wounds under marked tension. Because each throw is not tied off, however, it is important to adequately secure the knot.

Drawbacks and Cautions

As with other running dermal techniques, this approach leaves a fair amount of absorbable suture material in the dermis, and since this technique places two sets of purse-string sutures, it leaves even more suture material in place than the standard purse-string approach. Therefore, foreign-body reactions, suture abscess formation, and infection are possibilities. That said, since each suture line is secured with a single knot and since most of the bulk of any suture line is in the knots, rather than the lengths of suture material between knots, this technique may be less susceptible to suture abscess or suture spitting than others.

The pucker effect of this closure resolves rapidly in atrophic skin, though it can persist in other areas; patients should realize that some degree of residual puckering toward the center of the wound is to be expected.

Since the entire closure is held by two knots, this approach may be associated with a higher rate of wound dehiscence, as knot failure or failure in the suture material at any point leads to an immediate loss of tension on the closure. Given the concern regarding knot breakage, it may be helpful to attempt to better secure the knot. This may be done by paying particularly close attention to knot tying, tying an extra full knot, adding extra throws, or leaving a longer tail than would traditionally be executed.

This approach provides less wound eversion than vertically oriented approaches such as the set-back dermal or buried vertical mattress sutures. Therefore, consideration should be given to adding additional superficially placed everting sutures, such as the vertical mattress suture, in order to mitigate this problem. Still, since this approach is generally adopted when the surgeon has accepted that the cosmetic outcome may be less than ideal, it may be reasonable to use this approach as a solitary closure.

References

Cohen PR, Martinelli PT, Schulze KE, Nelson BR. Closure of round cutaneous postoperative wounds with the purse string suture. *South Med J*. 2006;99(12):1401-1402.

Cohen PR, Martinelli PT, Schulze KE, Nelson BR. The cuticular purse string suture: a modified purse string suture for the partial closure of round postoperative wounds. *Int J Dermatol*. 2007;46(7):746-753.

Cohen PR, Martinelli PT, Schulze KE, Nelson BR. The purse-string suture revisited: a useful technique for the closure of cutaneous surgical wounds. *Int J Dermatol*. 2007;46(4):341-347.

Davis JC, Baillis B, Love WE. Novel stacked double purse-string closure. *Dermatol Surg*. 2014;40(12):1409-1412.

Field LM. Inadvertent and undesirable sequelae of the stellate purse-string closure. *Dermatol Surg*. 2000;26(10):982.

Greenbaum SS, Radonich M. Closing skin defects with purse-string suture. *Plast Reconstr Surg*. 1998;101(6):1749-1751.

Harrington AC, Montemarano A, Welch M, Farley M. Variations of the pursestring suture in skin cancer reconstruction. *Dermatol Surg*. 1999;25(4):277-281.

Hoffman A, Lander J, Lee PK. Modification of the purse-string closure for large defects of the extremities. *Dermatol Surg*. 2008;34(2):243-245.

Joo J, Custis T, Armstrong AW, et al. Purse-string suture vs second intention healing: results of a randomized, blind clinical trial. *JAMA Dermatol*. 2015;151:265-270.

Ku BS, Kwon OE, Kim DC, et al. A case of erosive adenomatosis of nipple treated with total excision using purse-string suture. *Dermatol Surg*. 2006;32(8):1093-1096.

Nicholas L, Bingham J, Marquart J. Percutaneous buried modification of the purse-string closure. *Dermatol Surg*. 2014;40(9):1052-1054.

Patel KK, Telfer MR, Southee R. A "round block" purse-string suture in facial reconstruction after operations for skin cancer surgery. *Br J Oral Maxillofac Surg*. 2003;41(3):151-156.

Peled IJ, Zagher U, Wexler MR. Purse-string suture for reduction and closure of skin defects. *Ann Plast Surg*. 1985;14(5):465-469.

Randle HW. Modified purse string suture closure. *Dermatol Surg*. 2004;30(2 pt 1):237.

Romiti R, Randle HW. Complete closure by purse-string suture after Mohs micrographic surgery on thin, sun-damaged skin. *Dermatol Surg*. 2002;28(11):1070-1072.

Spencer JM, Malerich SA, Moon SD. A regional survey of purse-string sutures for partial and complete closure of Mohs surgical defects. *Dermatol Surg*. 2014;40(6):679-685.

Teitelbaum S. The purse-string suture. *Plast Reconstr Surg*. 1998;101(6):1748-1749.

Zhu JW, Wu XJ, Lu ZF, Cai SQ, Zheng M. Purse-string suture for round and oval defects: a useful technique in dermatologic surgery. *J Cutan Med Surg*. 2012;16(1):11-17.

The Bootlace Suture

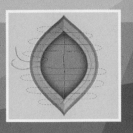

Application

Like traditional running buried sutures, this is a hybrid technique, combining the tension relief and lack of transepidermal suture placement of a classic buried suture with the rapidity of placement and lack of resilience of a superficial running technique. This is therefore a niche approach, since the running nature of the technique means that compromise at any point in the course of suture placement may result in wound dehiscence. It does afford the advantage of the knot resting in the center of the wound, which may reduce the tendency for the central portions of the wound to gape open. Still, unless truly needed, this approach should not be utilized as a solitary technique for the closure of most wounds.

Suture Material Choice

Suture choice is dependent in large part on location, though as always, the smallest gauge suture material appropriate for the anatomic location should be utilized. On the back and shoulders, 2-0 or 3-0 suture material is effective, though if there is marked tension across the wound, this approach would not be appropriate as the primary closure and would be used best for its pulley benefits. On the extremities, a 3-0 or 4-0 absorbable suture material may be used, and on the face and areas under minimal tension, a 5-0 absorbable suture is adequate. Since the technique requires easy pull through of suture material, monofilament absorbable suture is probably preferable.

Technique

1. At the midpoint of the wound, the wound edge is reflected back using surgical forceps or hooks.
2. While reflecting back the dermis, the suture needle is inserted at 90 degrees into the underside of the dermis 2 mm distant from the incised wound edge.
3. The first bite is executed by following the curvature of the needle and allowing the needle to exit in the incised wound edge. The size of this bite is based on the size of the needle, the thickness of the dermis, and the need for and tolerance of eversion. The needle's zenith with respect to the wound surface should be between the entry and exit points.
4. Keeping the loose end of suture between the surgeon and the patient, the dermis on the side of the first bite is released. The tissue on the opposite edge is then gently grasped with the forceps.
5. The second bite is executed by inserting the needle into the incised

wound edge at the level of the superficial papillary dermis. This bite should be completed by following the curvature of the needle and avoiding catching the undersurface of the epidermis that could result in epidermal dimpling. It then exits approximately 2 mm distal to the wound edge on the undersurface of the dermis. This should mirror the first bite taken on the contralateral side of the wound.

6. Instead of tying the suture, a tail is left protruding from this first set of sutures and may be secured with a hemostat.

7. Moving superiorly toward the distal pole of the wound, the procedure is then repeated sequentially, repeating steps (2) through (5) while moving distally toward the apex for as many throws as are desired, without placing any additional knots.

8. Once the superior-most set of throws is placed, the needle is passed beneath all of the previously placed sets of sutures until it exits proximal to the starting point at the midpoint of the wound. Only then are the ends of the suture material pulled to effect partial closure of the distal portion of the wound.

9. Starting at the inferior or proximal apex, steps (2) through (5) are then repeated, with the pairs of sutures moving upward toward the center of the wound.

10. Once the desired number of throws have been placed and the midpoint of the wound has been reached, the suture material is then pulled taut, leading to complete closure of the wound, and tied utilizing an instrument tie (Figures 4-37A through 4-37J).

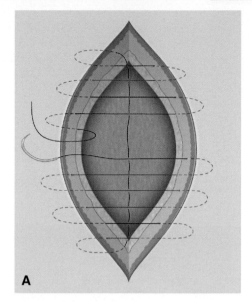

Figure 4-37A. Overview of the bootlace suture technique.

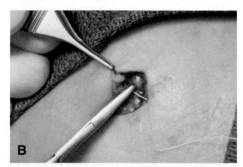

Figure 4-37B. The needle is inserted at the center of the wound through the dermis and exits at the incised wound edge.

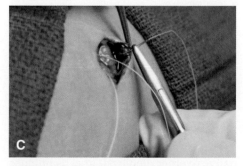

Figure 4-37C. The needle is then inserted on the contralateral side of the wound, still at the center of the wound, entering the incised wound edge and exiting in the dermis.

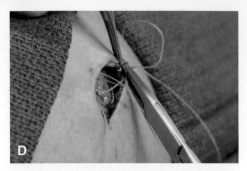

Figure 4-37D. Moving distally, similar bites are taken from alternating wound edges.

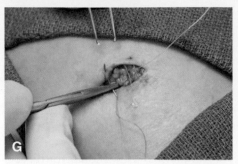

Figure 4-37G. Starting at the proximal wound apex, the needle is then again inserted through the incised wound edge, exiting in the dermis.

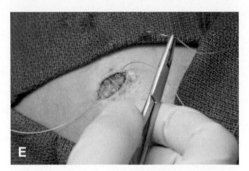

Figure 4-37E. When the distal apex of the wound is reached, the needle is reloaded on the needle driver.

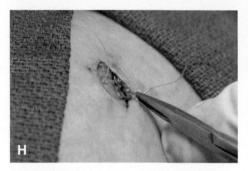

Figure 4-37H. Alternating bites are then taken, moving toward the center of the wound.

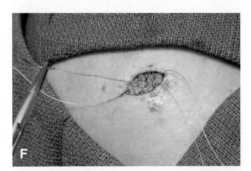

Figure 4-37F. The needle is then passed carefully under the already-placed loops of suture and reloaded on the needle driver.

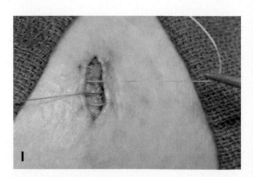

Figure 4-37I. The ends of the suture are then pulled gently, tightening the length of suture and bringing the wound edges together.

Tips and Pearls

This technique was designed as an alternative to other running dermal techniques that would solve one of their chief drawbacks, the tendency toward differential scar spread in the center of the wound as a function of the increased tension in this central area.

While originally described as a modification of the buried dermal suture, it may be easily modified as a buried vertical mattress or set-back suture technique as

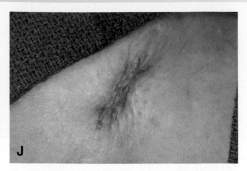

J

Figure 4-37J. Immediate postoperative appearance, after tying the suture in the center of the wound.

well, with the same principle that suture material is tied in the central portion of the wound.

Like other running dermal techniques, this technique may be used as a modified winch or pulley suture, since the multiple loops help minimize the tension across any one loop and permit closure of wounds under marked tension. Because each throw is not tied off, however, it is important to adequately secure the knot.

Given the theoretical susceptibility to suture material breakage or compromise, this is a technique that is probably best used in a layered fashion, either superficial to previously placed interrupted buried sutures or deep to a set of more superficially placed buried sutures.

It may be beneficial to place the running sutures closer together toward the center of the wound than at the poles of the incision, as this may foster a more pronounced pulley effect at the center of the wound where the tensile forces are greatest.

Given the concern regarding knot breakage, it may be helpful to attempt to better secure the central (and only) knot. This may be done by paying particularly close attention to knot tying, tying an extra full knot, adding extra throws, or leaving a longer tail than would traditionally be executed. An additional approach is to secure the final knot with the aid of a tacking knot, which may similarly provide extra security.

Drawbacks and Cautions

Unlike other running dermal techniques, this approach leaves an additional bolus of suture material in the wound from the suture material traversing from the superior apex to the inferior apex at the halfway point of the closure. This added foreign-body material increases the theoretical risk of foreign-body reaction, suture abscess formation, and infection. That said, these theoretical disadvantages should be weighed against the real benefit of tying the knot centrally and better securing the central, highest tension portion of the wound.

This approach should usually not be used as a solitary closure technique, since there is no redundancy in the closure. It may be useful as an adjunct when there is either minimal tension across a wound (and therefore interrupted buried sutures may be unnecessary) or as a pulley approach to bring recalcitrant wound edges together.

Like the standard buried dermal suture, this approach as originally described provides less wound eversion than other approaches such as the set-back dermal or buried vertical mattress; therefore, a bootlace variation of the latter two techniques, as discussed earlier, may often be preferred to a bootlace running dermal approach, since wound eversion may be associated with improved cosmesis over the long term.

Reference

Esdaile BA, Turner R. The bootlace suture: a novel buried running dermal continuous suture for primary closure of wounds. *Clin Exp Dermatol.* 2013;38(7):795-796.

The Buried Tip Stitch

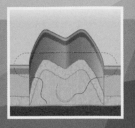

Synonym

Deep tip stitch

Video 4-38. Buried tip stitch
Access to video can be found via
mhprofessional.com/atlasofsuturingtechniques2e

Application

This technique is designed to bring three ends of tissue together and is often used in the context of a flap, where it permits the tip of tissue to be inset. The buried variation of the tip stitch can be conceptualized as a low-tension purse-string closure, since it utilizes a mild form of circumferential tissue advancement. Since it is used only when attempting to approximate three segments of skin, it is a niche technique.

Suture Material Choice

Suture choice is dependent in large part on location, though as always, the smallest gauge suture material appropriate for the anatomic location should be utilized. On the face, where this technique may be used for flap repairs, a 5-0 absorbable suture is appropriate. On the extremities and scalp, a 3-0 or 4-0 absorbable suture material may be used, and on the back and shoulders, 2-0 or 3-0 suture material is effective, though care should be taken with leaving the relatively thick 2-0 suture in the superficial dermis, as it may hydrolyze relatively slowly. Monofilament and braided suture materials may both be appropriate when utilizing this technique.

Technique

1. The flap is brought into place using buried sutures, allowing the tip to rest with only minimal tension in its desired position. The wound edge of the distal portion of nonflap skin is gently reflected back, permitting visualization of the dermis.

2. The needle is inserted into the underside of the dermis on the far right edge of the distal nonflap section of skin with a trajectory running parallel to an imaginary circle around the point where all three segments of skin will meet. Generally, this entry point in the dermis should be approximately 1-3 mm set back from the epidermal edge, depending on the thickness of the dermis and the anticipated degree of tension across the tip. The needle, and therefore the suture, should pass through the deep dermis at a uniform depth. Bite size is dependent on needle size, though in order to minimize the risk of necrosis, it may be prudent to restrict the size of each bite.

3. The needle is then grasped with the surgical pickups and simultaneously released by the hand holding the needle driver. As the needle is freed from the tissue with the pickups, the needle is grasped again by the needle driver in an appropriate position to repeat the preceding step on the flap tip to the left of the previously placed suture.

4. A small amount of suture material is pulled through, and the needle is inserted into the dermis in the flap tip, and the same movement is repeated.

5. The same technique is then repeated on the proximal nonflap edge of skin, keeping the needle parallel to the imaginary circle and moving in the same counterclockwise direction. The needle then exits close to the original entry point on the right side of the wound.

6. The suture material is then gently pulled taut and tied utilizing an instrument tie, burying the knot (Figures 4-38A through 4-38E).

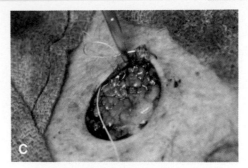

Figure 4-38C. The needle is then inserted through the dermis at the same depth on the tip.

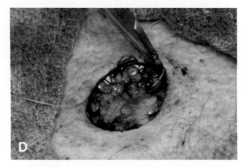

Figure 4-38D. The needle's course continues on the contralateral wound edge, remaining at the same depth and on the same axis.

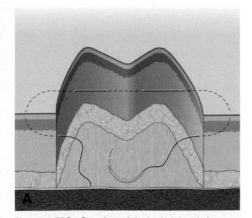

Figure 4-38A. Overview of the buried tip stitch.

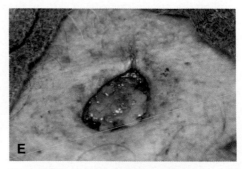

Figure 4-38E. Immediate appearance after suture placement. Note that the tip is brought into close approximation with the other wound edges.

Tips and Pearls

The buried tip stitch is very useful when bringing the tip of a flap into place. Importantly, this technique is designed to gently approximate the tissues so that the flap

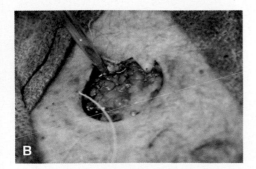

Figure 4-38B. The needle is inserted in the mid-dermis, parallel to the surface of the skin, on an axis following the curvature of an imaginary circle drawn between the two edges and the tip.

is properly inset in the surrounding skin. While it bears a technical resemblance to the buried purse-string approach, it is important to appreciate that the buried tip stitch is not designed to work under significant tension, as tension across the suture may lead to necrosis of the delicate and lightly vascularized tip of the flap.

Placing set-back dermal sutures, imbrication sutures, or suspension sutures prior to placement of the tip stitch will ensure that the tip itself is not under tension when it is approximated with the surrounding skin.

Depending on patient positioning, the three wound edges may be approximated in any order, so that a backhand approach could be used if desired or the bite through the flap tip could be executed as the first step in a closure. If this is done, however, the knot will be placed directly adjacent to the tip of the flap, which may not be ideal.

A downside of traditional tip stitch placement is the tendency for the tip to sit deeper than the surrounding tissues. This may be related to the relative upward pull on the nontip sections of skin by the transepidermal sutures in the standard tip stitch. Therefore, the problem of a depressed tip is not generally seen with the buried tip stitch approach, another significant advantage of this technique.

Drawbacks and Cautions

Since some absorbable suture material is left in the dermis, foreign-body reactions, suture abscess formation, and infections are possibilities. That said, this technique joins only three edges of tissue and, therefore, leaves only slightly more suture material in situ than a standard buried suture.

Flap tip necrosis is the greatest risk with this technique, since suture material traverses the dermis containing the tip's vascular supply. This risk may be mitigated by tying the suture together relatively loosely so that the tip is not overly constricted when the knot is tied. Additionally, if the bites of dermis are sufficiently set back from the wound edge, a small bite comprising less than half of the dermis in the tip could be taken. This would allow blood supply to the tip even in the context of a relatively tight loop running through the distal flap.

Finally, while flap tip necrosis is a risk, studies have suggested that the tip stitch provides less vascular constriction than other options, such as placing two vertically oriented sutures at the edges of the tip or a suture directly through the tip itself. Vascular compromise and ensuing necrosis of the flap tip are always a risk, even if no sutures are placed through the tip itself, and therefore, the buried tip stitch approach likely provides a reasonable balance between tissue approximation and adequate vascular supply.

Reference

Chan JL, Miller EK, Jou RM, Posten W. Novel surgical technique: placement of a deep tip stitch. *Dermatol Surg.* 2009;35(12):2001-2003.

The Backtracking Running Butterfly Suture

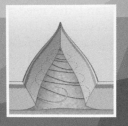

Synonyms

G suture, continuous buried backstitch

Video 4-39. Backtracking running butterfly suture
Access to video can be found via
mhprofessional.com/atlasofsuturingtechniques2e

Application

This is a niche hybrid technique, combining the tension relief, eversion, and lack of transepidermal suture placement of a butterfly suture with the locking ability of a running locking suture and the rapidity of placement and lack of resilience of a superficial running technique. This approach is infrequently used, since the running nature of the technique means that compromise at any point in the course of suture placement may result in wound dehiscence.

Suture Material Choice

Suture choice is dependent in large part on location, though as always, the smallest gauge suture material appropriate for the anatomic location should be utilized. On the back and shoulders, 2-0 or 3-0 suture material is effective, though if there is marked tension across the wound, this approach would not be appropriate as the primary closure and would be used best for its pulley benefits. On the extremities, a 3-0 or 4-0 absorbable suture material may be used, and while rarely utilized in these locations, on the face and areas under minimal tension, a 5-0 absorbable

suture is adequate. Braided absorbable suture has been advocated as ideal for this approach, as it helps lock each of the throws in place while still permitting sufficient slippage to take advantage of the pulley effect of the multiple throws.

Technique

1. After incising the wound with an inward bevel, the wound edge is reflected back using surgical forceps or hooks.
2. The suture is anchored to the undersurface of the dermis distal to the apex of the wound. This may be accomplished by taking a bite of dermis distal to the wound apex and tying off the suture material. A minimum of four throws is recommended to maximize knot security.
3. While reflecting back the dermis on the left side of the wound, the suture needle, loaded in a backhand fashion, is inserted parallel to the skin surface into the base of the beveled undersurface of the dermis 2 mm distant from the incised wound edge.
4. The needle is rotated through its arc, moving parallel to the skin surface toward the surgeon.
5. The first bite is completed by following the curvature of the needle and allowing the needle to exit in the incised wound edge. The size of this bite is based on the size of the needle, the thickness of the dermis,

and the need for and tolerance of eversion. The needle's zenith with respect to the wound surface should be between the entry and exit points.

6. Keeping the loose end of suture material distal to the preceding bite, the dermis on the side of the first bite is released. The tissue on the opposite edge is then gently grasped with the forceps.

7. The second bite is executed by inserting the needle into the incised wound edge, parallel to the skin surface and again at the level of the superficial papillary dermis. This bite should be completed by following the curvature of the needle and avoiding catching the undersurface of the epidermis, which could result in epidermal dimpling. It then exits approximately 2 mm distal to the wound edge on the undersurface of the dermis, distal to its entry point.

8. The procedure is then repeated sequentially, repeating steps (2) through (7) while moving proximally toward the surgeon for as many throws as are desired, without placing any additional knots until the desired number of loops have been placed. Each backstitch should overlap the preceding suture throw by approximately half of its radius.

9. The suture material is then tied utilizing an instrument tie (Figures 4-39A through 4-39H).

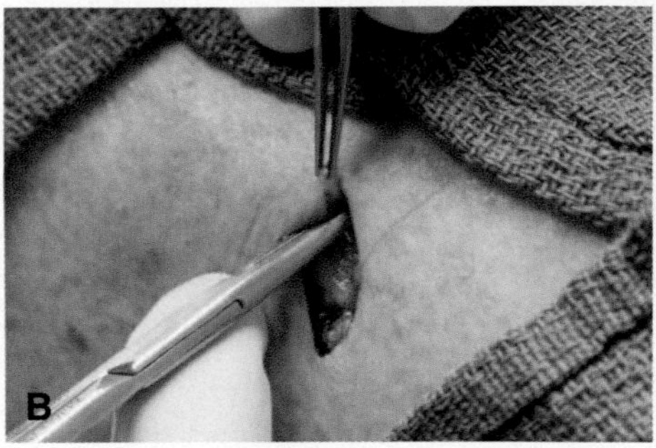

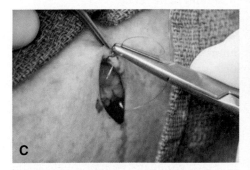

Figure 4-39B. Beginning of the anchoring suture. The needle is inserted through the underside of the dermis, exiting through the incised wound edge.

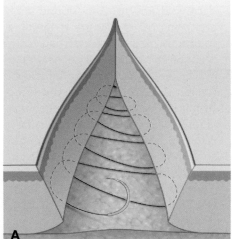

Figure 4-39A. Overview of the backtracking running butterfly suture.

Figure 4-39C. Second portion of the anchoring suture; the needle is inserted on the contralateral side through the incised wound edge, exiting at the undersurface of the wound.

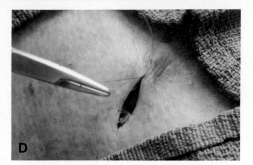

Figure 4-39D. The anchoring suture is tied.

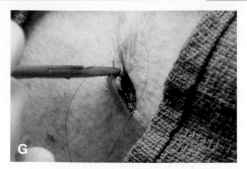

Figure 4-39G. The bites are repeated on alternating sides, each time with the needle exiting at the midpoint of its prior throw, so that a continuous backstitch is executed.

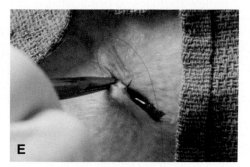

Figure 4-39E. With the needle driver held in a pencil-like fashion, the needle is rotated through the dermis, entering the deep dermis and taking a bite parallel to the incised wound edge, with the needle reaching its zenith at the center of the bite.

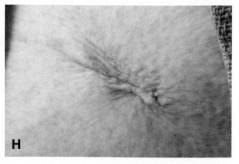

Figure 4-39H. Immediate postoperative appearance.

Tips and Pearls

This technique may be used as a modified winch or pulley suture, since the multiple loops help minimize the tension across any one loop and permit closure of wounds under marked tension. Because each throw is not tied off, however, it is important to adequately secure the first and final throws with a well-locked knot.

Like the butterfly suture, this technique is best used with a beveled incision. Indeed, the horizontal orientation of this suture may be conceptualized as a continuous butterfly suture with a backstitch component.

Given the theoretical susceptibility to suture material breakage or compromise, this is a technique that is probably best used in a layered fashion, either superficial

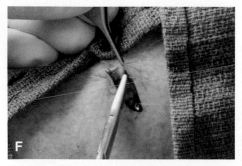

Figure 4-39F. A similar bite is taken on the contralateral wound edge, with the needle exiting the contralateral wound edge proximal to its exit point from the previous side, leading to a backstitch configuration.

to previously placed interrupted buried sutures or deep to a set of more superficially placed buried sutures.

If braided absorbable suture is used, the added friction between loops may help lock the suture material in place with each throw, but caution should be taken to pull sufficient suture material through with each throw, as this friction may impede the surgeon's ability to pull suture material through the course of multiple loops. Similarly, if monofilament suture is used, it may be easier to pull the additional suture material through, but it may make it more difficult to lock the suture in place before tying, and the running suture loops may gape open as the surgeon moves proximally through the different sets of throws.

It may be beneficial to place the running sutures closer together toward the center of the wound than at the poles of the incision, as this may foster a more pronounced pulley effect at the center of the wound where the tensile forces are greatest.

Given the concern regarding knot breakage, it may be helpful to attempt to better secure the first and final knots at the ends of the running series of loops. This may be done by paying particularly close attention to knot tying, tying an extra full knot, adding extra throws, or leaving a longer tail than would traditionally be executed. An additional approach is to secure the final knot with the aid of a tacking knot, which may similarly provide extra security.

This technique calls for horizontally oriented suture loops to be placed with a slight upward tilt at their apex (ie, when the suture material moves laterally away from the incised edge). This approach, in the context of a beveled incision, leads to a nicely everted wound edge, as is seen with the butterfly suture.

Drawbacks and Cautions

As noted previously, this approach should usually not be used as a solitary closure technique, since there is no redundancy in the closure. It may be useful either as an adjunct when there is minimal tension across a wound (and therefore interrupted buried sutures may be unnecessary) or as a pulley approach to bring recalcitrant wound edges together.

The central drawback of this approach is the fact that it is a running technique; therefore, suture material or knot compromise at any point will lead to potential wound dehiscence. While the locking effect of the backstitch when using braided suture material is somewhat helpful, it does not guarantee that the edges will remain locked in the absence of an anchoring suture.

Theoretically, the horizontal orientation of the suture loops may increase the risk of wound-edge necrosis, though this has not been reported as a significant problem. The backstitch component does result in a slightly larger quantity of suture material being left in the wound when compared with a standard running buried technique, theoretically increasing the risk of a foreign-body reaction or other complications.

Reference

Almuhammadi RA. The G-suture: continuous buried backstitch (CBB). An innovative aesthetic dermal suture technique. *J Dtsch Dermatol Ges.* 2011;9(12):1058-1061.

The Stacked Backing Out Subcuticular Suture Technique

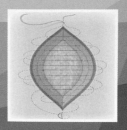

Synonym

Super loop suture

Video 4-40. Stacked backing out subcuticular suture
Access to video can be found via mhprofessional.com/atlasofsuturingtechniques2e

Application

This is a niche technique that may be conceptualized as a backing out subcuticular approach with the first row of subcuticular sutures placed in the deep dermis or as a variation of the stacked double purse-string technique. It is useful for wounds under mild to moderate tension and may be used overlying deeper tension-relieving sutures.

Suture Material Choice

As with any technique, it is best to utilize the thinnest suture possible for any given anatomic location. As this technique is not designed to hold marked tension irrespective of anatomic location, generally a 4-0 or 5-0 suture may be used. This is especially important since a large volume of suture material is left in situ when utilizing this approach. It is best to utilize a monofilament suture material to minimize the coefficient of friction at the time of suture removal, though this technique may also be finessed for use with absorbable suture material.

Technique

1. The needle is inserted at the far right corner of the wound, parallel to the incision line, beginning approximately 2-5 mm from the apex. The needle is passed from this point, which is lateral to the incision apex, directly through the epidermis, exiting into the interior of the wound just medial to the apex.

2. With the tail of the suture material resting lateral to the incision apex and outside the wound, the wound edge is gently reflected back, and the needle is inserted into the deep dermis or fascia on the far edge of the wound with a trajectory running parallel to the incision line. The needle, and therefore the suture, should pass through the deep dermis or fascia at a uniform depth. Bite size is dependent on needle size, though in order to minimize the risk of necrosis, it may be prudent to restrict the size of each bite. The needle should exit the deep dermis or fascia at a point equidistant from the cut edge from where it entered.

3. The needle is then grasped with the surgical pickups and simultaneously released by the hand holding the needle driver. As the needle is freed from the tissue with the pickups, the needle is grasped again by the needle driver in an appropriate position

to repeat the previously mentioned step on the contralateral edge of the incised wound edge.

4. A small amount of suture material is pulled through, and the needle is inserted into the deep dermis or fascia on the contralateral side of the incised wound edge after reflecting back the skin, and the same movement is repeated. The needle should enter slightly proximal (relative to the wound apex where the suture line began) to the exit point, thus introducing a small degree of backtracking to the snake-like flow of the suture material. This will help reduce the risk of tissue bunching.

5. The same technique is repeated on the contralateral side of the incision line, and alternating bites are then taken from each side of the incision line, continuing on until the end of the wound is reached. At this point, the needle's direction is changed to head in the opposite direction, toward the apex where the suture began.

6. Moving in the opposite direction, steps (1) through (5) are then repeated but now in the superficial dermis, with the suture material snaking an alternating course through the superficial dermis, using a backhand technique if desired.

7. The suture material may either be tied to the free end of suture at the original apex or, alternatively, be tied on the exterior of the wound (Figures 4-40A through 4-40J).

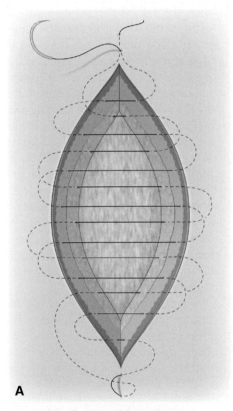

A

Figure 4-40A. Overview of the stacked backing out subcuticular suture.

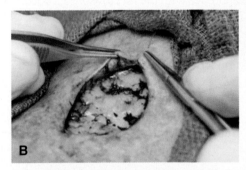

B

Figure 4-40B. The needle is inserted from outside the skin, lateral to the wound apex, exiting in the interior of the wound.

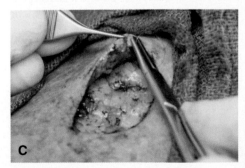

C

Figure 4-40C. The needle is passed through the deep dermis, parallel to the incised wound edge.

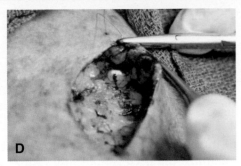

Figure 4-40D. This is repeated along the contralateral wound edge.

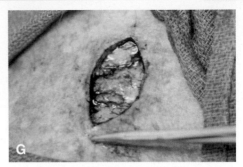

Figure 4-40G. The needle is reinserted lateral to the apex, entering the interior of the wound, now heading in the opposite direction.

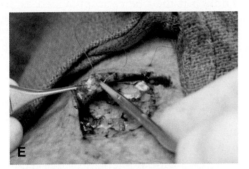

Figure 4-40E. Suture placement continues in the deep dermis parallel to the wound edge, alternating sides.

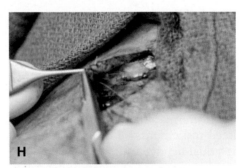

Figure 4-40H. The needle is passed through the superficial dermis parallel to the wound edge in the direction of the initial entry point.

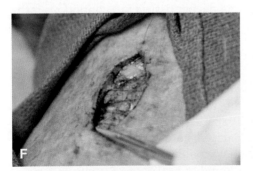

Figure 4-40F. Once the end of the wound is reached, the needle is passed through the deep dermis lateral to the wound apex, exiting the skin lateral to the apex.

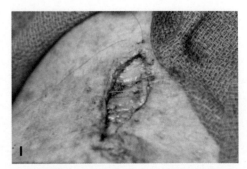

Figure 4-40I. After reaching the end of the wound by successively taking bites of the superficial dermis on alternating edges of the wound, the needle again exits lateral to the apex.

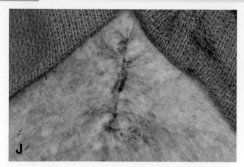

Figure 4-40J. Immediate postoperative appearance after the suture material has been pulled taut and tied. Note the bunching at the wound's poles, which may be mitigated by utilizing a bolster so that the downward pull of the suture loops does not lead to exaggerated dimpling.

Tips and Pearls

This is a niche technique, as the addition of a second row of subcuticular suture material in the wound may add only modest wound security, since it is a running technique, while it doubles the amount of suture material that will ultimately need to be removed or absorbed. This is a dual-depth closure that is otherwise similar to the more recently described cross-running intradermal suture.

As with the standard subcuticular technique, body positioning can be very helpful in maintaining an efficient and comfortable technique. Most surgeons are trained to work with the surgical site flat and perpendicular to their body. Since the motions associated with subcuticular suture placement are 90 degrees off from this, it may be useful to stand with the surgeon's body (shoulder to shoulder) parallel to the incision line. This allows for a flowing motion from right to left without the need to twist the shoulders or wrists.

Since this approach requires the surgeon to perform the second half of the closure moving in the opposite direction, it may be useful to use a backhand technique for many of the suture throws when moving back toward the original wound apex.

This may add significantly to the time needed to complete this closure.

A smooth, flowing technique is of paramount importance in executing this technique effectively and efficiently. Some authors have advocated adjusting the angle used to hold the needle in the needle driver from the traditional 90-135 degrees to increase the surgeon's comfort and minimize the need for physical contortion, though slightly adjusting the surgeon's body position helps significantly in this regard.

Drawbacks and Cautions

Though it may be conceptualized as a bidirectional, two-depth subcuticular closure, the extra row of sutures in this technique pulls the deep tissues together but also adds only modestly to wound security, as the entire suture line is secured with a single knot. Therefore, it is probably best not used as a solitary closure approach, but rather layered over the top of a deeper suturing technique.

While a central strength of this technique is its entirely intradermal placement, this may also represent one of its greatest drawbacks. This technique results in leaving a very significant quantity of foreign-body material in the dermis and deeper tissues in a continuous fashion. While this may not represent a major problem in areas with a thick dermis such as the back, in other anatomic locations, the large quantity of suture that is left in situ may result in concerns regarding infection, foreign-body reaction, and even the potential that the suture material itself could present a physical barrier that would impinge on the ability of the wound to heal appropriately.

The extra row of deep sutures used in this technique raises further concern regarding the possibility of tissue strangulation along the wound margin that could theoretically be associated with tightly placed subcuticular sutures. Therefore, it should be reserved for areas with an outstanding vascular supply, such as the face.

If nonabsorbable suture material is used, removal of long-standing suture entails a theoretical risk that a potential space—albeit a thin and long one—is created on the removal of the suture material. This theoretical risk may be mitigated by utilizing the thinnest possible suture material.

References

Bolander L. The super loop suture: a way of suturing skin and subcutaneous tissue. *Plast Reconstr Surg.* 1992;89(4):766.

Xiong L, Sun J, Pan Q, Yang J. The cross-running intradermal suture: a novel method for incision closure. *Facial Plast Surg.* 2012;28(5):541-542.

CHAPTER 4.41

The Running Locked Intradermal Suture

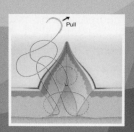

Video 4-41. Running locked intradermal suture
Access to video can be found via
mhprofessional.com/atlasofsuturingtechniques2e

Application

This is a niche hybrid technique, combining the tension relief and lack of transepidermal suture placement of a classic buried suture with the rapidity of placement and lack of resilience of a superficial running technique and the locking benefit of a running locked suture. The locking loops of suture add significantly to the volume of retained suture material and also make suture placement more challenging to learn than other techniques.

Suture Material Choice

Suture choice is dependent in large part on location, though as always, the smallest gauge suture material appropriate for the anatomic location should be utilized. On the back and shoulders, a 3-0 suture material is effective, though if there is marked tension across the wound, this approach would not be appropriate as the primary closure. On the extremities, a 3-0 or 4-0 absorbable suture material may be used, and on the face and areas under minimal tension, a 5-0 absorbable suture is adequate.

Technique

1. The wound edge is reflected back using surgical forceps or hooks.

2. While reflecting back the dermis, the suture needle is inserted at 90 degrees into the underside of the dermis 2 mm distant from the incised wound edge.

3. The first bite is executed by following the curvature of the needle and allowing the needle to exit in the incised wound edge. The needle's zenith with respect to the wound surface should be between the entry and exit points.

4. Keeping the loose end of the suture between the surgeon and the patient, the dermis on the side of the first bite is released. The tissue on the opposite edge is then gently grasped with the forceps.

5. The second bite is executed by inserting the needle into the incised wound edge at the level of the superficial papillary dermis. This bite should be completed by following the curvature of the needle and avoiding catching the undersurface of the epidermis. It then exits approximately 2 mm distal to the wound edge on the undersurface of the dermis. This should mirror the first bite taken on the contralateral side of the wound.

6. This first anchoring set of sutures is then tied with an instrument tie.

7. Moving proximally toward the surgeon, steps (1) through (5) are then repeated, leaving a loop of suture material created between the

anchor suture and the start of this second dermal suture protruding from the wound center.

8. The needle is inserted beneath the loop of suture and then looped again around the loop, creating a secondary loop of suture material.

9. The needle is then pulled through this secondary loop and gently pulled upward, securing the loop in place.

10. The needle is then inserted through the center of the wound underneath the newly formed loop.

11. The procedure is then repeated sequentially, repeating steps (7) through (10) while moving proximally toward the surgeon for as many throws as are desired, without placing any additional knots until the desired number of loops have been placed.

12. The suture material is then tied utilizing an instrument tie. Alternatively, a hand tie may be used if desired (Figures 4-41A through 4-41K).

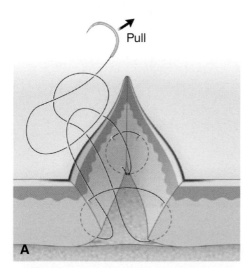

Figure 4-41A. Overview of the running locked intradermal suture.

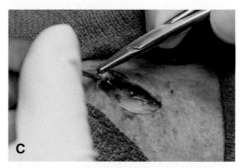

Figure 4-41C. The needle then enters the incised wound edge on the contralateral side, exiting in the dermis. The suture is then tied, and the loose end of suture material is trimmed.

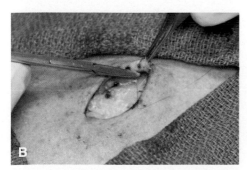

Figure 4-41B. Placement of the anchoring suture; the first bite enters from the dermis, exiting in the incised wound edge.

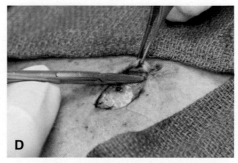

Figure 4-41D. Moving proximally toward the surgeon, a loop of suture is left as the needle is passed through the dermis, exiting the incised wound edge.

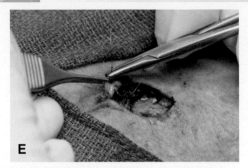

Figure 4-41E. This is repeated on the contralateral side, with the needle exiting between the wound apex and the newly placed portion of suture material.

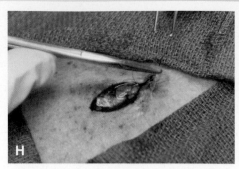

Figure 4-41H. The needle is then passed again through this loop of suture.

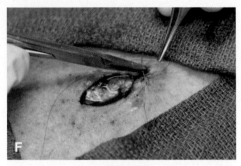

Figure 4-41F. The needle is then passed through the loop left on the contralateral side.

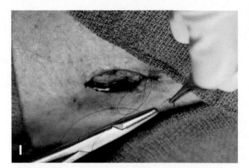

Figure 4-41I. The needle is then passed through the newly created secondary loop of suture material.

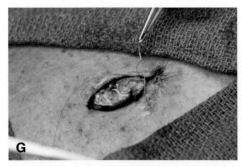

Figure 4-41G. The needle may be gently grasped with surgical forceps.

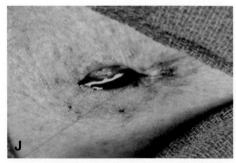

Figure 4-41J. The suture material is then pulled taut, locking the suture in place. This procedure is then repeated sequentially along the length of the wound.

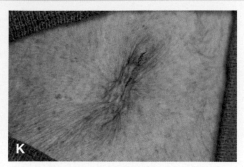

Figure 4-41K. Immediate postoperative appearance.

Tips and Pearls

This is a complex technique and takes some time to master. Its chief advantage is that although each individual dermal suture is not fully tied, it is locked so securely that compromise along the line of sutures will likely not lead to a complete loss of security in the suture line.

As with other techniques, if braided absorbable suture is used, the added friction between loops may help lock the suture material in place with each throw, but caution should be taken to pull sufficient suture material through with each throw, as this friction may impede the surgeon's ability to pull suture material through the course of multiple loops. Similarly, if monofilament suture is used, it may be easier to pull the additional suture material through, but it may make it more difficult to lock the suture in place before tying.

It may be helpful to attempt to better secure the first and final knots at the ends of the running series of loops. This may be done by paying particularly close attention to knot tying, tying an extra full knot, adding extra throws, or leaving a longer tail than would traditionally be executed.

Drawbacks and Cautions

The major drawback of this technique is that it may be challenging to learn. Once mastered, this technique presents a viable option for securing deep sutures, though as with all techniques, it does have some limitations.

This approach leaves a sizable quantity of suture material in place along the incised wound edge. Since this material may serve as a barrier to healing and may also increase the risk of suture spitting, this is a disadvantage. Moreover, since some of the suture material is placed fairly superficially and extends laterally along the incised wound edge, if suture spitting or suture abscess formation becomes a problem, this may be particularly troublesome as it may affect a greater proportion of the wound rather than the single punctate area, as is seen with interrupted sutures.

The added time needed to effectively lock each throw also means that one of the greatest advantages of the running approach—that it is faster than interrupted sutures—is minimized, since the differential between the time needed to tie individual sutures and to effectively lock the line of sutures may not be that great.

Like the standard buried dermal suture, this approach provides less wound eversion than other approaches such as the set-back dermal or buried vertical mattress; therefore, a running locking variation of the latter two techniques may be preferred to a running locking dermal approach, since wound eversion may be associated with improved cosmesis over the long term.

Reference

Wong NL. The running locked intradermal suture. A cosmetically elegant continuous suture for wounds under light tension. *J Dermatol Surg Oncol.* 1993;19(1):30-36.

The Buried Dog-Ear Tip Stitch

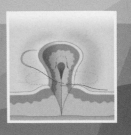

 Video 4-42. The buried dog-ear tip stitch
Access to video can be found via mhprofessional.com/atlasofsuturingtechniques2e

Application

This is a niche technique used for reducing the appearance of dog ears, or standing cones, at the ends of elliptical excisions or local flaps. While dog-ear minimization is generally accomplished by excising lesions with fusiform incisions, this often extends the length of the wound significantly, which is undesirable. This technique was designed as an approach to mitigate the raised dog-ear appearance of the standing cone while concomitantly avoiding unnecessarily extending the length of the wound.

Suture Material Choice

Suture choice is dependent in large part on location. On the back and extremities, a 2-0, 3-0, or 4-0 absorbable suture material may be used, and on the face and other areas under minimal tension, a 4-0 or 5-0 absorbable suture is adequate.

Technique

1. The suture needle is inserted at 90 degrees into the underside of the dermis on the far side of the wound, 4-6 mm distant from the apex.
2. The first bite is executed by traversing the dermis following the curvature of the needle as with a buried dermal suture.
3. The needle is reloaded, and a horizontally oriented bite is taken through the base of the dog ear.
4. The needle is again reloaded, and the needle is inserted through the underside of the dermis, exiting at the dermal-epidermal junction on the opposite side of the wound from the first throw, in a mirror image of the first throw.
5. The suture material is then tied utilizing an instrument tie (Figures 4-42A through 4-42G).

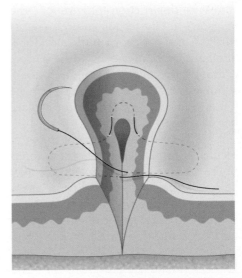

Figure 4-42A. Overview of the buried dog-ear tip stitch.

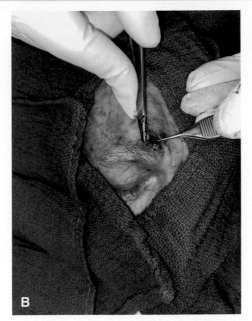

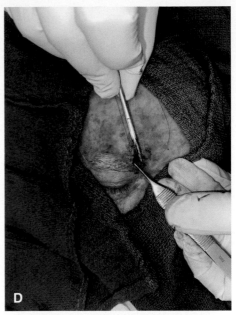

Figure 4-42B. The suture needle is inserted at 90 degrees into the underside of the dermis on the far side of the wound, 4-6 mm distant from the apex. The first bite is executed by traversing the dermis following the curvature of the needle as with a buried dermal suture. The needle is then reloaded.

Figure 4-42D. The needle exits running along the base of the dog ear and is again reloaded.

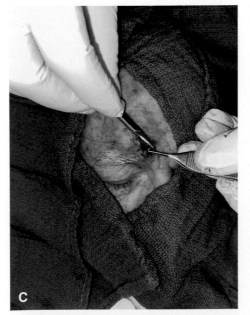

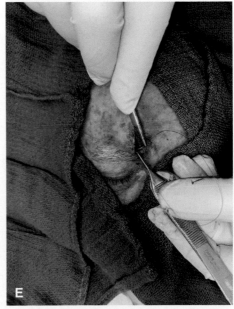

Figure 4-42C. A horizontally oriented bite is taken through the base of the dog ear.

Figure 4-42E. The needle is inserted through the dermal-epidermal junction.

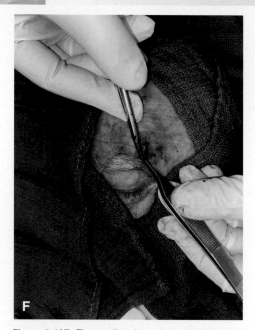

Figure 4-42F. The needle exits at the underside of the dermis on the opposite side of the wound from the first throw, in a mirror image of the first throw.

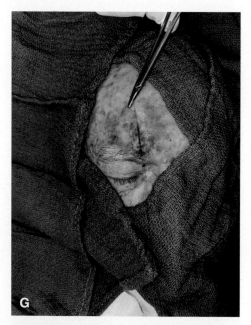

Figure 4-42G. The suture material is then tied utilizing an instrument tie.

Tips and Pearls

In some locations, such as convexities over the forehead, even defects repaired with a 4:1 ellipse may still display residual standing cones at the apices; therefore, this approach may be used as an adjunct in such cases as well.

This approach can be conceptualized a hybrid between a buried tip stitch and a purse-string suture, since it is designed to pull the dog ear inward and reduce its appearance.

Some experience is helpful in deciding what degree of residual standing cone appearance is acceptable. Wounds on the lower legs, for example, often heal well, and residual standing cones may smooth out spontaneously, likely due to the tension over bony prominences. Conversely, standing cones over cheeks and other areas with abundant soft tissue often resolve only minimally over time, and therefore, leaving significant dog ears in these locations should be assiduously avoided if possible.

This approach, when used in concert with a technique such as the fascial plication suture that causes a round or oval defect to appear more fusiform, may permit closure of wounds with significantly less standing cone removal, leading to shorter—and therefore more cosmetically appealing—scars.

Drawbacks and Cautions

As with any suspension suture, since the underside of the dermis is tacked to periosteum, this technique may result in an area of depression at the site of suture placement.

The anchoring portion of this suture technique carries the risk of damage to an underlying vascular or neural plexus. Familiarity with the underlying bony anatomy is therefore of paramount importance, as it also permits the surgeon to select appropriate locations for dog-ear tacking suture placement.

As suture material is tacked to the periosteum—and traverses muscle and fascia—patients should be warned that they may experience more pain with this approach than would be experienced with a typical bilayered closure.

When tacking to the underlying fascia, since the anchoring point is not entirely immobile, it is possible that the degree of standing cone reduction will be only modest. Therefore, such cases may require a greater degree of standing cone excision than those overlying bony prominences.

The residual focal rippling of the epidermis caused by tissue redundancy will generally resolve with time, though in areas with significant actinic damage and solar elastosis, the lack of underlying elasticity may lead to residual textural changes that do not resolve. In these unusual cases, surgical revision may be useful to excise the residual area, as would be done for a dog-ear removal, thus leading to a more acceptable cosmetic outcome.

The Buried Leveling Suture

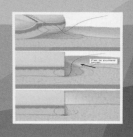

 Video 4-43. Buried leveling suture
Access to video can be found via
mhprofessional.com/atlasofsuturingtechniques2e

Application

This technique is used to reduce the step-off between the wound edge and an area that is left open to granulate. It is a niche technique used, for example, when repairing a defect that involves the thin lower eyelid skin, where it is sometimes beneficial to allow granulation to occur while also minimizing the step-off between cheek skin and the granulated area.

Suture Choice

Since this technique is used to fine-tune the relationship between the epidermal edge and an area that will heal secondarily, it is not designed to hold tension, and a 5-0 or 6-0 absorbable suture is often appropriate.

Technique

1. The needle is inserted through the underside of the dermis, exiting at the dermal-epidermal junction following the needle's curvature. The needle is then reloaded.
2. A bite is then taken through the center of the wound.
3. The suture material is then tied off gently, with care being taken to minimize tension and avoid any pull on free margins such as the eyelid (Figures 4-43A through 4-43D).

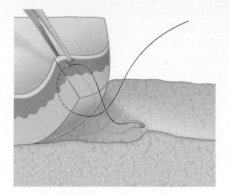

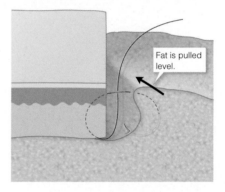

Fat is pulled level.

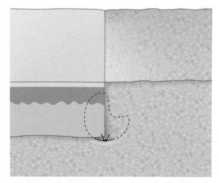

Figure 4-43A. Overview of the leveling suture technique.

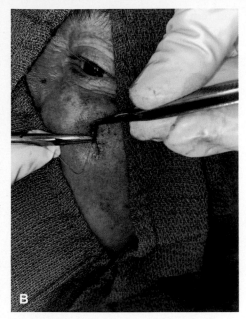

Figure 4-43B. The needle is inserted through the underside of the dermis. The needle exits at the dermal-epidermal junction following the needle's curvature. The needle is then reloaded.

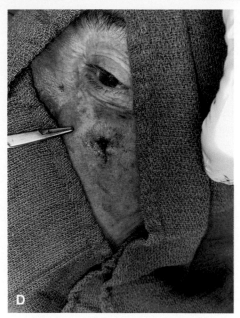

Figure 4-43D. The suture material is then tied off gently, with care being taken to minimize tension and avoid any pull on free margins such as the eyelid.

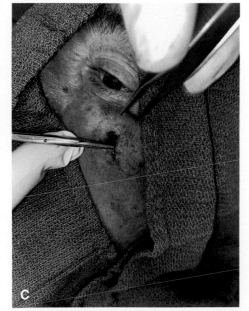

Figure 4-43C. A bite is then taken through the center of the wound.

Tips and Pearls

This suture technique is useful when repairing defects that arise from tumors that bridge the thin skin of the lower eyelid and the thicker skin of the cheek. In such cases, either linear repairs or advancement flaps (including island pedicle flaps) may be performed, but the repairs should not, ideally, bridge the boundary between the infraorbital and maxillary cheek. Therefore, it may be best to allow a small portion of the defect on the infraorbital cheek/lower eyelid skin to heal secondarily, while also obviating an overly dramatic step-off between the repaired area and the area permitted to heal secondarily.

This approach may also be useful when performing any closure that heals in part secondarily, since it may result in faster healing times and less risk of scarring or contraction. A series of leveling sutures can be placed (and the technique can also be used in a running fashion) circumferentially around a defect, as long as the bulk of the repair has already been fixed in place ensuring that there is no tension across the free margin.

Drawbacks and Cautions

This is a niche technique that is generally used when an area is left to heal secondarily. Caution should be exercised to avoid oversewing areas, with the goal of correcting slight imbalances and reducing the step-off between the epidermal edge and the bed of a granulating wound, since even deep wounds will often heal without the assistance of leveling sutures. Indeed, overuse of leveling sutures could theoretically introduce added foreign-body material to a wound and induce an inflammatory response that could ultimately result in slower healing.

Reference

Davis JC, Tsai S, Bordeaux JS. Modified V-Y advancement flap with "directed" granulation and leveling sutures for defects of the lid-cheek junction. *Dermatol Surg.* 2017;43(10):1298-1300.

Suture Techniques for Superficial Structures: Transepidermal Approaches

The Simple Interrupted Suture

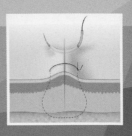

Video 5-1. Simple interrupted suture
Access to video can be found via
mhprofessional.com/atlasofsuturingtechniques2e

Application

This is the standard benchmark suture used for closure and epidermal approximation. It may be used alone in the context of small wounds under minimal to no tension, such as those formed by either a small bunch biopsy or a traumatic laceration. It is also frequently used as a secondary layer to aid in the approximation of the epidermis when the dermis has been closed using a dermal or other deep suturing technique.

Suture Material Choice

With all techniques, it is best to use the thinnest suture possible in order to minimize the risk of track marks and foreign-body reactions. Suture choice will depend largely on anatomic location and the goal of suture placement. Simple interrupted sutures may be placed with the goal of (1) accomplishing epidermal approximation in a wound under moderate tension, such as a laceration or punch biopsy, or (2) fine-tuning the epidermal approximation of a wound where the tension has already been shifted deep utilizing a deeper dermal or fascial suturing technique.

On the face and eyelids, a 6-0 or 7-0 monofilament suture may be utilized for epidermal approximation. When the goal of simple interrupted suture placement is solely epidermal approximation, this suture material may be used on the extremities as well. Otherwise, 5-0 monofilament suture material can be used if there is minimal tension, and 4-0 monofilament suture may be used in areas under moderate tension where the goal of suture placement is relieving tension as well as epidermal approximation. In select high-tension areas, 3-0 monofilament suture may be utilized as well, particularly in the context of a multimodality approach, for example, when mattress sutures are placed in the center of the wound to maximize tension relief and eversion, and simple interrupted sutures are placed at the lateral edges of the wound to minimize dog-ear formation.

Technique

1. The needle is inserted perpendicular to the epidermis, approximately one-half the radius of the needle distant to the wound edge. This will allow the needle to exit the wound on the contralateral side at an equal distance from the wound edge by simply following the curvature of the needle.

2. With a fluid motion of the wrist, the needle is rotated through the dermis, taking the bite wider at the deep margin than at the surface, and the needle tip exits the skin on the contralateral side.

3. The needle body is grasped with surgical forceps in the left hand, with

care being taken to avoid grasping the needle tip, which can be easily dulled by repetitive friction against the surgical forceps. It is gently grasped and pulled upward with the surgical forceps as the body of the needle is released from the needle driver. Alternatively, the needle may be released from the needle driver, and the needle driver itself may be used to grasp the needle from the contralateral side of the wound to complete its rotation through its arc, obviating the need for surgical forceps.

4. The suture material is then tied off gently, with care being taken to minimize tension across the epidermis and avoid overly constricting the wound edges (Figures 5-1A through 5-1D).

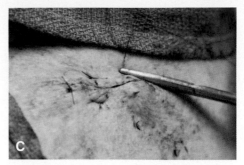

Figure 5-1C. Completion of the simple interrupted suture. Note that the needle now exits the skin at a 90-degree angle.

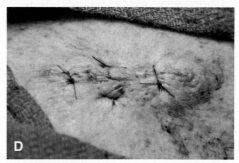

Figure 5-1D. Appearance after placement of the simple interrupted suture. Note the presence of the adjacent horizontal mattress suture and the depth-correcting simple interrupted suture, whose postoperative appearance is identical to that of the simple interrupted suture.

Tips and Pearls

It is important to enter the epidermis at 90 degrees, allowing the needle to travel slightly laterally away from the wound edge before fully following the curvature of the needle when utilizing this technique. This will allow for maximal wound eversion and accurate wound-edge approximation. The final cross-sectional appearance of the needle's course should be a flask-like shape, wider at the base than at the surface.

The simple interrupted suture may also be used layered over the top of another suture in order to fine-tune epidermal approximation. For example, if a vertical mattress suture was placed to facilitate

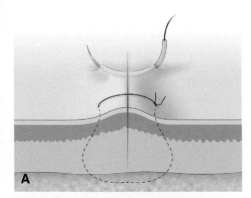

Figure 5-1A. Overview of the simple interrupted suture technique.

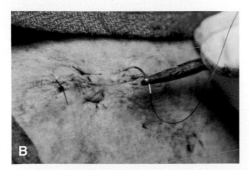

Figure 5-1B. Beginning of the simple interrupted suture. Note that the needle enters the skin at a 90-degree angle before curving slightly away from the wound edge to take a flask-like bite of tissue.

eversion, occasionally the wound edges may not be fully approximated. A small simple interrupted suture, placed at the point where the wound edges are farthest apart, may be used to solve this problem and effect accurate approximation of the wound edges.

Care should be taken to avoid skimming the needle superficially beneath the epidermis. This results from failing to enter the skin at a perpendicular angle and to follow the curvature of the needle. This may result in wound inversion as the tension vector of the shallow bite pulls the wound edges outward and down.

This approach can also be used to correct the so-called sandwiching phenomenon that is seen occasionally after placement of mattress sutures, where the approximation of the deep tissues leads the epidermal edges to paradoxically separate. In such cases, placing a simple interrupted suture over the area that is exaggeratingly separated—directly superficial to the mattress suture—can simply solve this problem.

Drawbacks and Cautions

With any suturing technique, knowledge of the relevant anatomy is critical. When placing a simple interrupted suture, it is important to recall that the structures deep to the epidermis may be compromised by the passage of the needle and suture material. For example, the needle may pierce a vessel, leading to increased bleeding.

Similarly, particularly if the knot is tied relatively tightly, structures deep to the defect may be constricted. This can lead to necrosis due to vascular compromise or even, theoretically, superficial nerve damage.

The potential to constrict deeper structures may be used to the surgeon's advantage in the event that a small vessel deep to the incision line is oozing; rather than opening the wound, localizing the source of the bleed, and tying off the individual vessel, it may be possible to simply place an interrupted suture incorporating the culprit vessel within its arc, tie it tightly, and thus indirectly ligate the vessel. This should only be used in the event that the offending vessel is relatively small, since otherwise there is a significant risk that this indirect ligation will not be sufficiently resilient. Moreover, tying the suture too tightly may increase the risk of developing track marks or superficial necrosis.

This technique may result in an increased risk of track marks, necrosis, and other complications when compared with techniques that do not entail suture material traversing the scar line, such as buried or subcuticular approaches. Therefore, sutures should be removed as early as possible to minimize these complications, and consideration should be given to adopting other closure techniques in the event that sutures will not be able to be removed in a timely fashion. Some studies have also demonstrated an increased rate of dehiscence when utilizing interrupted sutures alone without underlying dermal tension-relieving sutures, highlighting that this technique should be used either for wounds under minimal tension or in concert with deeper tension-relieving sutures.

Reference

Blattner CM, Markus B, Lear W. Correction of "sandwiching phenomenon" following horizontal mattress suture. *J Am Acad Dermatol.* 2018;78(4):e87-88.

CHAPTER 5.2

The Depth-Correcting Simple Interrupted Suture

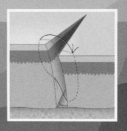

Synonym

Step-off correction suture

 Video 5-2. Depth-correcting simple interrupted suture
Access to video can be found via mhprofessional.com/atlasofsuturingtechniques2e

Application

This technique is used to correct depth disparities when the elevation of the epidermis on each side of an incised wound edge is significantly different. This problem usually stems from inaccurate placement of deeper sutures, though it may also occur as the result of differential dermal thicknesses in certain anatomic locations, such as the boundary of the lateral nose and medial cheek.

Suture Choice

With all techniques, it is best to use the thinnest suture possible in order to minimize the risk of track marks and foreign-body reactions. Since this technique is used to fine-tune epidermal depth and is therefore not designed to hold a significant amount of tension, a 6-0 monofilament suture is often appropriate. In areas under greater tension, such as the trunk and extremities, a 5-0 monofilament suture material may be used as well.

Technique

1. The needle is inserted perpendicular to the epidermis, approximately one-half the radius of the needle distant to the wound edge.

2. If the side of the wound where the needle is first inserted is higher than the contralateral side, a shallow bite is taken, with the needle skimming the dermal-epidermal junction and exiting in the center of the wound. If the side where the needle first enters is lower than the contralateral side, a deep bite is taken, with the needle exiting through the deep dermis or into the undersurface of the dermis, depending on the degree of desired correction.

3. The needle body is grasped with surgical forceps in the left hand and pulled medially with the surgical forceps as the body of the needle is released from the needle driver.

4. The needle is reloaded on the needle driver, and the contralateral wound edge is gently reflected back with the forceps.

5. If the second side of the wound is deeper than the first, then depending on the required degree of depth correction, the needle is inserted either through the underside of the dermis or laterally through the deep dermis on the contralateral side of the wound. If the second side is higher than the first, a superficial bite is taken, through the dermal-epidermal junction if needed, to permit correction.

6. The needle is rotated and exits through the epidermis, equidistant from the incised wound edge relative to the first bite.

201

7. The suture material is then tied off gently, with care being taken to minimize tension across the epidermis and avoid overly constricting the wound edges (Figures 5-2A through 5-2E).

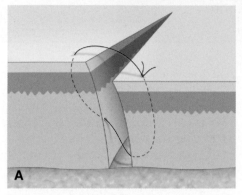

Figure 5-2A. Overview of the depth-correcting simple interrupted suture technique.

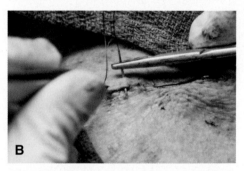

Figure 5-2B. First throw of the depth-correcting simple interrupted suture technique. The side where the needle exits was superficial relative to the contralateral wound edge. Thus, the needle passes superficially through the dermis on this side, exiting in the center of the wound.

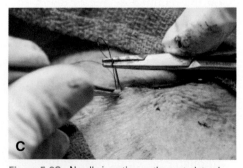

Figure 5-2C. Needle insertion on the contralateral, deeper side. Note that the skin is reflected upward to permit insertion of the needle through the deep undersurface of the dermis.

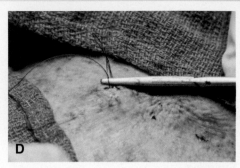

Figure 5-2D. The needle exits the skin at a 90-degree angle.

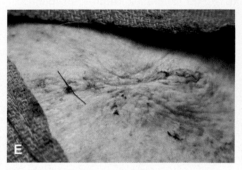

Figure 5-2E. Final appearance after suture placement. Note that the wound edges are now of equal depth.

Tips and Pearls

This suture technique is very useful for correcting depth disparities between the two sides of a wound. This may be helpful as it is often far easier to fine-tune depth disparities by adding this suturing technique than it is to remove a less than ideally placed deeper suture.

The depth-correcting simple interrupted suture may be used layered over the top of another suture in order to fine-tune the depth of epidermal approximation. For example, if a vertical mattress suture were placed to facilitate eversion, occasionally the wound edges remain at slightly different depths. A small depth-correcting simple interrupted suture, placed at the point where the wound edges are most unequal, may be used to solve this problem and effect accurate approximation of the wound edges. A variant of this approach, the leveling suture (see Chapter 5.3), can be used to adjust the depth of a defect when it is left open to heal secondarily.

This technique may also be used in the context of a simple running suture technique, as it can be placed over the top of the simple running sutures to equalize the depth or can be incorporated into the running sutures themselves so that interspersed between traditional simple running bites (entering and exiting lateral to the wound at 90 degrees) some depth-correcting bites are taken as well to equalize the relative depths of the epidermis on either side of the wound. This allows the surgeon to minimize the number of ties necessary, although it should only be used when the wound is under minimal tension, since the security of the depth-correcting bite may be compromised by an increase in laxity across the wound surface over time and the unpredictability of suture material stretch.

Drawbacks and Cautions

This technique can be very useful in correcting slight imperfections in the equality of the depth of wound edges. Ideally, however, this technique should be employed infrequently because, as long as the deeper sutures are placed accurately

and appropriately, it should only rarely be necessary.

Therefore, caution should be exercised to avoid utilizing this technique as a crutch; as long as the surgeon appreciates that the use of this approach should be the exception, rather than the rule, it is acceptable, but it should not be utilized in lieu of attention to detail and precise placement of deeper sutures.

Some anatomic locations, however, may intrinsically present the surgeon with areas of differential dermal thickness, in which case, unless the dermal sutures were placed differentially, depth-correcting simple interrupted sutures may be needed. This includes areas such as the nasal sidewall, the cheek-eyelid junction, and nasofacial sulcus, as well as other skinfold areas.

Finally, caution should be exercised to avoid oversewing areas with the goal of correcting slight imbalances in epidermal depth. While one or two depth-correcting sutures may be necessary, moderation is key as each suture introduces additional foreign-body material and has the potential to induce an inflammatory response.

Reference

Moy RL, Waldman B, Hein DW. A review of sutures and suturing techniques. *J Dermatol Surg Oncol.* 1992;18(9):785-795.

The Leveling Suture

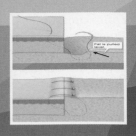

Video 5-3. Leveling suture
Access to video can be found via
mhprofessional.com/atlasofsuturingtechniques2e

Application

This technique is used to reduce the step-off between the wound edge and an area that is left open to granulate. It is a niche technique used, for example, when repairing a defect that involves the thin lower eyelid skin, where it is sometimes beneficial to allow granulation to occur while also minimizing the step-off between cheek skin and the granulated area.

Suture Choice

Since this technique is used to fine-tune the relationship between the epidermal edge and an area that will heal secondarily, it is not designed to hold a significant amount of tension, and a 5-0 or 6-0 fast-absorbing suture is often appropriate.

Technique

1. The needle is inserted perpendicular to the epidermis, approximately one-half the radius of the needle distant from the wound edge.
2. A shallow bite is taken, with the needle skimming the dermal-epidermal junction and exiting in the center of the wound.
3. The needle body is grasped with surgical forceps in the left hand and pulled medially with the surgical forceps as the body of the needle is released from the needle driver.

4. The needle is reloaded on the needle driver, and the needle is inserted into the open portion of the defect directly adjacent to the epidermal edge, and a small bite of the deep portion of the wound is taken.
5. The suture material is then tied off gently, with care being taken to minimize tension across the epidermis and avoid any pull on free margins such as the eyelid (Figures 5-3A through 5-3E).

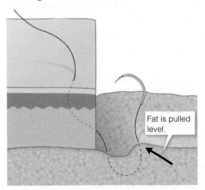

Fat is pulled level.

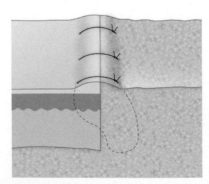

Figure 5-3A. Overview of the leveling suture technique.

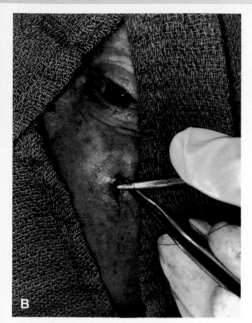

Figure 5-3B. First throw of the leveling suture technique. The needle passes superficially through the epidermis.

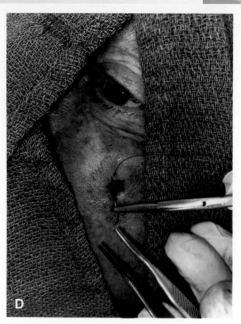

Figure 5-3D. The needle is reloaded.

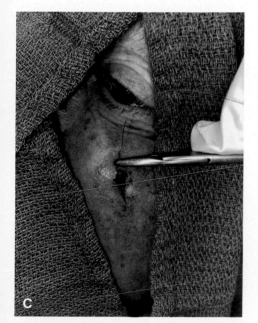

Figure 5-3C. The needle exits in the center of the wound.

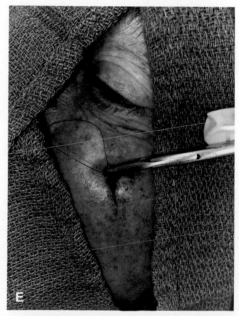

Figure 5-3E. The needle is inserted into the open portion of the wound.

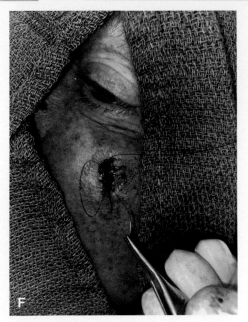

Figure 5-3F. The needle exits the deep portion of the wound and is regrasped.

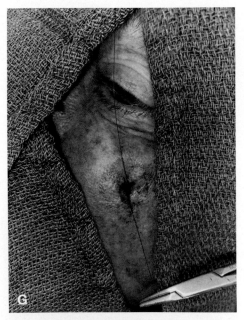

Figure 5-3G. The suture is tied with an instrument tie. Note that there is reduced discrepancy between the depth of the defect and the epidermal edge.

Tips and Pearls

This suture technique is useful when repairing defects that arise from tumors that bridge the thin skin of the lower eyelid and the thicker skin of the cheek. In such cases, either linear repairs or advancement flaps (including island pedicle flaps) may be performed, but the repairs should not, ideally, bridge the boundary between the infraorbital and maxillary cheek. Therefore, it may be best to allow a small portion of the defect on the infraorbital cheek/lower eyelid skin to heal secondarily, while also obviating an overly dramatic step-off between the repaired area and the area permitted to heal secondarily.

This approach may also be useful when performing any closure that heals in part secondarily, since it may result in faster healing times and less risk of scarring or contraction. A series of leveling sutures can be placed (and the technique can also be used in a running fashion) circumferentially around a defect, as long as the bulk of the repair has already been fixed in place, ensuring that there is no tension across the free margin.

Drawbacks and Cautions

This is a niche technique that is generally used when an area is left to heal secondarily. Caution should be exercised to avoid oversewing areas with the goal of correcting slight imbalances and reducing the step-off between the epidermal edge and the bed of a granulating wound, since even deep wounds will often heal without the assistance of leveling sutures. Indeed, overuse of leveling sutures could theoretically introduce added foreign-body material to a wound and induce an inflammatory response that could ultimately result in slower healing.

Reference

Davis JC, Tsai S, Bordeaux JS. Modified V-Y advancement flap with "directed" granulation and leveling sutures for defects of the lid-cheek junction. *Dermatol Surg.* 2017;43(10):1298-1300.

The Simple Running Suture

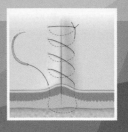

Application

This is the standard running suture used for epidermal approximation. It may be used alone in the context of small wounds under minimal to no tension, such as those formed by a traumatic laceration. It is generally used as a secondary layer to aid in the approximation of the epidermis when the dermis has been closed using a dermal or other deep suturing technique.

Suture Material Choice

With all techniques, it is best to use the thinnest suture possible in order to minimize the risk of track marks and foreign-body reactions. Suture choice will depend largely on anatomic location and the goal of suture placement. Simple running sutures may be placed with the goal of (1) accomplishing epidermal approximation in a wound under mild to moderate tension, such as a laceration, or, more frequently, (2) fine-tuning the epidermal approximation of a wound where the tension has already been shifted deep utilizing a deeper dermal or fascial suturing technique.

On the face and eyelids, a 6-0 or 7-0 monofilament suture is useful for epidermal approximation. When the goal of the simple running suture layer is solely epidermal approximation, 6-0 monofilament

may be used on the extremities as well. Otherwise, 5-0 monofilament suture material may be used if there is minimal tension, and 4-0 monofilament suture may be utilized in areas under moderate tension where the goal of suture placement is relieving tension as well as epidermal approximation.

Technique

1. The needle is inserted perpendicular to the epidermis, approximately one-half the radius of the needle distant to the wound edge. This will allow the needle to exit the wound on the contralateral side at an equal distance from the wound edge by simply following the curvature of the needle.
2. With a fluid motion of the wrist, the needle is rotated through the dermis, taking the bite wider at the deep margin than at the surface, and the needle tip exits the skin on the contralateral side.
3. The needle body is grasped with surgical forceps in the left hand, with care being taken to avoid grasping the needle tip, which can be easily dulled by repetitive friction against the surgical forceps. It is gently grasped and pulled upward with the surgical forceps as the body of the needle is released from the needle driver. Alternatively, the needle may be released from the needle driver and the needle driver itself may be used to grasp the needle from the contralateral side of

the wound to complete its rotation through its arc, obviating the need for surgical forceps.

4. The suture material is then tied off gently, with care being taken to minimize tension across the epidermis and avoid overly constricting the wound edges. This forms the first anchoring knot for the running line of sutures. The loose tail is trimmed, and the needle is reloaded.

5. Starting proximal to the prior knot relative to the surgeon, steps (1) through (3) are then repeated.

6. Instead of tying a knot, steps (1) through (3) are then sequentially repeated until the end of the wound is reached.

7. For the final throw at the inferior apex of the wound, the needle is loaded with a backhand technique and inserted into the skin at a 90-degree angle in a mirror image of the other throws, entering just proximal to the exit point relative to the surgeon on the same side of the incision line and exiting on the contralateral side.

8. The suture material is only partly pulled through, leaving a loop of suture material on the side of the incision opposite to the needle.

9. The suture material is then tied to the loop using an instrument tie (Figures 5-4A through 5-4I).

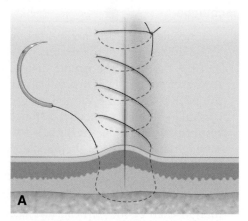

Figure 5-4A. Overview of the simple running suture technique.

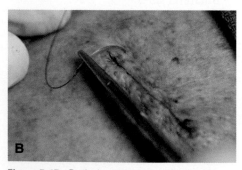

Figure 5-4B. Beginning of the first anchoring throw of the simple running suture technique. Note that the needle enters the skin at 90 degrees prior to moving laterally away from the wound edge.

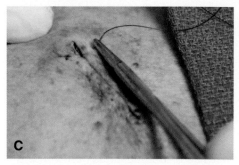

Figure 5-4C. Completion of the first anchoring throw of suture. Note that the needle has taken a wide bite of dermis.

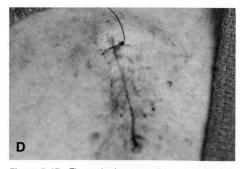

Figure 5-4D. The anchoring suture has now been tied off.

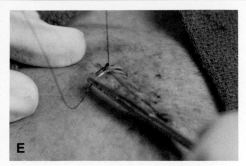

Figure 5-4E. The running portion of the suture commences. Note again that needle entry is at 90 degrees.

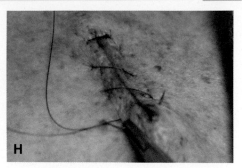

Figure 5-4H. The final throw is performed with a backhand technique.

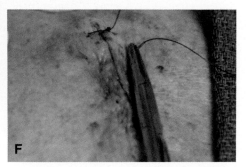

Figure 5-4F. Completion of the first running suture. Note that the needle exits again at 90 degrees.

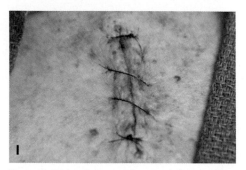

Figure 5-4I. Appearance of the wound after a series of simple running sutures.

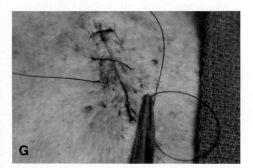

Figure 5-4G. Subsequent throws continue in a similar pattern.

Tips and Pearls

As with the simple interrupted suture, it is important to enter the epidermis at 90 degrees, allowing the needle to travel slightly laterally away from the wound edge before fully following the curvature of the needle when utilizing this technique. This will allow for maximal wound eversion and accurate wound-edge approximation.

The simple running suture is generally used layered over the top of another suture in order to fine-tune epidermal approximation. For example, if set-back dermal sutures were placed to facilitate eversion, occasionally the wound edges may not be fully approximated. A layer of simple running sutures may be used to solve this problem and effect accurate approximation of the wound edges.

Care should be taken to avoid skimming the needle superficially beneath the epidermis. This results from failing to enter the skin at a perpendicular angle and failing to follow the curvature of the needle. This may result in wound inversion as the tension vector of the shallow bite pulls the wound edges outward and down.

In order to maintain uniformity in the length of the visible running sutures and to allow the suture loops to remain parallel, it is important to take uniform bites with each throw of the simple running suture technique. Therefore, each subsequent loop should begin at the same point lateral to the incised wound edge and at a uniform distance closer to the surgeon than the preceding entry point.

Some surgeons prefer to finesse their running closures so that the loops of suture appear to run perpendicular to the incision line. This approach, however, requires that each loop of running suture be placed at a uniform angle across the incised wound edge, rather than perpendicular to the incised wound edge. Since this affects the force vectors across the wound and since a row of parallel diagonally oriented sutures is also aesthetically pleasing, this approach is a reasonable option but is not necessary.

It is critical to permit sufficient laxity between the epidermis and the suture material when using this technique in order to minimize the risk of track marks or an exaggerated inflammatory response. Recalling that this technique is designed exclusively for epidermal approximation and that some postoperative wound edema is expected will help with conceptualizing the need to keep the throws of suture material loose.

Drawbacks and Cautions

The central drawback of this approach is that, as with all running techniques, the integrity of the entire suture line rests on two knots. Moreover, suture material compromise at any point may lead to a complete loss of the integrity of the line of sutures. Since this technique is

designed for low-tension environments, however, even in the face of suture material breakage, the remaining throws of suture may permit some residual epidermal approximation.

Since all loops of suture are placed in succession, this technique does not permit the same degree of fine-tuning of the epidermal approximation as a simple interrupted suture. This must be weighed against the benefit of the increased speed of placement of a line of running sutures versus interrupted suture placement, where each throw is secured with its own set of three or more knots.

Moreover, since each loop of the running suture material is designed to hold an equal amount of tension, it follows that areas of the wound under greater tension, such as its central portion, may tend to gape or potentially exist under greater tension, leading to an increased risk of track marks.

With any suturing technique, knowledge of the relevant anatomy is critical. When placing simple running sutures, it is important to recall that the structures deep to the epidermis may be compromised by the passage of the needle and suture material. For example, the needle may pierce a vessel, leading to increased bleeding.

Similarly, particularly if the knot is tied relatively tightly, structures deep to the defect may be constricted. This can lead to necrosis due to vascular compromise or even, theoretically, superficial nerve damage; again, this risk may be mitigated by maintaining some laxity in the suture throws.

This technique may elicit an increased risk of track marks, necrosis, inflammation, and other complications when compared with techniques that do not entail suture material traversing the scar line, such as buried or subcuticular approaches.

Therefore, sutures should be removed as early as possible to minimize these complications, and consideration should be given to adopting other closure techniques in the event that sutures will not be able to be removed in a timely fashion.

References

Adams B, Levy R, Rademaker AE, Goldberg LH, Alam M. Frequency of use of suturing and repair techniques preferred by dermatologic surgeons. *Dermatol Surg*. 2006;32(5):682-689.

Gurusamy KS, Toon CD, Allen VB, Davidson BR. Continuous versus interrupted skin sutures for non-obstetric surgery. *Cochrane Database Syst Rev*. 2014;2:CD010365.

McLean NR, Fyfe AH, Flint EF, Irvine BH, Calvert MH. Comparison of skin closure using continuous and interrupted nylon sutures. *Br J Surg*. 1980;67(9):633-635.

Orozco-Covarrubias ML, Ruiz-Maldonado R. Surgical facial wounds: simple interrupted percutaneous suture versus running intradermal suture. *Dermatol Surg*. 1999;25(2):109-112.

Pauniaho SL, Lahdes-Vasama T, Helminen MT, et al. Non-absorbable interrupted versus absorbable continuous skin closure in pediatric appendectomies. *Scand J Surg*. 2010;99(3):142-146.

The Running Locking Suture

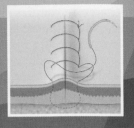

Video 5-5. Running locking suture

Access to video can be found via mhprofessional.com/atlasofsuturingtechniques2e

Application

This is a locking variation of the standard running suture used for epidermal approximation. It may be used alone in the context of small wounds under minimal to no tension, such as those formed by a traumatic laceration. It is generally used as a secondary layer to aid in the approximation of the epidermis when the dermis has been closed using a dermal or other deep suturing technique.

It is used for three central reasons: (1) to aid in hemostasis, (2) to provide improved eversion over the standard running suture, and (3) to provide equal tension across all loops of the running suture.

Suture Material Choice

With all techniques, it is best to use the thinnest suture possible in order to minimize the risk of track marks and foreign-body reactions. Suture choice will depend largely on anatomic location and the goal of suture placement. On the face and eyelids, a 6-0 or 7-0 monofilament suture is useful for epidermal approximation. When the goal of the running locking suture layer is solely epidermal approximation, 6-0 monofilament may be used on the extremities as well. Otherwise, 5-0 monofilament suture material may be used if there is minimal tension,

and 4-0 monofilament suture is useful in areas under moderate tension where the goal of suture placement is relieving tension or hemostasis as well as epidermal approximation.

Technique

1. The needle is inserted perpendicular to the epidermis, approximately one-half the radius of the needle distant to the wound edge. This will allow the needle to exit the wound on the contralateral side at an equal distance from the wound edge by simply following the curvature of the needle.

2. With a fluid motion of the wrist, the needle is rotated through the dermis, taking the bite wider at the deep margin than at the surface, and the needle tip exits the skin on the contralateral side.

3. The needle body is grasped with surgical forceps in the left hand and pulled upward with the surgical forceps as the body of the needle is released from the needle driver. Alternatively, the needle may be released from the needle driver and the needle driver itself may be used to grasp the needle from the contralateral side of the wound to complete its rotation through its arc, obviating the need for surgical forceps.

4. The suture material is then tied off gently, with care being taken to minimize tension across the epidermis and avoid overly constricting the

wound edges. This forms the first anchoring knot for the running line of sutures. The loose tail is trimmed, and the needle is reloaded.

5. Starting proximal to the prior knot relative to the surgeon, steps (1) through (3) are then repeated, but rather than pulling all of the suture material through after completing the throw, a loop of suture is left from the beginning of the throw, and the needle is then passed through the loop of suture, locking the suture in place.

6. Instead of tying a knot, step (5) is then sequentially repeated until the end of the wound is reached.

7. For the final throw at the inferior apex of the wound, the needle is loaded with a backhand technique and inserted into the skin at a 90-degree angle in a mirror image of the other throws, entering just proximal to the exit point relative to the surgeon on the same side of the incision line and exiting on the contralateral side.

8. The suture material is only partly pulled through, leaving a loop of suture material on the side of the incision opposite to the needle.

9. The suture material is then tied to the loop using an instrument tie (Figures 5-5A through 5-5L).

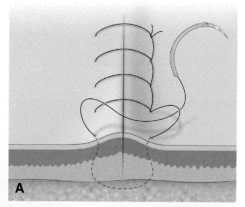

Figure 5-5A. Overview of the running locking suture technique.

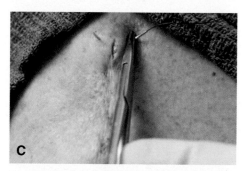

Figure 5-5C. Completed first anchoring throw of the running locking suture technique. This is essentially a simple interrupted suture used for anchoring the set of running sutures.

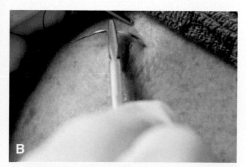

Figure 5-5B. Beginning of the first throw of the running locking suture technique. Note the needle enters the skin at 90 degrees.

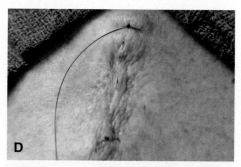

Figure 5-5D. Knot tied after placing the anchoring suture.

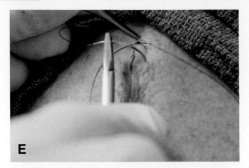

Figure 5-5E. Beginning of running suture placement.

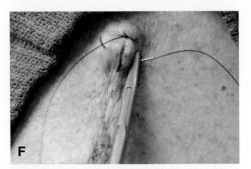

Figure 5-5F. Completion of first running throw.

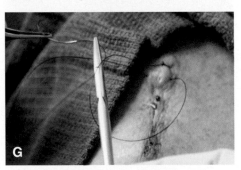

Figure 5-5G. Locking the suture. Note the needle driver is inserted through the loop of suture created by the prior throw before grasping the needle, permitting the locking effect of this technique.

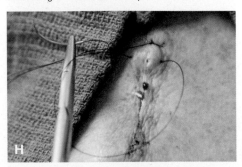

Figure 5-5H. The needle is grasped.

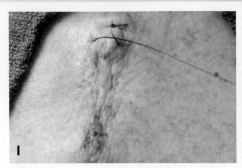

Figure 5-5I. The suture and needle are pulled laterally, locking the suture.

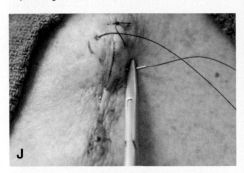

Figure 5-5J. The running technique continues.

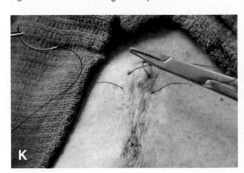

Figure 5-5K. The suture is locked with each successive throw.

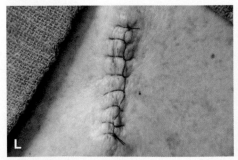

Figure 5-5L. Appearance of the completed running locking suture.

Tips and Pearls

The running locking technique permits better hemostasis than the standard simple running technique, and therefore, it is sometimes used with traumatic lacerations (when a small amount of oozing may be present) or as a secondary layer in repairs on patients who are on aspirin or otherwise may have a small amount of oozing even after placement of deeper sutures. Importantly, the hemostatic effect of the locking should not be used as a replacement for properly tying off deeper vessels or cauterizing small vessels.

This technique also affords improved eversion over the standard simple running suture approach, since the locked edges of suture have an almost horizontal mattress-like effect on the epidermis, leading sometimes to the formation of a ridge along the wound.

Standard simple running sutures may lead to gaping at the central portions of the wound, since the equal tension across each loop in the context of unequal lateral forces over the course of the length of the wound means that the areas under greatest tension—those in the central wound—may pull laterally while areas under only minimal tension at the apices do not exert a similar effect. This tendency is obviated with the running locking technique, as the amount of tension across each loop of suture is individually controlled.

An assistant may be helpful in keeping each of the loops under a small degree of tension before the needle and suture material are passed through the loops. This helps with maintaining a uniform degree of tension across the loops of suture and aids in permitting each throw of suture to be easily locked.

As with the simple running suture, it is important to enter the epidermis at 90 degrees, allowing the needle to travel slightly laterally away from the wound edge before fully following the curvature of the needle when utilizing this technique. This will allow for maximal wound eversion and accurate wound-edge approximation.

Care should be taken to avoid skimming the needle superficially beneath the epidermis. This results from failing to enter the skin at a perpendicular angle and following the curvature of the needle. This may result in wound inversion as the tension vector of the shallow bite pulls the wound edges outward and down.

In order to maintain uniformity in the length of the visible running sutures and to allow all of the suture loops to remain parallel, it is important to take uniform bites with each throw of the running locking suture technique. Therefore, each subsequent loop should begin at the same point lateral to the incised wound edge and at a uniform distance closer to the surgeon than the preceding entry point.

As with the simple running technique, it is critical to permit sufficient laxity between the epidermis and the suture material when using this technique in order to minimize the risk of track marks or an exaggerated inflammatory response. Recalling that this technique is designed exclusively for epidermal approximation and that some postoperative wound edema is expected will help with conceptualizing the need to keep the throws of suture material loose.

Drawbacks and Cautions

The central drawback of this approach is that, as with all running techniques, the integrity of the entire suture line rests on two knots. Moreover, suture material compromise at any point may lead to a complete loss of the integrity of the line of sutures. Since this technique is designed for low-tension environments, however, and the locked loops of suture may hold in place due to pressure from the skin against the suture, this problem is less pronounced with this technique than with many other running approaches.

In order to avoid wound-edge necrosis, it is important not to be overzealous with tightening the locking loops of suture. While it may be tempting to pull each loop tight to maximize the hemostatic effect of this approach, this should be avoided. This is particularly important as postoperative edema may lead the sutures to be even tighter after time has passed, increasing the risk of tissue strangulation.

Since all loops of suture are placed in succession, this technique does not permit the same degree of fine-tuning of epidermal approximation as a simple interrupted suture. This must be weighed against the benefit of the increased speed of placement of a line of running locking sutures versus interrupted suture placement, where each throw is secured with its own set of three or more knots.

While this technique may help minimize some of the potential risk of track marks associated with running techniques—the differential pull across different areas of the wound—overly tight throws may actually increase this risk, since the locked loops lead to a secondary row of suture material running parallel to the incision line.

With any suturing technique, knowledge of the relevant anatomy is critical. When placing running locking sutures, it is important to recall that the structures

deep to the epidermis may be compromised by the passage of the needle and suture material.

Similarly, particularly if the throws are locked relatively tightly, structures deep to the defect may be constricted. This can lead to necrosis due to vascular compromise or even, theoretically, superficial nerve damage; again, this risk may be mitigated by maintaining some laxity in the locked suture throws.

This technique may elicit an increased risk of track marks, necrosis, inflammation, and other complications when compared with techniques that do not entail suture material traversing the scar line, such as buried or subcuticular approaches. Therefore, sutures should be removed as early as possible to minimize these complications, and consideration should be given to adopting other closure techniques in the event that sutures will not be able to be removed in a timely fashion.

References

Joshi AS, Janjanin S, Tanna N, Geist C, Lindsey WH. Does suture material and technique really matter? Lessons learned from 800 consecutive blepharoplasties. *Laryngoscope.* 2007;117(6):981-984.

MacDougal BA. Locking a continuous running suture. *J Am Coll Surg.* 1995;181(6):563-564.

Schlechter B, Guyuron B. A comparison of different suture techniques for microvascular anastomosis. *Ann Plast Surg.* 1994;33(1):28-31.

Wong NL. The running locked intradermal suture. A cosmetically elegant continuous suture for wounds under light tension. *J Dermatol Surg Oncol.* 1993;19(1):30-36.

The Horizontal Mattress Suture

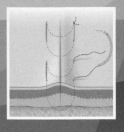

 Video 5-6. Horizontal mattress suture
Access to video can be found via
mhprofessional.com/atlasofsuturingtechniques2e

Application

This is a frequently used everting technique employed for closure and epidermal approximation. As with many interrupted techniques, it may be used alone for wounds under minimal tension, such as those formed by either a small punch biopsy or a traumatic laceration. It is also frequently used as a secondary layer to aid in everting the wound edges when the dermis has been closed using a deep suturing technique. This technique may also be used in the context of atrophic skin, as the broader anchoring bites may help limit tissue tear-through that may be seen with a simple interrupted suture.

Suture Material Choice

With all techniques, it is best to use the thinnest suture possible in order to minimize the risk of track marks and foreign-body reactions. Suture choice will depend largely on anatomic location and the goal of suture placement. Horizontal mattress sutures may be placed with the goal of (1) effecting eversion or (2) adding an additional layer of closure for wound stability and dead-space minimization.

On the face and eyelids, a 6-0 or 7-0 monofilament suture may be used, though fast-absorbing gut may be used on the eyelids and ears to obviate the

need for suture removal. When the goal of the horizontal mattress suture placement is solely to encourage wound-edge eversion, fine-gauge suture material may be used on the extremities as well. Otherwise, 5-0 monofilament suture material is useful if there is minimal tension, and 4-0 monofilament suture may be used in areas under moderate tension where the goal of suture placement is relieving tension as well as epidermal approximation. In select high-tension areas, 3-0 monofilament suture may be utilized as well, sometimes in the context of a multimodality approach, for example, when mattress sutures are placed in the center of the wound to maximize tension relief and eversion and to obviate any dead space beneath a large wound.

Technique

1. The needle is inserted perpendicular to the epidermis, approximately one-half the radius of the needle distant to the wound edge. This will allow the needle to exit the wound on the contralateral side at an equal distance from the wound edge by simply following the curvature of the needle.

2. With a fluid motion of the wrist, the needle is rotated through the dermis, taking the bite wider at the deep margin than at the surface, and the needle tip exits the skin on the contralateral side.

3. The needle body is grasped with surgical forceps in the left hand and

217

pulled upward as the body of the needle is released from the needle driver. Alternatively, the needle may be released from the needle driver, and the needle driver itself may be used to grasp the needle from the contralateral side of the wound to complete its rotation through its arc, obviating the need for surgical forceps.

4. The needle is then reloaded in a backhand fashion and inserted at 90 degrees perpendicular to the epidermis proximal (relative to the surgeon)

to its exit point along the length of the wound on the same side of the incision line as the exit point.

5. The needle is rotated through its arc, exiting on the right side of the wound (relative to the surgeon) in a mirror image of steps (2) and (3).

6. The suture material is then tied off gently, with care being taken to minimize tension across the epidermis and avoid overly constricting the wound edges (Figures 5-6A through 5-6F).

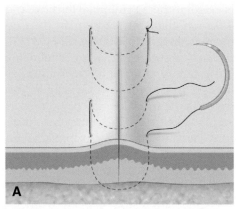

Figure 5-6A. Overview of the horizontal mattress suture technique.

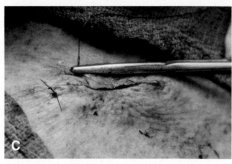

Figure 5-6C. Completion of the first throw of the horizontal mattress suture technique. Note that the needle now exits the skin on the contralateral wound edge at a 90-degree angle.

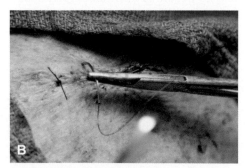

Figure 5-6B. Beginning of the first throw of the horizontal mattress suture technique. Note that the needle enters the skin at a 90-degree angle.

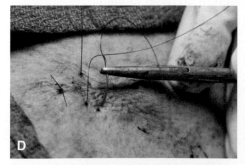

Figure 5-6D. Beginning of the second throw of the horizontal mattress suture technique. Note that the needle again enters the skin at a 90-degree angle, now distal to its exit point.

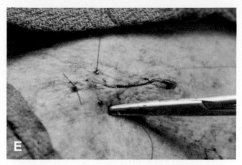

Figure 5-6E. Completion of the second throw of the horizontal mattress suture technique. Note that the needle again exits the skin on the contralateral wound edge at a 90-degree angle.

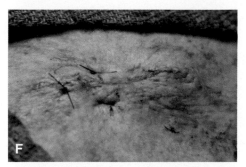

Figure 5-6F. Wound appearance after placement of a horizontal mattress suture. Note the pronounced eversion of the wound edges.

Tips and Pearls

It is important to enter the epidermis at 90 degrees, allowing the needle to travel slightly laterally away from the wound edge before fully following the curvature of the needle when utilizing this technique. This will allow for maximal wound eversion and accurate wound-edge approximation.

As with the simple interrupted suture, care should be taken to avoid skimming the needle superficially beneath the epidermis. This results from failing to enter the skin at a perpendicular angle and failing to follow the curvature of the needle. This may result in wound inversion as the tension vector of the shallow bite pulls the wound edges outward and down.

Since a wide bite of dermis and epidermis is included in the suture arc, it is particularly important to avoid tying the suture material too tight, as this could lead to wound-edge necrosis. Some surgeons utilize bolsters when utilizing this technique under high tension, such as when a 3-0 suture is used on the back, in an attempt to avoid track marks and reduce the risk of tissue necrosis. A wide array of materials may be used for the bolster, including gauze, dental rolls, or plastic tubing. In practice, bolsters are rarely needed with this technique as long as the bulk of the wound tension has been shifted deep using fascial or dermal buried sutures.

The placement of a horizontal mattress suture can sometimes lead to what has been termed the sandwich phenomenon, where the tight dermal wound approximation leads to hypereversion of the wound edges and to a raised ridge with epidermal gaping at the center of the wound. If this occurs, placing a simple interrupted suture (see Chapter 5.1) directly over the offending horizontal mattress suture can solve this problem.

Drawbacks and Cautions

This technique does not typically permit the same degree of wound-edge apposition as can be accomplished with other transepidermal sutures, since the everting effect of the suture technique may be associated with a small degree of gaping at the center of the horizontal mattress suture. In the event that deeper sutures were carefully placed, this may not be a significant drawback, since the wound edges may be well aligned from the placement of these deeper sutures. If not, or if there is a need for improved wound-edge apposition even after placing the horizontal mattress suture, a small simple interrupted suture may be placed centrally over the horizontal mattress suture to bring the wound edges together more precisely.

Suture removal with this technique may be more involved than with simple interrupted sutures, particularly if sutures are left in situ for an extended period of time and some of the suture material has been overgrown by the healing epidermis, as the knot may be somewhat buried in the context of a ridged everted repair.

With any suturing technique, knowledge of the relevant anatomy is critical. When placing a horizontal mattress suture, it is important to recall that the structures deep to the epidermis may be compromised by the passage of the needle and suture material. For example, the needle may pierce a vessel, leading to increased bleeding.

Similarly, particularly if the knot is tied relatively tightly, structures deep to the defect may be constricted. This can lead to necrosis due to vascular compromise or even, theoretically, superficial nerve damage. These concerns are more acute with the horizontal mattress suture than with the simple interrupted suture, since the wide arc of the suture material and its horizontal component incorporate more skin and underlying structures, thus increasing the risk of strangulation.

The potential to constrict deeper structures may be used to the surgeon's advantage in the event that a small vessel deep to the incision line is oozing; rather than opening the wound, localizing the source of the bleed, and tying off the individual vessel, it may be possible to simply place a horizontal mattress suture incorporating the culprit vessel within its arc, tie it tightly, and thus indirectly ligate the vessel. This should only be used in the event that the offending vessel is relatively small, since otherwise, there is a significant risk that this indirect ligation will not be sufficiently resilient. Moreover, tying the suture too tightly may increase the risk of developing track marks or superficial necrosis.

This technique may elicit an increased risk of track marks, necrosis, and other complications when compared with techniques that do not entail suture material traversing the scar line, such as buried or subcuticular approaches. Therefore, sutures should be removed as early as possible to minimize these complications, and consideration should be given to adopting other closure techniques in the event that sutures will not be able to be removed in a timely fashion.

References

Blattner CM, Markus B, Lear W. Correction of "sandwiching phenomenon" following horizontal mattress suture. *J Am Acad Dermatol.* 2018;78(4):e87-88.

Zuber TJ. The mattress sutures: vertical, horizontal, and corner stitch. *Am Fam Physician.* 2002;66(12):2231-2236.

The Locking Horizontal Mattress Suture

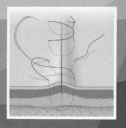

Synonym

Modified locking horizontal mattress

Video 5-7. Locking horizontal mattress suture
Access to video can be found via
mhprofessional.com/atlasofsuturingtechniques2e

Application

This is a modification of the horizontal mattress suture. As with many interrupted techniques, it may be used alone for wounds under minimal tension, such as those formed by a small punch biopsy or a traumatic laceration. It is also frequently used as a secondary layer to aid in everting the wound edges when the dermis has been closed using a deep suturing technique. This technique may also be used in the context of atrophic skin, as the broader anchoring bites may help limit the tissue tear-through that may be seen with a simple interrupted suture. This locking variation confers two advantages over the traditional horizontal mattress suture: better ease of suture removal and improved wound-edge apposition.

Suture Material Choice

With all techniques, it is best to use the thinnest suture possible in order to minimize the risk of track marks and foreign-body reactions. Suture choice will depend largely on anatomic location and the goal of suture placement. Locking horizontal mattress sutures may be placed with the goal of (1) effecting eversion or (2) adding an additional layer of closure for wound stability and dead-space minimization.

On the face, a 6-0 or 7-0 monofilament suture may be used, though fast-absorbing gut may be used on the eyelids and ears to obviate the need for suture removal; in these cases, standard horizontal mattress sutures are probably preferable to their locking counterparts. When the goal of the horizontal mattress suture placement is solely to encourage wound-edge eversion, fine-gauge suture material may be used on the extremities as well. Otherwise, 5-0 monofilament suture material is useful if there is minimal tension, and 4-0 monofilament suture may be used in areas under moderate tension where the goal of suture placement is relieving tension as well as epidermal approximation. In select high-tension areas, 3-0 monofilament suture may be utilized as well.

Technique

1. The needle is inserted perpendicular to the epidermis, approximately one-half the radius of the needle distant to the wound edge. This will allow the needle to exit the wound on the contralateral side at an equal distance from the wound edge by simply following the curvature of the needle.
2. With a fluid motion of the wrist, the needle is rotated through the dermis, taking the bite wider at the deep margin than at the surface, and the needle tip exits the skin on the contralateral side.

3. The needle body is grasped with surgical forceps in the left hand, with care being taken to avoid grasping the needle tip, which can be easily dulled by repetitive friction against the surgical forceps. It is gently grasped and pulled upward with the surgical forceps as the body of the needle is released from the needle driver. Alternatively, the needle may be released from the needle driver, and the needle driver itself may be used to grasp the needle from the contralateral side of the wound to complete its rotation through its arc, obviating the need for surgical forceps.

4. The needle is then reloaded in a backhand fashion and inserted at 90-degrees perpendicular to the epidermis proximal (relative to the surgeon) to its exit point on the same side of the incision line as the exit point. Importantly, a loop of suture material is left protruding from the wound from where the needle exited on the prior throw to where it enters on this throw.

5. The needle is rotated through its arc, exiting on the right side of the wound (relative to the surgeon) in a mirror image of steps (2) and (3).

6. The needle is then passed under the loop of suture material on the contralateral side.

7. The suture material is then tied off gently, with care being taken to minimize tension across the epidermis and avoid overly constricting the wound edges (Figures 5-7A through 5-7F).

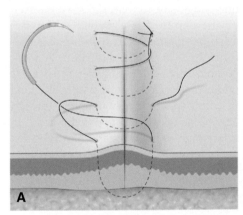

Figure 5-7A. Overview of the locking horizontal mattress suture.

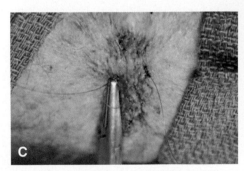

Figure 5-7C. The needle is then reinserted from the same side as the entry point, slightly further along the wound edge, exiting back on the side where the suture began.

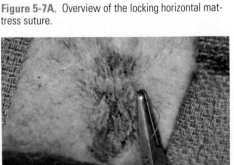

Figure 5-7B. The needle is inserted perpendicular to the skin, exiting on the contralateral side of the wound edge.

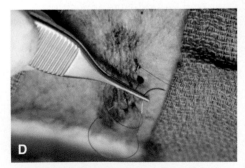

Figure 5-7D. The needle is then passed under the newly formed loop.

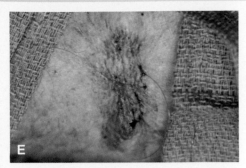

Figure 5-7E. This has the effect of locking the suture material under the loop.

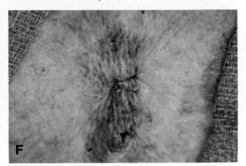

Figure 5-7F. Immediate postoperative appearance.

Tips and Pearls

The locking technique confers two important advantages over the traditional horizontal mattress suture. First, the standard horizontal mattress suture does not typically permit the same degree of wound-edge apposition as can be accomplished with other transepidermal sutures, since the everting effect of the suture technique may be associated with a small degree of gaping at the center of the horizontal mattress suture. Locking the suture material brings the knot, as well as the two parallel external rows of suture, to the center of the wound, thus improving wound-edge approximation.

Second, suture removal with the standard horizontal mattress technique may be challenging, particularly if sutures are left in situ for an extended period of time and some of the suture material has been overgrown by the healing epidermis, as the knot may be buried in the context of a ridged everted repair. Bringing the knot, along with the parallel rows of external suture material, centrally with the locking technique allows the knot to be more easily grasped at the time of suture removal.

A modification of this technique has also been described, where instead of passing the needle under the loop of suture, the loop is instead incorporated into the knot, thus increasing economy of motion. For this modification, a loop is left as described previously, and all steps are followed through step (5). Then, the end of the suture with the needle attached is looped twice around the needle driver, and the tip of the needle driver is passed through the loop to grasp the tail of the suture. Once the suture tail is pulled, the horizontal mattress suture becomes locked.

As with most transepidermal techniques, it is important to enter the epidermis at 90 degrees, allowing the needle to travel slightly laterally away from the wound edge before fully following the curvature of the needle when utilizing this technique. This will allow for maximal wound eversion and accurate wound-edge approximation.

As with the simple interrupted suture, care should be taken to avoid skimming the needle superficially beneath the epidermis. This results from failing to enter the skin at a perpendicular angle and failing to follow the curvature of the needle. This may result in wound inversion as the tension vector of the shallow bite pulls the wound edges outward and down.

Drawbacks and Cautions

With any suturing technique, knowledge of the relevant anatomy is critical. When placing a locking horizontal mattress suture, it is important to recall that the structures deep to the epidermis may be compromised by the passage of the needle and suture material. For example, the needle may pierce a vessel, leading to increased bleeding.

Similarly, particularly if the knot is tied relatively tightly, structures deep to the defect may be constricted. This can lead to necrosis due to vascular compromise or even, theoretically, superficial nerve damage. These concerns are more acute with the locking horizontal mattress suture than with the simple interrupted suture, since the wide arc of the suture material and its horizontal component incorporate more skin and underlying structures, thus increasing the risk of strangulation.

The potential to constrict deeper structures may be used to the surgeon's advantage in the event that a small vessel deep to the incision line is oozing; rather than opening the wound, localizing the source of the bleed, and tying off the individual vessel, it may be possible to simply place a locking horizontal mattress suture incorporating the culprit vessel within its arc, tie it tightly, and thus indirectly ligate the vessel. This should only be used in the event that the offending vessel is relatively small, since otherwise there is a significant risk that this indirect ligation will not be sufficiently resilient. Moreover, tying the suture too tightly may increase the risk of developing track marks or superficial necrosis.

This technique may elicit an increased risk of track marks, necrosis, and other complications when compared with techniques that do not entail suture material traversing the scar line, such as buried or subcuticular approaches. Therefore, sutures should be removed as early as possible to minimize these complications, and consideration should be given to adopting other closure techniques in the event that sutures will not be able to be removed in a timely fashion.

References

Hanasono MM, Hotchkiss RN. Locking horizontal mattress suture. *Dermatol Surg.* 2005;31(5):572-573.

Niazi ZB. Two novel and useful suturing techniques. *Plast Reconstr Surg.* 1997;100(6):1617-1618.

Olson J, Berg D. Modified locking horizontal mattress suture. *Dermatol Surg.* 2014;40(1):72-74.

Zuber TJ. The mattress sutures: vertical, horizontal, and corner stitch. *Am Fam Physician.* 2002;66(12):2231-2236.

The Inverting Horizontal Mattress Suture

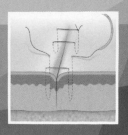

Video 5-8. Inverting horizontal mattress suture
Access to video can be found via
mhprofessional.com/atlasofsuturingtechniques2e

Application

This is a niche technique designed to encourage wound-edge inversion and is useful primarily to recreate a natural crease. It may be used to recreate the alar creases as well as to better define the helical rim and may also be useful when recreating the mental crease.

Suture Material Choice

Using the thinnest suture possible in order to minimize the risk of track marks and foreign-body reactions is wise. Generally, this suture is used on the face and ears, and therefore, a 6-0 or 7-0 monofilament suture may be best, though fast-absorbing gut may be used to obviate the need for suture removal.

Technique

1. The needle is inserted perpendicular to the epidermis in a direction parallel to the incised wound edge, approximately 5 mm from the wound edge. The needle is rotated, following its curvature, through the dermis, exiting proximal relative to the surgeon but still on the ipsilateral side of the incised wound edge.
2. The needle is then reloaded in a backhand fashion and inserted on the contralateral side of the incision

directly across from its exit point, perpendicular to the epidermis and parallel to the incised wound, now facing in the opposite direction. With a fluid motion of the wrist, the needle is rotated through the dermis, and the needle tip exits the skin on the ipsilateral side, across the wound edge from the original insertion point.
3. The suture material is then tied off gently, with care being taken to minimize tension across the epidermis and avoid overly constricting the wound edges (Figures 5-8A through 5-8F).

Tips and Pearls

This approach is very useful when attempting to recreate a natural crease, especially since traditional everting sutures have a tendency to blunt natural creases. Since the eye is naturally drawn to skin folds and creases, this small change may have a dramatic effect on the ultimate outcome of the repair.

Unlike the traditional horizontal mattress, this technique does not result in significant compression of the underlying vascular plexus, and in fact, it results in only modest tension across the wound surface.

A gap remains between the suture material and the incised wound edge, since the inversion of the wound edges causes them to be depressed relative to the surrounding skin. Therefore, track marks are unlikely with this technique.

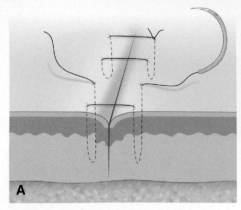

Figure 5-8A. Overview of the inverting horizontal mattress technique.

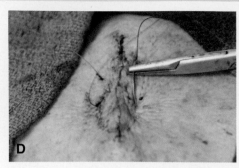

Figure 5-8D. The needle is then inserted lateral to the contralateral wound edge, across from its exit point on the other wound edge, again on a trajectory parallel to the incised wound edge.

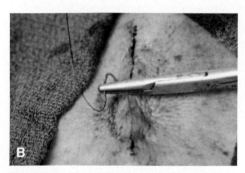

Figure 5-8B. The needle is inserted at 90 degrees, on a trajectory parallel to the wound edge.

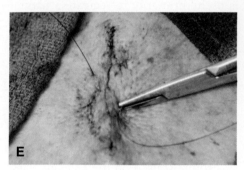

Figure 5-8E. The needle then exits further along its trajectory, directly across from its original insertion point.

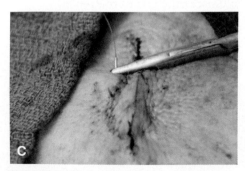

Figure 5-8C. The needle exits further along its trajectory along the wound but the same distance from the wound edge.

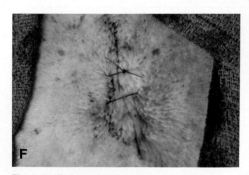

Figure 5-8F. Immediate postoperative appearance.

It is helpful to take the bites of the inverting horizontal mattress suture approximately 5 mm lateral to the incised wound edge, as this leads to a relative lift on the skin lateral to the wound edge, helping to accentuate the desired wound inversion.

Drawbacks and Cautions

This technique may lead to dramatic wound inversion, and therefore, it should only be used when the goal is recreating a natural crease. Moreover, since wound inversion may be associated with inferior cosmesis over the long term, the benefit of accentuated inversion should be weighed against the possibility that the long-term cosmetic outcome of the suture scar may be less than ideal. The overinversion of the wound edges caused by the suturing technique relaxes somewhat after suture removal, allowing the wound edges to meet and heal.

This technique also does not consistently lead to full wound-edge apposition, which is again an important consideration when choosing this approach. Therefore, it is best used when the deep sutures have resulted in acceptable wound-edge approximation.

Reference

Wentzell JM, Lund JJ. The inverting horizontal mattress suture: applications in dermatologic surgery. *Dermatol Surg.* 2012;38(9):1535-1539.

The Running Horizontal Mattress Suture

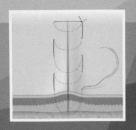

 Video 5-9. Running horizontal mattress suture
Access to video can be found via
mhprofessional.com/atlasofsuturingtechniques2e

Application

This is a frequently used running everting technique employed for closure and epidermal approximation. It is useful, especially on the face, to aid in everting the wound edges when the dermis has been closed using a deep suturing technique. This technique may also be used in patients with atrophic skin, as the broader anchoring bites may help limit tissue tear-through that may be seen with a simple interrupted suture.

Suture Material Choice

With all techniques, it is best to use the thinnest suture possible in order to minimize the risk of track marks and foreign-body reactions. On the face and eyelids, a 6-0 or 7-0 monofilament suture may be used, though fast-absorbing gut may be used on the eyelids and ears to obviate the need for suture removal. Since the goal of the running horizontal mattress suture placement is primarily to encourage wound-edge eversion, fine-gauge suture material may be used on the extremities as well.

Technique

1. The needle is inserted perpendicular to the epidermis, approximately one-half the radius of the needle distant to the wound edge. This will allow the needle to exit the wound on the contralateral side at an equal distance from the wound edge by simply following the curvature of the needle.

2. With a fluid motion of the wrist, the needle is rotated through the dermis, taking the bite wider at the deep margin than at the surface, and the needle tip exits the skin on the contralateral side.

3. The needle body is grasped with surgical forceps in the left hand, with care being taken to avoid grasping the needle tip, which can be easily dulled by repetitive friction against the surgical forceps. It is gently grasped and pulled upward with the surgical forceps as the body of the needle is released from the needle driver. Alternatively, the needle may be released from the needle driver, and the needle driver itself may be used to grasp the needle from the contralateral side of the wound to complete its rotation through its arc, obviating the need for surgical forceps.

4. The suture material is then tied off gently, with care being taken to minimize tension across the epidermis and avoid overly constricting the wound edges.

5. Starting proximal relative to the surgeon, the needle is then reinserted perpendicular to the epidermis,

approximately one-half the radius of the needle distant to the wound edge.

6. With a fluid motion of the wrist, the needle is rotated through the dermis, taking the bite wider at the deep margin than at the surface, and the needle tip exits the skin on the contralateral side.

7. The needle body is grasped with surgical forceps in the left hand and pulled upward with the surgical forceps as the body of the needle is released from the needle driver.

8. The needle is then reloaded in a backhand fashion and inserted at 90 degrees perpendicular to the epidermis proximal (relative to the surgeon) to its exit point on the same side of the incision line as the exit point.

9. The needle is rotated through its arc, exiting on the right side of the wound (relative to the surgeon) in a mirror image of step (6).

10. Moving proximally relative to the surgeon, steps (5) through (9) are then sequentially repeated, until the end of the wound is reached. At that point, a loop is left in the penultimate throw, and the suture material is then tied off gently, with care being taken to minimize tension across the epidermis and avoid overly constricting the wound edges (Figures 5-9A through 5-9H).

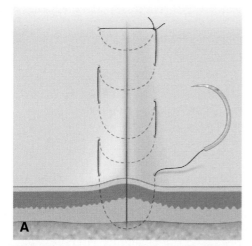

Figure 5-9A. Overview of the running horizontal mattress technique.

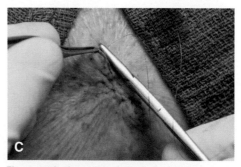

Figure 5-9C. Completion of the first pass of the needle, now exiting at 90 degrees.

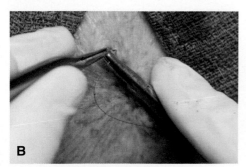

Figure 5-9B. Initiation of the anchoring suture of the running horizontal mattress suture technique. Note the needle entry at 90 degrees.

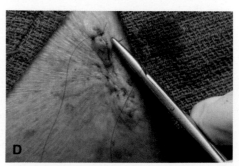

Figure 5-9D. The anchoring suture is tied off, and the running component of the suture begins.

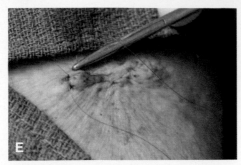

Figure 5-9E. Completion of the first pass of the running component.

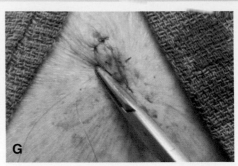

Figure 5-9G. The needle exits on the contralateral wound edge.

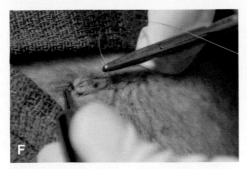

Figure 5-9F. The needle is then reinserted in a back-hand fashion on the ipsilateral wound edge, just proximal to its exit point.

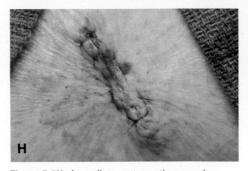

Figure 5-9H. Immediate postoperative wound appearance.

Tips and Pearls

This technique is frequently used on the face, as it aids with dramatic wound eversion. Generally, if the dermis was closed using the set-back dermal suture, no additional eversion is needed; however, when the buried dermal suture or even the buried vertical mattress suture is used, occasionally the wound edges do not evert to the desired degree.

This approach also helps minimize cross-hatched railroad track marks, since the suture material does not cross over the incised wound edge. Similarly, this technique can sometimes yield a tidier immediate postoperative appearance because, even if bite sizes are not uniform, this is not apparent to the observer, as only the portions of suture material parallel to the incision line are visible.

As always, it is important to enter the epidermis at 90 degrees, allowing the needle to travel slightly laterally away from the wound edge before fully following the curvature of the needle when utilizing this technique. This will allow for maximal wound eversion and accurate wound-edge approximation.

As with the simple interrupted suture, care should be taken to avoid skimming the needle superficially beneath the epidermis. This results from failing to enter the skin at a perpendicular angle and failing to follow the curvature of the needle. This may result in wound inversion as the tension vector of the shallow bite pulls the wound edges outward and down.

Drawbacks and Cautions

This technique does not typically permit the same degree of wound-edge apposition as can be accomplished with other running transepidermal sutures, since the everting effect of the suture technique may even be associated with a small degree of gaping at the center of the horizontal mattress suture and suture material does not cross over the incised wound edge. In the event that deeper sutures were carefully placed, this may not be a significant drawback, since the wound edges may be well aligned from the placement of these deeper sutures. If not, or if there is a need for improved wound-edge apposition even after placing the running horizontal mattress suture, a small simple interrupted suture may be placed intermittently over the horizontal mattress suture to bring the wound edges together more precisely.

Suture removal with this technique may be more involved than with simple interrupted sutures, particularly if sutures are left in situ for an extended period of time and some of the suture material has been overgrown by the healing epidermis, and the knot may be somewhat buried in the context of a ridged everted repair. Moreover, since this is a running technique, it may be difficult to locate a portion of suture easily amenable to cutting at the time of suture removal, as it is best to minimize the length of pulled through suture material at the time of removal.

As with any suturing technique, knowledge of the relevant anatomy is critical. When placing a running horizontal mattress suture, it is important to recall that the structures deep to the epidermis may be compromised by the passage of the needle and suture material.

Similarly, structures deep to the defect may be constricted. This can lead to necrosis due to vascular compromise or even, theoretically, superficial nerve damage. These concerns are more acute with the running horizontal mattress suture than with the simple running suture, since the wide arc of the suture material and its horizontal component incorporate more skin and underlying structures, thus increasing the risk of strangulation.

This technique may elicit an increased risk of track marks, necrosis, and other complications when compared with techniques that do not entail suture material traversing the scar line, such as buried or subcuticular approaches. Therefore, sutures should be removed as early as possible to minimize these complications, and consideration should be given to adopting other closure techniques or utilizing fast-absorbing gut suture material in the event that the sutures will not be able to be removed in a timely fashion.

Reference

Moody BR, McCarthy JE, Linder J, Hruza GJ. Enhanced cosmetic outcome with running horizontal mattress sutures. *Dermatol Surg.* 2005;31(10):1313-1316.

The Running Horizontal Mattress Suture with Intermittent Simple Loops

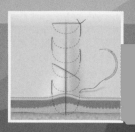

Video 5-10. Running horizontal mattress suture with intermittent simple loops
Access to video can be found via mhprofessional.com/atlasofsuturingtechniques2e

Application

Like the standard running horizontal mattress suture, this is a running everting technique used for closure and epidermal approximation. It is useful, especially on the face, to aid in everting the wound edges when the dermis has been closed using a deep suturing technique. This technique may also be used in patients with atrophic skin, as the broader anchoring bites may help limit tissue tear-through that may be seen with a simple interrupted suture.

Suture Material Choice

With all techniques, it is best to use the thinnest suture possible in order to minimize the risk of track marks and foreign-body reactions. On the face and eyelids, a 6-0 or 7-0 monofilament suture may be used, though fast-absorbing gut may be used on the eyelids and ears to obviate the need for suture removal. Since the goal of this technique is primarily to encourage wound-edge eversion, fine-gauge suture material may be used on the extremities as well.

Technique

1. The needle is inserted perpendicular to the epidermis, approximately one-half the radius of the needle distant to the wound edge. This will allow the needle to exit the wound on the contralateral side at an equal distance from the wound edge by simply following the curvature of the needle.

2. With a fluid motion of the wrist, the needle is rotated through the dermis, taking the bite wider at the deep margin than at the surface, and the needle tip exits the skin on the contralateral side.

3. The needle body is grasped with surgical forceps in the left hand, with care being taken to avoid grasping the needle tip, which can be easily dulled by repetitive friction against the surgical forceps. It is gently grasped and pulled upward with the surgical forceps as the body of the needle is released from the needle driver. Alternatively, the needle may be released from the needle driver, and the needle driver itself may be used to grasp the needle from the contralateral side of the wound to complete its rotation through its arc, obviating the need for surgical forceps.

4. The suture material is then tied off gently, with care being taken to minimize tension across the epidermis and avoid overly constricting the wound edges. The trailing end of suture is then trimmed.

5. Starting proximal relative to the surgeon, the needle is then reinserted perpendicular to the epidermis, approximately one-half the radius of the needle distant to the wound edge.

6. With a fluid motion of the wrist, the needle is rotated through the dermis, taking the bite wider at the deep margin than at the surface, and the needle tip exits the skin on the contralateral side.

7. The needle body is grasped with surgical forceps in the left hand and pulled upward with the surgical forceps as the body of the needle is released from the needle driver.

8. The needle is then reloaded in a backhand fashion and inserted at 90 degrees perpendicular to the epidermis proximal (relative to the surgeon) to its exit point on the same side of the incision line as the exit point.

9. The needle is rotated through its arc, exiting on the right side of the wound (relative to the surgeon) in a mirror image of step (6).

10. Steps (5) through (9) are then repeated.

11. Moving proximally, the needle is then reinserted perpendicular to the epidermis on the right side of the wound, approximately one-half the radius of the needle distant to the wound edge.

12. With a fluid motion of the wrist, the needle is rotated through the dermis, taking the bite wider at the deep margin than at the surface, and the needle tip exits the skin on the contralateral side.

13. Again moving proximally, the needle is reinserted perpendicular to the epidermis on the right side of the wound, approximately one-half the radius of the needle distant to the wound edge.

14. With a fluid motion of the wrist, the needle is rotated through the dermis, taking the bite wider at the deep margin than at the surface, and the needle tip exits the skin on the contralateral side.

15. The needle is then reloaded in a backhand fashion and inserted at 90 degrees perpendicular to the epidermis proximal (relative to the surgeon) to its exit point on the same side of the incision line as the exit point.

16. The needle is rotated through its arc, exiting on the right side of the wound (relative to the surgeon) in a mirror image of step (6).

17. Moving proximally relative to the surgeon, these steps are sequentially repeated, occasionally inserting simple interrupted throws between the running horizontal mattress throws, until the end of the wound is reached. At that point, a loop is left in the penultimate throw, and the suture material is then tied off gently, with care being taken to minimize tension across the epidermis and avoid overly constricting the wound edges (Figures 5-10A through 5-10I).

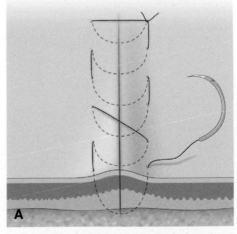

Figure 5-10A. Overview of the running horizontal mattress suture with intermittent simple loops.

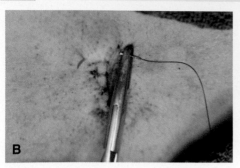

Figure 5-10B. The anchoring suture is placed.

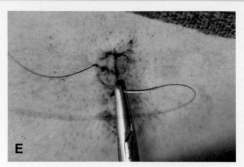

Figure 5-10E. The needle is reloaded in a backhand fashion and again inserted into the skin at 90 degrees.

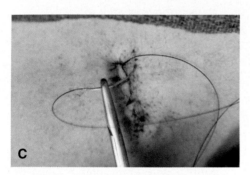

Figure 5-10C. The anchoring suture knot has been tied, and the first running horizontal mattress suture is begun. Note the 90-degree entry angle.

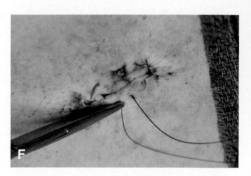

Figure 5-10F. The needle is reloaded in a standard fashion and passed through the skin.

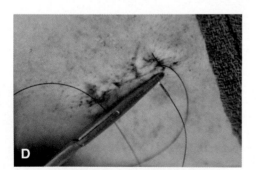

Figure 5-10D. The first running horizontal mattress suture continues.

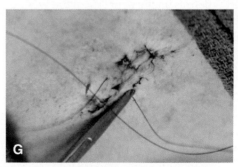

Figure 5-10G. This process is repeated to place a simple running loop.

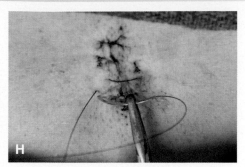

Figure 5-10H. The horizontal mattress component then continues.

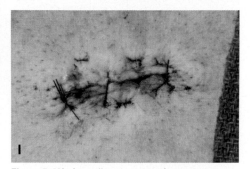

Figure 5-10I. Immediate postoperative appearance.

Tips and Pearls

The ratio of horizontal mattress to simple running throws can be greater than 1:1; many surgeons favor a ratio of 2:1, while the original published description of this approach advocates a ratio of 4:1. On relatively short repairs on the face, a simple running interrupted loop may be placed at the center of the wound.

This approach helps mitigate the problem of challenging suture removal that is associated with the running horizontal mattress approach. The simple running loops are easily accessible at the time of suture removal and may be cut, thus allowing the suture material to be pulled through. An additional benefit is that the intermittent simple running loops help with wound-edge apposition, as the horizontal mattress components tend to

evert the edges but do not always bring the wound edges together as elegantly as would otherwise be desired.

This technique is frequently used on the face, as it aids with dramatic wound eversion. Generally, if the dermis was closed using the set-back dermal suture, no additional eversion is needed; however, when the buried dermal suture or even the buried vertical mattress suture is used, occasionally the wound edges do not evert to the desired degree.

This approach also helps minimize cross-hatched railroad track marks, since most of the suture material does not cross over the incised wound edge. Similarly, this technique can sometimes yield a neater immediate postoperative appearance because even if bite sizes are not uniform, this is not apparent to the observer, as only the portions of suture material parallel to the incision line are visible.

As always, it is important to enter the epidermis at 90 degrees, allowing the needle to travel slightly laterally away from the wound edge before fully following the curvature of the needle when utilizing this technique. This will allow for maximal wound eversion and accurate wound-edge approximation.

As with the simple interrupted suture, care should be taken to avoid skimming the needle superficially beneath the epidermis. This results from failing to enter the skin at a perpendicular angle and failing to follow the curvature of the needle. This may result in wound inversion as the tension vector of the shallow bite pulls the wound edges outward and down.

Drawbacks and Cautions

Even with the placement of intermittent simple running loops, this technique does not uniformly permit the same degree of wound-edge apposition as can be accomplished with other running transepidermal sutures, since the everting effect of the suture technique may even be associated with a small degree of gaping at the center of the horizontal mattress suture and suture material does not cross over the incised wound edge. In the event that deeper sutures were carefully placed, this may not be a significant drawback, since the wound edges may be well aligned from the placement of these deeper sutures.

With any suturing technique, knowledge of the relevant anatomy is critical. When placing a running horizontal mattress suture with intermittent simple loops, it is important to recall that the structures deep to the epidermis may be compromised by the passage of the needle and suture material.

As always, structures deep to the defect may be constricted. This can lead to necrosis due to vascular compromise or even, theoretically, superficial nerve damage. These concerns are more acute with the running horizontal mattress suture than with the simple running suture, since the wide arc of the suture material and its horizontal component incorporate more skin and underlying structures, thus increasing the risk of strangulation.

This technique may elicit an increased risk of track marks, necrosis, and other complications when compared with techniques that do not entail suture material traversing the scar line, such as buried or subcuticular approaches. Therefore, sutures should be removed as early as possible to minimize these complications, and consideration should be given to adopting other closure techniques or utilizing rapidly absorbing suture material in the event that the sutures will not be able to be removed in a timely fashion.

Reference

Wang SQ, Goldberg LH. Surgical pearl: running horizontal mattress suture with intermittent simple loops. *J Am Acad Dermatol.* 2006;55(5):870-871.

The Running Alternating Simple and Horizontal Mattress Suture

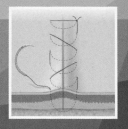

Synonym

Running combined mattress suture

 Video 5-11. Running alternating simple and horizontal mattress suture
Access to video can be found via
mhprofessional.com/atlasofsuturingtechniques2e

Application

This is a hybrid running everting technique used for closure and epidermal approximation. It incorporates a horizontal mattress component, which encourages wound eversion, and a simple running component, which encourages wound-edge apposition. This technique may also be used in patients with atrophic skin, as the broader anchoring bites of the horizontal mattress component may help limit the tissue tear-through that may be seen with a simple running suture.

Suture Material Choice

With all techniques, it is best to use the thinnest suture possible in order to minimize the risk of track marks and foreign-body reactions. On the face and eyelids, a 6-0 or 7-0 monofilament suture is useful. Since the goal of this technique is primarily to encourage wound-edge eversion, fine-gauge suture material may be used on the extremities as well, though if the wound is under significant tension or if the simple running component of the technique is being used to approximate wound edges under significant tension, then 5-0 suture material may be used on the extremities and neck, and thicker suture material, including 3-0, may be used on the trunk if the anticipated tension is marked.

Technique

1. The needle is inserted perpendicular to the epidermis, approximately one-half the radius of the needle distant to the wound edge. This will allow the needle to exit the wound on the contralateral side at an equal distance from the wound edge by simply following the curvature of the needle.

2. With a fluid motion of the wrist, the needle is rotated through the dermis, taking the bite wider at the deep margin than at the surface, and the needle tip exits the skin on the contralateral side.

3. The needle body is grasped with surgical forceps in the left hand, with care being taken to avoid grasping the needle tip, which can be easily dulled by repetitive friction against the surgical forceps. It is gently grasped and pulled upward with the surgical forceps as the body of the needle is released from the needle driver. Alternatively, the needle may be released from the needle driver, and the needle driver itself may be used to grasp the needle from the contralateral side of the wound to complete its rotation through its arc, obviating the need for surgical forceps.

4. The suture material is then tied off gently, with care being taken to minimize tension across the epidermis and avoid overly constricting the wound edges. The trailing end of suture is trimmed.

5. Starting proximal relative to the surgeon, the needle is then reinserted perpendicular to the epidermis, approximately one-half the radius of the needle distant to the wound edge.

6. With a fluid motion of the wrist, the needle is rotated through the dermis, taking the bite wider at the deep margin than at the surface, and the needle tip exits the skin on the contralateral side.

7. The needle body is grasped with surgical forceps in the left hand and pulled upward with the surgical forceps as the body of the needle is released from the needle driver.

8. The needle is then reloaded in a backhand fashion and inserted at 90 degrees perpendicular to the epidermis proximal (relative to the surgeon) to its exit point on the same side of the incision line as the exit point.

9. The needle is rotated through its arc, exiting on the right side of the wound (relative to the surgeon) in a mirror image of step (6).

10. Starting proximal relative to the surgeon, the needle is then reinserted perpendicular to the epidermis, approximately one-half the radius of the needle distant to the wound edge.

11. With a fluid motion of the wrist, the needle is rotated through the dermis, taking the bite wider at the deep margin than at the surface, and the needle tip exits the skin on the contralateral side.

12. The needle body is grasped with surgical forceps in the left hand and pulled upward with the surgical forceps as the body of the needle is released from the needle driver.

13. Starting proximal relative to the surgeon, the needle is then reinserted perpendicular to the epidermis, approximately one-half the radius of the needle distant to the wound edge.

14. With a fluid motion of the wrist, the needle is rotated through the dermis, taking the bite wider at the deep margin than at the surface, and the needle tip exits the skin on the contralateral side.

15. The needle body is grasped with surgical forceps in the left hand and pulled upward with the surgical forceps as the body of the needle is released from the needle driver.

16. The needle is then reloaded in a backhand fashion and inserted at 90 degrees perpendicular to the epidermis proximal (relative to the surgeon) to its exit point on the same side of the incision line as the exit point.

17. The needle is rotated through its arc, exiting on the right side of the wound (relative to the surgeon) in a mirror image of step (6).

18. Moving proximally relative to the surgeon, the previously mentioned steps are then sequentially repeated, alternating the placement of a simple running suture with a running horizontal mattress suture, until the end of the wound is reached. At that point, a loop is left in the penultimate throw, and the suture material is then tied off gently, with care being taken to minimize tension across the epidermis and avoid overly constricting the wound edges (Figures 5-11A through 5-11G).

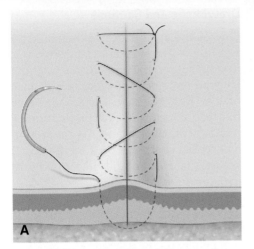

Figure 5-11A. Overview of the running alternating simple and horizontal mattress suture.

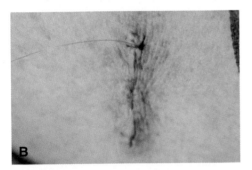

Figure 5-11B. The anchoring suture is tied.

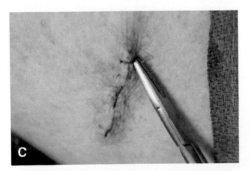

Figure 5-11C. The needle is then inserted through the skin and rotated diagonally across the wound, exiting on the contralateral side.

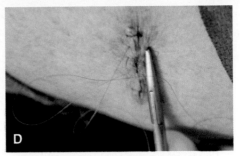

Figure 5-11D. The needle is then reloaded and inserted, again from the contralateral side of the wound, with a trajectory perpendicular to the wound edge.

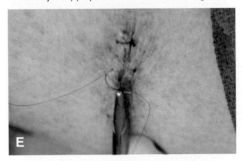

Figure 5-11E. Using a backhand technique, the needle is then reinserted from the ipsilateral side, again with a course directly across the incised wound edge.

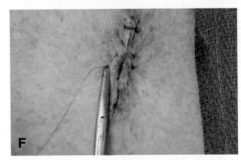

Figure 5-11F. The needle is then inserted, again from same side, and rotated diagonally across the wound. This pattern is continued along the course of the wound.

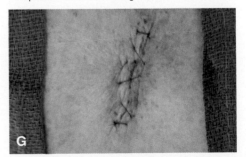

Figure 5-11G. Immediate postoperative appearance.

Tips and Pearls

Since this technique entails alternating between a simple running and a running horizontal mattress suture, two bites should be taken from each side of the wound in succession in order to effectively combine these techniques.

This technique addresses a shortcoming in the running horizontal mattress suture, which tends to effectively evert the skin edges but may be unreliable at wound-edge apposition and coaptation. By combining these two approaches, this technique encourages excellent wound-edge eversion with its horizontal component while concomitantly permitting wound-edge apposition with the simple running component.

Moreover, a shortcoming of the traditional running horizontal mattress suture is that suture removal may be challenging. Since this technique entails alternating the mattress sutures with their simple running counterparts, suture removal is straightforward as the simple running loops are easily visualized and grasped at the time of suture removal.

As always, it is important to enter the epidermis at 90 degrees, allowing the needle to travel slightly laterally away from the wound edge before fully following the curvature of the needle when utilizing this technique. This will allow for maximal wound eversion and accurate wound-edge approximation.

Again, care should be taken to avoid skimming the needle superficially beneath the epidermis. This results from failing to enter the skin at a perpendicular angle and failing to follow the curvature of the needle. This may result in wound inversion as the tension vector of the shallow bite pulls the wound edges outward and down.

Drawbacks and Cautions

One of the advantages of the standard running horizontal mattress suture is that no suture material crosses over the incision line and, therefore, the chance of leaving track marks is small. Since this technique includes a simple running component, track marks may represent a potential complication, and therefore, suture material should be removed as early as possible.

As with any suturing technique, knowledge of the relevant anatomy is critical. Similarly, structures deep to the defect may be constricted. This can lead to necrosis due to vascular compromise or even, theoretically, superficial nerve damage. These concerns are more acute with the running alternating simple and horizontal mattress suture than with the simple running suture, since the wide arc of the suture material and its horizontal component incorporate more skin and underlying structures, thus increasing the risk of strangulation.

This technique may elicit an increased risk of track marks, necrosis, and other complications when compared with techniques that do not entail suture material traversing the scar line, such as buried or subcuticular approaches. Therefore, sutures should be removed as early as possible to minimize these complications, and consideration should be given to adopting other closure techniques in the event that the sutures will not be able to be removed in a timely fashion.

Reference

Niazi ZB. Two novel and useful suturing techniques. *Plast Reconstr Surg.* 1997;100(6):1617-1618.

The Running Locking Horizontal Mattress Suture

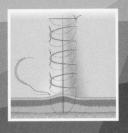

Synonym

Running looped mattress suture

Video 5-12. Running locking horizontal mattress suture

Access to video can be found via
mhprofessional.com/atlasofsuturingtechniques2e

Application

This is a modification of the running horizontal mattress suture, an everting technique used for closure and epidermal approximation. It is best used as a secondary layer when deeper sutures have been previously placed. This technique may be particularly useful in the context of atrophic skin, as the broader anchoring bites may help limit tissue tear-through. This locking variation confers two advantages over the traditional horizontal mattress suture: (1) better ease of suture removal, and (2) improved wound-edge apposition.

Suture Material Choice

With all techniques, it is best to use the thinnest suture possible in order to minimize the risk of track marks and foreign-body reactions. Suture choice will depend largely on anatomic location and the goal of suture placement.

On the face, a 6-0 or 7-0 monofilament suture may be used, though fast-absorbing gut may be used on the eyelids and ears to obviate the need for suture removal; in these cases, standard running horizontal mattress sutures are probably preferable to their locking counterparts. When the goal of the running locking horizontal mattress suture placement is solely to encourage wound-edge eversion, fine-gauge suture material may be used on the extremities as well. Otherwise, 5-0 monofilament suture material may be used if there is minimal tension, and 4-0 monofilament suture is useful in areas under moderate tension where the goal of suture placement is relieving tension as well as epidermal approximation. In select high-tension areas, 3-0 monofilament suture may be utilized as well.

Technique

1. The needle is inserted perpendicular to the epidermis, approximately one-half the radius of the needle distant to the wound edge. This will allow the needle to exit the wound on the contralateral side at an equal distance from the wound edge by simply following the curvature of the needle.

2. With a fluid motion of the wrist, the needle is rotated through the dermis, taking the bite wider at the deep margin than at the surface, and the needle tip exits the skin on the contralateral side.

3. The needle body is grasped with surgical forceps in the left hand and pulled upward with the surgical forceps as the body of the needle is released from the needle driver.

4. The suture material is then tied off gently, with care being taken to minimize tension across the epidermis and avoid overly constricting the wound edges. Only the loose end of suture is trimmed.

5. Moving proximally toward the surgeon, the needle is again inserted perpendicular to the epidermis, approximately one-half the radius of the needle distant to the wound edge.

6. With a fluid motion of the wrist, the needle is rotated through the dermis, taking the bite wider at the deep margin than at the surface, and the needle tip exits the skin on the contralateral side.

7. The needle body is grasped with surgical forceps in the left hand and pulled upward with the surgical forceps as the body of the needle is released from the needle driver.

8. The needle is then reloaded in a backhand fashion and inserted at 90 degrees perpendicular to the epidermis proximal (relative to the surgeon) to its exit point on the same side of the incision line as the exit point. Importantly, a loop of suture material is left protruding from the wound from where the needle exited on the prior throw to where it enters on this throw.

9. The needle is rotated through its arc, exiting on the right side of the wound (relative to the surgeon) in a mirror image of steps (6) and (7).

10. The needle is then passed under the loop of suture material on the contralateral side.

11. Steps (5) through (10) are then sequentially repeated, moving proximally toward the surgeon.

12. The suture material is then tied off gently, with care being taken to minimize tension across the epidermis and avoid overly constricting the wound edges (Figures 5-12A through 5-12G).

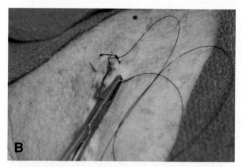

Figure 5-12B. After the anchoring suture is placed, the needle is again inserted at 90 degrees through the epidermis, exiting on the contralateral wound edge.

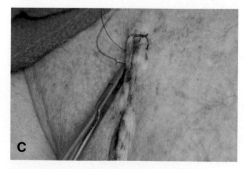

Figure 5-12C. The needle is then reloaded in a backhand fashion and enters the skin on the ipsilateral wound edge, exiting on the contralateral side.

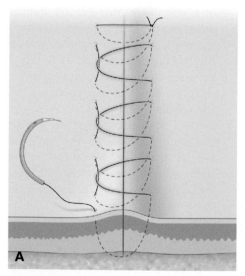

Figure 5-12A. Overview of the running locking horizontal mattress technique.

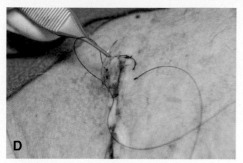

Figure 5-12D. The needle is then passed through the loop formed by the horizontal mattress suture.

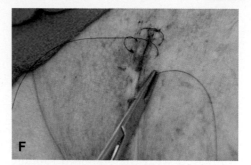

Figure 5-12F. The pattern continues, moving along the course of the wound.

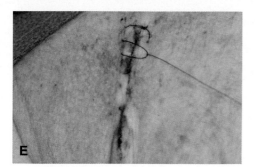

Figure 5-12E. The needle is then pulled laterally, securing the locking loop.

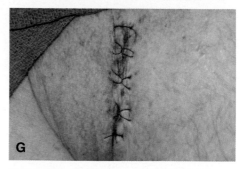

Figure 5-12G. Immediate postoperative appearance.

Tips and Pearls

The running locking technique confers two important advantages over the traditional running horizontal mattress suture. First, the standard horizontal mattress suture does not typically permit the same degree of wound-edge apposition as can be accomplished with other transepidermal sutures, since the everting effect of the suture technique may even be associated with a small degree of gaping at the center of the horizontal mattress suture. Locking the suture material brings the knot, as well as the two parallel external rows of suture, to the center of the wound, thus improving wound-edge approximation.

Second, suture removal with the standard running horizontal mattress technique may be challenging, particularly if sutures are left in place for an extended period of time and some of the suture material has been overgrown by the healing epidermis, as the knot may be buried in the context of a ridged everted repair. Bringing the knot, along with the parallel rows of external suture material, centrally with the locking technique allows the knot to be more easily grasped at the time of suture removal.

As with most transepidermal techniques, it is important to enter the epidermis at 90 degrees, allowing the needle to travel slightly laterally away from the wound edge before fully following the curvature of the needle when utilizing this technique. This will allow for maximal wound eversion and accurate wound-edge approximation.

As with the simple interrupted suture, care should be taken to avoid skimming the needle superficially beneath the epidermis. This results from failing to enter the skin at a perpendicular angle and to follow the curvature of the needle. This may result in wound inversion as the tension vector of the shallow bite pulls the wound edges outward and down.

Drawbacks and Cautions

This variation has a disadvantage when compared with the standard running horizontal mattress technique, in that locking each throw means that there is suture material passing over the incision line with every throw. As suture material passing over the center of the wound may be associated with track-like scarring, this disadvantage needs to be weighed carefully against any perceived advantages of this technique.

Moreover, particularly if the suture material is under significant tension, structures deep to the defect may be constricted. This can lead to necrosis due to vascular compromise or even, theoretically, superficial nerve damage. These concerns are more acute with the running locking horizontal mattress suture than with the simple running suture, since the wide arc of the suture material and its horizontal component incorporate more skin and underlying structures, thus increasing the risk of strangulation.

The potential to constrict deeper structures may be used to the surgeon's advantage in the context of a slowly oozing surgical wound, since this technique may indirectly ligate the culprit vessels. This should only be used in the event that the offending vessel is relatively small, since otherwise there is a significant risk that this indirect ligation will not be sufficiently resilient. Moreover, tying the suture too tightly may increase the risk of developing track marks or superficial necrosis.

This technique may elicit an increased risk of track marks, necrosis, and other complications when compared with techniques that do not entail suture material traversing the scar line, such as buried or subcuticular approaches. Therefore, sutures should be removed as early as possible to minimize these complications, and, as noted previously, consideration should be given to adopting other closure techniques in the event that the sutures will not be able to be removed in a timely fashion.

References

Hanasono MM, Hotchkiss RN. Locking horizontal mattress suture. *Dermatol Surg.* 2005;31(5):572-573.

Niazi ZB. Running looped mattress suturing technique. *Plast Reconstr Surg.* 1998;101(1):248-249.

Niazi ZB. Two novel and useful suturing techniques. *Plast Reconstr Surg.* 1997;100(6):1617-1618.

Olson J, Berg D. Modified locking horizontal mattress suture. *Dermatol Surg.* 2014;40(1):72-74.

Zuber TJ. The mattress sutures: vertical, horizontal, and corner stitch. *Am Fam Physician.* 2002;66(12):2231-2236.

The Cruciate Mattress Suture

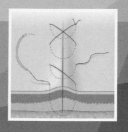

Synonym

Figure of 8 suture

Video 5-13. Cruciate mattress suture
Access to video can be found via
mhprofessional.com/atlasofsuturingtechniques2e

Application

This is an infrequently used technique that is a hybrid between a simple interrupted suture, a mattress suture, and a simple running suture. It is useful when the benefits of interrupted sutures—especially the frequent knot placement leading to a more secure closure—are desired. It may also be used if the wound length is slightly too long for a single simple interrupted suture. This approach entails taking two simple interrupted bites in succession and then tying off the suture, leaving an "x" of suture material over the wound edge.

This approach may be used alone in the context of small wounds under minimal to no tension, such as those formed by a punch biopsy or a traumatic laceration. It may also be used as a secondary layer to aid in the approximation of the epidermis when the dermis has been closed using a dermal or other deep suturing technique. This technique may also be used for vessel ligation and hemostasis, where it is classically referred to as the figure of 8 suture.

Suture Material Choice

With all techniques, it is best to use the thinnest suture possible in order to minimize the risk of track marks and foreign-body reactions. Suture choice will depend largely on anatomic location and the goal of suture placement. This technique is rarely used on the face, but if it is used on the face, a 6-0 or 7-0 monofilament suture may be used for epidermal approximation. On the extremities, a 5-0 monofilament suture may be used if there is minimal tension, and a 4-0 monofilament suture can be used in areas under moderate tension where the goal of suture placement is relieving tension or hemostasis as well as epidermal approximation. In select high-tension areas, a 3-0 monofilament suture may be utilized as well. When used for hemostasis on the interior of a wound, a 4-0 absorbable suture may be used.

Technique

1. The needle is inserted perpendicular to the epidermis, approximately one-half the radius of the needle distant to the wound edge. This will allow the needle to exit the wound on the contralateral side at an equal distance from the wound edge by simply following the curvature of the needle.
2. With a fluid motion of the wrist, the needle is rotated through the dermis, taking the bite wider at the deep

margin than at the surface, and the needle tip exits the skin on the contralateral side.

3. The needle body is grasped with surgical forceps in the left hand, with care being taken to avoid grasping the needle tip, which can be easily dulled by repetitive friction against the surgical forceps. It is gently grasped and pulled upward with the surgical forceps as the body of the needle is released from the needle driver. Alternatively, the needle may be released from the needle driver, and the needle driver itself may be used to grasp the needle from the contralateral side of the wound to complete its rotation through its arc, obviating the need for surgical forceps.

4. Starting proximally relative to the surgeon, steps (1) through (3) are then repeated.

5. The suture material is then tied off gently (Figures 5-13A through 5-13E).

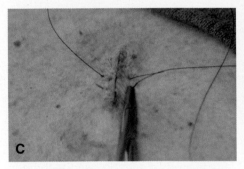

Figure 5-13C. Second step of the cruciate mattress technique. The needle is again rotated through the skin, repeating the first step.

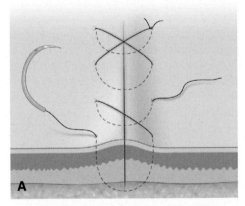

Figure 5-13A. Overview of the cruciate mattress technique. Note that this essentially represents a simple running suture with two loops.

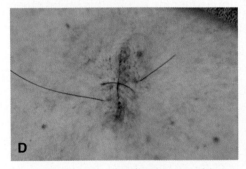

Figure 5-13D. Appearance after placement of the two sutures.

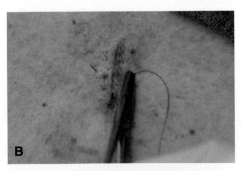

Figure 5-13B. First step of the cruciate mattress suture. The needle is inserted at 90 degrees to the epidermis and rotated through to the contralateral side of the wound, again exiting at 90 degrees.

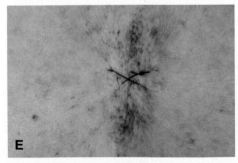

Figure 5-13E. Immediate postoperative appearance after tying the suture. Note the characteristic cruciate appearance.

Tips and Pearls

This technique is useful when attempting to obtain hemostasis in a punch biopsy site or when some superficial oozing remains in a patient on aspirin or anticoagulant therapy. It can be conceptualized as a transepidermal figure of 8 suture, as it has the potential to loosely ligate small vessels in the dermis and subcutis. This approach is, interestingly, fairly popular in the veterinary literature.

As always, it is important to enter the epidermis at 90 degrees, allowing the needle to travel slightly laterally away from the wound edge before fully following the curvature of the needle when utilizing this technique. This will allow for maximal wound eversion and accurate wound-edge approximation.

Care should be taken to avoid skimming the needle superficially beneath the epidermis. This results from failing to enter the skin at a perpendicular angle and to follow the curvature of the needle. This may result in wound inversion as the tension vector of the shallow bite pulls the wound edges outward and down.

Drawbacks and Cautions

The larger amount of suture material traversing the skin in this technique translates into an increased risk of track marks over comparable techniques. Instead of the single section of suture material that traverses the skin with a simple interrupted suture, the cruciate mattress leaves an "x" of suture material taut against the skin; all of this material has the tendency to bury itself in the underlying epidermis during healing, and this phenomenon may be exacerbated during the course of postoperative wound edema, leading to an increased risk of unsightly track marks if the suture material is not removed promptly.

As with any suturing technique, knowledge of the relevant anatomy is critical. When placing a cruciate mattress suture, it is important to recall that the structures deep to the epidermis may be compromised by the passage of the needle and suture material. For example, the needle may pierce a vessel, leading to increased bleeding.

While this may occasionally represent an advantage of this technique, particularly if the knot is tied relatively tightly, structures deep to the defect may be constricted. This can lead to necrosis due to vascular compromise or even, theoretically, superficial nerve damage.

The potential to constrict deeper structures may be used to the surgeon's advantage in the event that a small vessel deep to the incision line is oozing; rather than opening the wound, localizing the source of the bleed, and tying off the individual vessel, it may be possible to simply place a cruciate mattress suture incorporating the culprit vessel within its arc, tie it tightly, and thus indirectly ligate the vessel. This should only be used in the event that the offending vessel is relatively small, since otherwise there is a significant risk that this indirect ligation will not be sufficiently resilient. Moreover, tying the suture too tightly may increase the risk of developing track marks or superficial necrosis.

This technique may elicit an increased risk of track marks, necrosis, and other complications when compared with techniques that do not entail suture material traversing the scar line, such as buried or subcuticular approaches. Therefore, sutures should be removed as early as possible to minimize these complications, and consideration should be given to adopting other closure techniques in the event that the sutures will not be able to be removed in a timely fashion.

The Running Oblique Mattress Suture

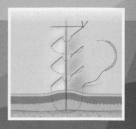

Synonym

Continuous oblique mattress suture

Video 5-14. Running oblique mattress suture

Access to video can be found via mhprofessional.com/atlasofsuturingtechniques2e

Application

This is a hybrid running everting technique used for closure and epidermal approximation. It incorporates an oblique mattress component, which encourages both wound eversion and wound-edge apposition. This technique may be useful for patients with atrophic skin, as the broader anchoring bites of the oblique mattress technique may help limit the tissue tear-through that may be seen with a simple running suture, while concomitantly providing improved wound-edge eversion.

Suture Material Choice

With all techniques, it is best to use the thinnest suture possible in order to minimize the risk of track marks and foreign-body reactions. This technique was originally described for the trunk and extremities, where a 2-0 nonabsorbable suture was advocated. Unless there is marked tension across the wound, smaller gauge suture material is preferable. Indeed, since the goal of the continuous oblique mattress suture is primarily to encourage wound-edge eversion, fine-gauge suture material may be used on

the extremities as well, though if the wound is under significant tension, then 5-0 suture material may be used on the extremities and neck, and thicker suture material, including 3-0, may be used on the trunk if the anticipated tension is marked.

Technique

1. The needle is inserted perpendicular to the epidermis, approximately 6 mm distant to the wound edge.
2. With a fluid motion of the wrist, the needle is rotated through the dermis, taking the bite wider at the deep margin than at the surface, and the needle tip exits the skin on the contralateral side.
3. The needle body is grasped with surgical forceps in the left hand, with care being taken to avoid grasping the needle tip, which can be easily dulled by repetitive friction against the surgical forceps. It is gently grasped and pulled upward with the surgical forceps as the body of the needle is released from the needle driver. Alternatively, the needle may be released from the needle driver, and the needle driver itself may be used to grasp the needle from the contralateral side of the wound to complete its rotation through its arc, obviating the need for surgical forceps.
4. The suture material is then tied off gently, with care being taken to minimize tension across the epidermis

and avoid overly constricting the wound edges. The trailing end of suture is trimmed.

5. Starting approximately 2 mm proximal relative to the surgeon, the needle is then reinserted perpendicular to the epidermis, 3 mm from the wound edge on the right side of the wound.

6. With a fluid motion of the wrist, the needle is rotated through the dermis, and the needle tip exits the skin on the contralateral side, again approximately 3 mm set back from the incised wound edge.

7. The needle is then reloaded in a backhand fashion and inserted 3 mm proximal and approximately 6 mm distant from the incised wound edge on the same side of the incision line as the exit point.

8. The needle is rotated through its arc, exiting on the contralateral side of the wound, again approximately 6 mm distant from the incised wound edge.

9. Moving proximally relative to the surgeon, steps (5) through (8) are then sequentially repeated, until the end of the wound is reached. At that point, a loop is left in the penultimate

throw, and the suture material is then tied off gently, with care being taken to minimize tension across the epidermis and avoid overly constricting the wound edges (Figures 5-14A through 5-14F).

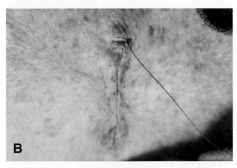

B

Figure 5-14B. The anchoring knot is tied.

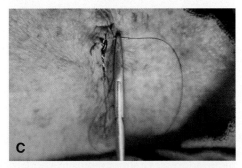

C

Figure 5-14C. The needle is then inserted at 90 degrees through the skin near to the incision line, exiting on the contralateral side near to the incision line.

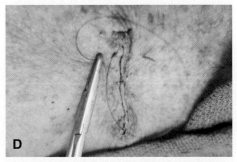

D

Figure 5-14D. The needle is reloaded in a backhand fashion and inserted just distal to its exit point and further away from incision line, following a course perpendicular to the incision line and exiting far from the incision line.

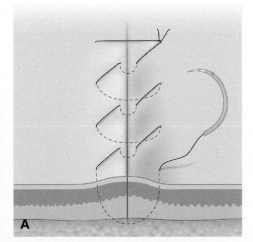

A

Figure 5-14A. Overview of the running oblique mattress suture.

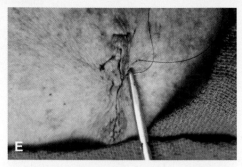

Figure 5-14E. The needle is then inserted distal to its exit point, near to the incision line, exiting on the contralateral side near to the incision line. This pattern is then repeated along the course of the wound.

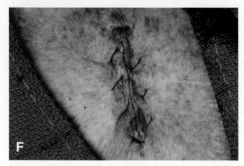

Figure 5-14F. Immediate postoperative appearance.

Tips and Pearls

Like the running alternating simple and horizontal mattress approach, this technique addresses a shortcoming in standard mattress sutures, which tend to effectively evert the skin edges but may be unreliable at wound-edge apposition and coaptation. As a hybrid approach, this technique encourages excellent wound-edge eversion with its mattress component while concomitantly permitting slightly improved wound-edge apposition.

Suture removal with this approach is easier than with a running horizontal or vertical mattress approach, as there is less of a tendency for the transepidermal portion of the sutures to become quickly overgrown with healing epidermis.

In the context of atrophic skin, the modest bites of epidermis taken with a traditional running suture may be insufficient and result in suture tear-through. The larger bites taken with the continuous oblique mattress suture may help mitigate some of these concerns in the context of atrophic skin.

Drawbacks and Cautions

As with the running horizontal mattress suture, no suture material crosses over the incision line, and therefore, the chance of leaving track marks is small. The oblique portions of the suture may tend to constrict with postoperative edema, which may result in obliquely oriented short track marks if sutures are not removed in a timely fashion.

As always, knowledge of the relevant anatomy is critical. Structures deep to the defect may be constricted. This can lead to necrosis due to vascular compromise or even, theoretically, superficial nerve damage. These concerns are more acute with the continuous oblique mattress suture than with the simple running suture, since the wide arc of the suture material and its oblique component incorporate more skin and underlying structures, thus increasing the risk of strangulation.

This technique may elicit an increased risk of track marks, necrosis, and other complications when compared with techniques that do not entail suture material traversing the scar line, such as buried or subcuticular approaches. Therefore, as noted previously, sutures should be removed as early as possible to minimize these complications, and consideration should be given to adopting other closure techniques in the event that the sutures will not be able to be removed in a timely fashion.

Reference

Sonanis SV, Gholve PA. Continuous oblique mattress suture. *Plast Reconstr Surg.* 2003;111(7): 2472-2473.

The Double Locking Horizontal Mattress Suture

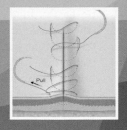

Synonym

Double loop mattress suture

Video 5-15. Double locking horizontal mattress suture
Access to video can be found via mhprofessional.com/atlasofsuturingtechniques2e

Application

This is a modification of the locking horizontal mattress suture, which adds an extra one-half horizontal mattress suture and then is locked through each of the resultant loops. As with many interrupted techniques, it may be used alone for wounds under minimal tension, such as those formed by a small punch biopsy or a traumatic laceration. It is useful in cleft palate repair and may be used as a transepidermal suture when deeper structures have already been closed. This technique may also be used in the context of atrophic skin, as the broader anchoring bites may help limit tissue tear-through that may be seen with a simple interrupted suture. The double locking variation confers three advantages over the traditional horizontal mattress suture: (1) better ease of suture removal, (2) improved wound-edge apposition, and (3) improved strength under tension.

Suture Material Choice

With all techniques, it is best to use the thinnest suture possible in order to minimize the risk of track marks and foreign-body reactions. Suture choice will depend largely on anatomic location and the goal of suture placement.

On the face and eyelids, though this technique is rarely used, a 6-0 or 7-0 monofilament suture may be used; in these cases, standard horizontal mattress sutures are probably preferable to their locking counterparts. Elsewhere, 5-0 monofilament suture material may be used if there is minimal tension, and 4-0 monofilament suture is used in areas under moderate tension where the goal of suture placement is relieving tension as well as epidermal approximation. In select high-tension areas, 3-0 monofilament suture may be utilized as well.

Technique

1. The needle is inserted perpendicular to the epidermis, approximately one-half the radius of the needle distant to the wound edge. This will allow the needle to exit the wound on the contralateral side at an equal distance from the wound edge by simply following the curvature of the needle.

2. With a fluid motion of the wrist, the needle is rotated through the dermis, taking the bite wider at the deep margin than at the surface, and the needle tip exits the skin on the contralateral side.

3. The needle body is grasped with surgical forceps in the left hand, with care being taken to avoid grasping the needle tip, which can

251

be easily dulled by repetitive friction against the surgical forceps. It is gently grasped and pulled upward with the surgical forceps as the body of the needle is released from the needle driver. Alternatively, the needle may be released from the needle driver, and the needle driver itself may be used to grasp the needle from the contralateral side of the wound to complete its rotation through its arc, obviating the need for surgical forceps.

4. The needle is then reloaded in a backhand fashion and inserted at 90 degrees perpendicular to the epidermis proximal (relative to the surgeon) to its exit point on the same side of the incision line as the exit point. Importantly, a loop of suture material is left protruding from where the needle exited on the prior throw to where it enters on this throw.

5. The needle is rotated through its arc, exiting on the right side of the wound (relative to the surgeon) in a mirror image of steps (2) and (3).

6. The needle is then reloaded in a standard fashion and inserted perpendicular to the epidermis proximal (relative to the surgeon) to its exit point on the same side of the incision line as the exit point. Again, a loop of suture material is left protruding from where the needle exited on the prior throw to where it enters on this throw.

7. The needle is rotated through its arc, exiting on the left side of the wound (relative to the surgeon).

8. The needle driver is then passed through the first loop, and the tail of the suture material is then grasped and gently pulled through the loop, temporarily locking it in place. The tail of the suture material is then released.

9. The needle driver is then passed through the second loop of suture material, and the needle is grasped with the needle driver and gently pulled through the loop, similarly locking it into place. At this point, both the leading and trailing strands of suture material are on the same side of the incision line.

10. The suture material is then tied off gently (Figures 5-15A through 5-15J).

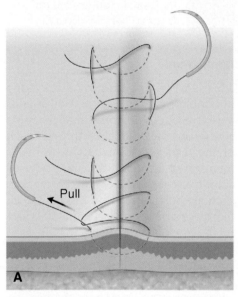

Figure 5-15A. Overview of the double locking horizontal mattress suture.

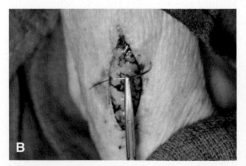

Figure 5-15B. The needle is inserted perpendicularly through the skin.

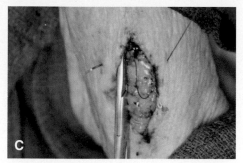

Figure 5-15C. The needle is reinserted through the undersurface of the dermis, exiting on the contralateral side. Note that for small wounds, the preceding two steps may be combined.

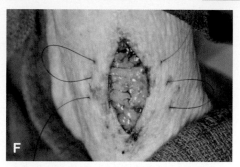

Figure 5-15F. Another horizontal mattress loop is then again placed, with the needle exiting back on the contralateral side.

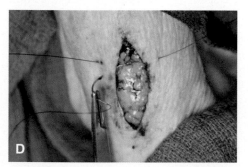

Figure 5-15D. The needle is then inserted on the ipsilateral side at 90 degrees, exiting in the open wound space.

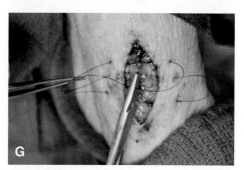

Figure 5-15G. The trailing end of suture is then pulled through the loop closest to its location.

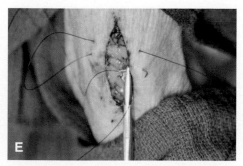

Figure 5-15E. The needle is inserted through the undersurface of the dermis, exiting on the contralateral wound edge.

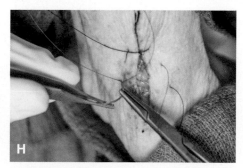

Figure 5-15H. The leading edge of suture with the needle is then pulled through the other loop.

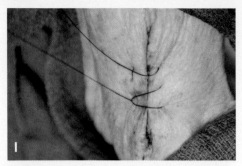

Figure 5-15I. Appearance after pulling through both loops.

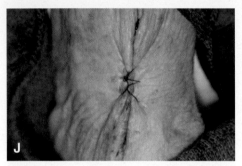

Figure 5-15J. Immediate postoperative appearance after tying the ends of suture together.

Tips and Pearls

This double locking technique allows for some wound eversion while concomitantly taking advantage of the pulley effect of spreading the wound tension over multiple loops. Its central advantage is the increased strength of this approach over the standard locking horizontal mattress suture, and therefore, it is best used in closures under significant tension, such as on the back and shoulders, or when a transepidermal approach is desired and no deeper sutures have been placed, such as the closure of punch biopsy sites.

The double locking technique confers three important advantages over the traditional horizontal mattress suture. First, the standard horizontal mattress suture does not typically permit the same degree of wound-edge apposition as can be

accomplished with other transepidermal sutures, since the everting effect of the suture technique may even be associated with a small degree of gaping at the center of the horizontal mattress suture. Double locking the suture material brings the knot, as well as the parallel external rows of suture, to the center of the wound, thus improving wound-edge approximation.

Second, suture removal with the standard horizontal mattress technique may be challenging, particularly if sutures are left in situ for an extended period of time and some of the suture material has been overgrown by the healing epidermis, as the knot may be buried in the context of a ridged everted repair. Bringing the knot, along with the parallel rows of external suture material, centrally with the locking technique allows the knot to be more easily grasped at the time of suture removal.

Finally, the double locking approach adds a pulley effect, thus increasing the strength of the suture and permitting closure under higher-tension environments. As an added benefit, the double locking technique incorporates an extra throw of the horizontal mattress suture, meaning that each suture extends further along the wound, thus necessitating fewer knot ties for a given incision length.

As with most transepidermal techniques, it is important to enter the epidermis at 90 degrees, allowing the needle to travel slightly laterally away from the wound edge before fully following the curvature of the needle when utilizing this technique. This will allow for maximal wound eversion and accurate wound-edge approximation.

As with the simple interrupted suture, care should be taken to avoid skimming the needle superficially beneath the epidermis. This results from failing to enter the skin at a perpendicular angle and to follow the curvature of the needle.

This may result in wound inversion as the tension vector of the shallow bite pulls the wound edges outward and down.

Drawbacks and Cautions

This technique incorporates three strands of suture crossing the wound, along with a significant amount of suture material resting parallel to the wound, and therefore, it may be associated with a higher risk of track marks than many other techniques. In addition, the double locking component and the change in the tension vectors markedly reduce the everting effect of the horizontal mattress technique, thus negating one of the major benefits of this approach.

Additionally, the tension vectors associated with this suture are not uniformly perpendicular to the incision line, theoretically increasing the chances of tissue bunching.

Moreover, structures deep to the defect may be constricted or may be perforated by the multiple passes of suture. This can lead to necrosis due to vascular compromise, bleeding, or even, theoretically,

superficial nerve damage. These concerns are more acute with the double locking horizontal mattress suture than with the simple interrupted suture, since the wide arc of the suture material and its horizontal component incorporate more skin and underlying structures, thus increasing the risk of strangulation.

As noted previously, this technique may elicit an increased risk of track marks, necrosis, and other complications when compared with techniques that do not entail suture material traversing the scar line, such as buried or subcuticular approaches. Therefore, this technique is best used when the closure is under significant tension. Regardless, sutures should be removed as early as possible to minimize these complications, and consideration should be given to adopting other closure techniques in the event that the sutures will not be able to be removed in a timely fashion.

Reference

Biddlestone J, Samuel M, Creagh T, Ahmad T. The double loop mattress suture. *Wound Repair Regen.* 2014;22(3):415-423.

The Running Diagonal Mattress Suture

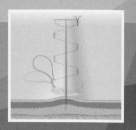

Synonyms

Victory stitch, running V mattress

Video 5-16. Running diagonal mattress suture
Access to video can be found via
mhprofessional.com/atlasofsuturingtechniques2e

Application

This is a modification of the running horizontal mattress suture, where suture material crosses the wound on a diagonal. It is useful in low-tension environments when additional wound eversion is desired, such as the face and extremities, as it leads to marked eversion of the wound edges.

Suture Material Choice

With all techniques, it is best to use the thinnest suture possible in order to minimize the risk of track marks and foreign-body reactions. On the face and eyelids, a 6-0 or 7-0 monofilament suture may be used, though fast-absorbing gut may be used on the eyelids and ears to obviate the need for suture removal. Since the goal of the running diagonal mattress suture placement is primarily to encourage wound-edge eversion, fine-gauge suture material may be used on the extremities as well.

Technique

1. The needle is inserted perpendicular to the epidermis, approximately one-half the radius of the needle distant to the wound edge. This will allow the needle to exit the wound on the contralateral side at an equal distance from the wound edge by simply following the curvature of the needle.

2. With a fluid motion of the wrist, the needle is rotated through the dermis, taking the bite wider at the deep margin than at the surface, and the needle tip exits the skin on the contralateral side.

3. The needle body is grasped with surgical forceps in the left hand, with care being taken to avoid grasping the needle tip, which can be easily dulled by repetitive friction against the surgical forceps. It is gently grasped and pulled upward with the surgical forceps as the body of the needle is released from the needle driver. Alternatively, the needle may be released from the needle driver, and the needle driver itself may be used to grasp the needle from the contralateral side of the wound to complete its rotation through its arc, obviating the need for surgical forceps.

4. The suture material is then tied off gently, with care being taken to minimize tension across the epidermis and avoid overly constricting the wound edges. The trailing end of suture is then trimmed.

5. Starting proximal relative to the surgeon, the needle is then reinserted

perpendicular to the epidermis, approximately one-half the radius of the needle distant to the wound edge. The trajectory of the needle, however, is designed to be on a 45- to 60-degree angle relative to the incision line, pointed away from the starting apex.

6. With a fluid motion of the wrist, the needle is rotated through the dermis, and the needle tip exits the skin on the contralateral side, further along the incision line than its entry point.

7. The needle body is grasped with surgical forceps in the left hand as the body of the needle is released from the needle driver.

8. The needle is then reloaded in a backhand fashion and inserted at 90 degrees perpendicular to the epidermis just proximal (relative to the surgeon) to its exit point on the same side of the incision line as the exit point. The trajectory of the needle, however, is designed to be on a 45- to 60-degree angle relative to the incision line, pointed away from the starting apex.

9. The needle is rotated through its arc, exiting on the contralateral side of the wound (relative to the surgeon) further along the incision line.

10. Moving proximally relative to the surgeon, steps (5) through (9) are then sequentially repeated, until the end of the wound is reached. At that point, a loop is left in the penultimate throw, and the suture material is then tied off gently, with care being taken to minimize tension across the epidermis and avoid overly constricting the wound edges (Figures 5-16A through 5-16F).

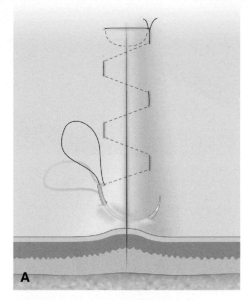

Figure 5-16A. Overview of the running diagonal mattress technique.

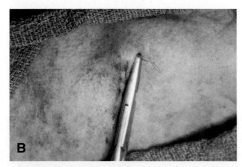

Figure 5-16B. The anchoring suture is placed.

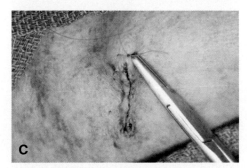

Figure 5-16C. After tying off the anchoring suture, the needle is then reinserted adjacent to the anchoring suture at a 90-degree angle and passed across the wound at a 45-degree angle relative to the incision line.

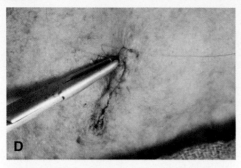

Figure 5-16D. Moving along the length of the wound, the needle is then again inserted adjacent to its exit point at a 90-degree angle and passed across the wound at a 45-degree angle relative to the incision line.

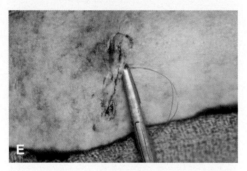

Figure 5-16E. This pattern continues along the length of the wound.

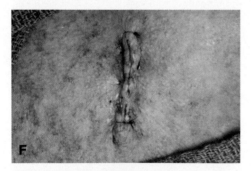

Figure 5-16F. Immediate postoperative appearance.

Tips and Pearls

This technique ostensibly provides the benefit of decreased risk of tissue necrosis when compared with the running horizontal mattress technique, since the watershed area at risk for vascular

compromise is smaller when the bites are taken at a diagonal than when they are perpendicular to the incision line. That said, in clinical experience, loosely tied mattress sutures almost never result in wound necrosis.

This technique does, however, have the advantage of taking very short bites parallel to the incision line, so that if any track marks are left, they will be very short and inconspicuous. This approach is therefore well suited to utilizing a rapidly absorbable suture, such as fast-absorbing gut, since there is little risk that a slowly degraded suture will leave track marks.

This technique is sometimes used on the face, as it aids with dramatic wound eversion. Generally, if the dermis was closed using the set-back dermal suture, no additional eversion is needed; however, when the buried dermal suture or even the buried vertical mattress suture is used, occasionally the wound edges do not evert to the desired degree.

This approach also helps minimize cross-hatched railroad track marks, since the suture material does not cross over the incised wound edge. Similarly, this technique can sometimes yield a neater immediate postoperative appearance because even if bite sizes are not uniform, this is not apparent to the observer, as only the portions of suture material parallel to the incision line are visible.

Drawbacks and Cautions

Since the suture material traverses the wound on a diagonal, it introduces a force vector across the surface of the wound that is not perpendicular to the incised wound edge. In wounds under only minimal tension due to the proper placement of deeper sutures, this is not a significant issue, since the running diagonal mattress suture is utilized largely to evert the wound edges, rather than to reduce tension across the incision line. However, if the wound is under tension, the running horizontal mattress suture may be preferable as it has the theoretical advantage of maintaining tension perpendicular to the incision line.

Like the running horizontal mattress technique, this suture does not typically permit the same degree of wound-edge apposition as can be accomplished with other running transepidermal sutures. The everting effect of the suture technique may even be associated with a small degree of gaping, and suture material does not cross over the incised wound edge. In the event that deeper sutures were carefully placed, this may not be a significant drawback, since the wound edges may be well aligned from the placement of these deeper sutures. If not, or if there is a need for improved wound-edge apposition even after placing the running diagonal mattress suture, a small simple interrupted suture may be placed intermittently over the mattress suture to bring the wound edges together more precisely.

Suture removal with this technique may be more involved than with simple interrupted sutures, particularly if sutures are left in situ for an extended period of time and some of the suture material has been overgrown by the healing epidermis. Moreover, since this is a running technique, it may be difficult to locate a portion of suture easily amenable to cutting at the time of suture removal, since it is best to minimize the length of pulled through suture material at the time of removal. For this reason, if nonabsorbable suture material is utilized, an intermittent simple running throw may be used every 1-3 cm to aid in suture removal.

As with any suturing technique, knowledge of the relevant anatomy is critical. When placing a running diagonal mattress suture, it is important to recall that the structures deep to the epidermis may be compromised by the passage of the needle and suture material.

Reference

Eleftheriou LI, Weinberger CH, Endrizzi BT, et al. The victory stitch: a novel running V-shaped horizontal mattress suturing technique. *Dermatol Surg.* 2011;37(11):1663-1665.

The Vertical Mattress Suture

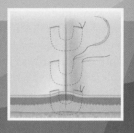

Synonyms

Donati suture, Allgöwer-Donati suture

Video 5-17. Vertical mattress suture

Access to video can be found via mhprofessional.com/atlasofsuturingtechniques2e

Application

This is a frequently used everting technique used for closure and epidermal approximation. As with many interrupted techniques, it may be used alone for wounds under minimal tension, such as those formed by either a small punch biopsy or a traumatic laceration. Like its horizontal counterpart, it is also frequently used as a secondary layer to aid in everting the wound edges when the dermis has been closed using a deep suturing technique.

Suture Material Choice

With all techniques, it is best to use the thinnest suture possible in order to minimize the risk of track marks and foreign-body reactions. Suture choice will depend largely on anatomic location and the goal of suture placement.

On the face, a 6-0 or 7-0 monofilament suture may be used, though fast-absorbing gut may be used on the eyelids and ears to obviate the need for suture removal. When the goal of the vertical mattress suture placement is solely to encourage wound-edge eversion, fine-gauge suture material may be used on

the extremities as well. Otherwise, 5-0 monofilament suture material is used if there is minimal tension, and 4-0 monofilament suture is useful in areas under moderate tension where the goal of suture placement is relieving tension as well as epidermal approximation. In select high-tension areas, 3-0 monofilament suture may be utilized as well.

Technique

1. The needle is inserted perpendicular to the epidermis, approximately 6 mm distant to the wound edge.
2. With a fluid motion of the wrist, the needle is rotated through the dermis, taking the bite wider at the deep margin than at the surface, and the needle tip exits the skin on the contralateral side. If the needle radius is too small to complete this arc in one movement, this first step may be divided into two, with the needle first exiting between the incised wound edges and then reloaded and reinserted to exit on the contralateral side.
3. The needle body is grasped with surgical forceps in the left hand and pulled upward with the surgical forceps as the body of the needle is released from the needle driver. Alternatively, the needle may be released from the needle driver, and the needle driver itself may be used to grasp the needle from the contralateral side of the wound to complete

its rotation through its arc, obviating the need for surgical forceps.

4. The needle is then reloaded in a backhand fashion and inserted at 90 degrees perpendicular to the epidermis approximately 3 mm from the wound edge on the same side of the incision line as the exit point, between the exit point and the incised wound edge.

5. The needle is rotated superficially through its arc, exiting on the contralateral side of the wound 3 mm from the incised wound edge.

6. The suture material is then tied off gently, with care being taken to minimize tension across the epidermis and avoid overly constricting the wound edges (Figures 5-17A through 5-17F).

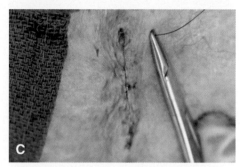

Figure 5-17C. The needle curves deep under the wound, exiting on the contralateral side. Note that in larger wounds or when working with smaller needles, the needle may exit through the center of the wound prior to being reinserted.

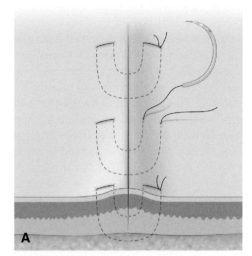

Figure 5-17A. Overview of the vertical mattress suture.

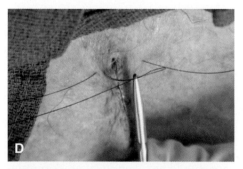

Figure 5-17D. The needle is then reinserted on the ipsilateral side, closer to the wound margin, again entering at 90 degrees to the wound surface.

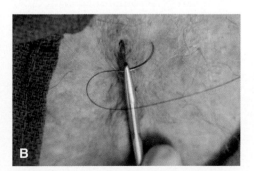

Figure 5-17B. The needle is inserted at 90 degrees to the skin, prior to angling slightly outward after it pierces the epidermis.

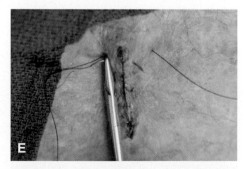

Figure 5-17E. The needle follows a more superficial course, exiting on the contralateral side, closer to the wound margin than the original suture entry point.

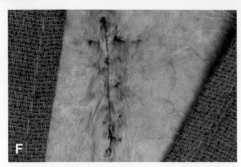

Figure 5-17F. Immediate postoperative appearance.

Tips and Pearls

This technique is generally used for its pronounced effect on wound eversion. Therefore, while it is appropriate for most skin closures, it should be avoided when either inversion is desired or when exaggerated eversion has already been accomplished with a buried suture.

As with most transepidermal techniques, it is important to enter the epidermis at 90 degrees, allowing the needle to travel slightly laterally away from the wound edge before fully following the curvature of the needle when utilizing this technique. This will allow for maximal wound eversion and accurate wound-edge approximation.

As with the simple interrupted suture, care should be taken to avoid skimming the needle superficially beneath the epidermis. This results from failing to enter the skin at a perpendicular angle and to follow the curvature of the needle. This may result in wound inversion as the tension vector of the shallow bite pulls the wound edges outward and down.

An advantage of this approach is that no suture material traverses the incised wound edge and that the suture similarly does not cross the surface of the wound. While this may be less than desirable when attempting to fine-tune epidermal apposition, it is helpful in minimizing the risk of unsightly track marks.

This technique is sometimes referred to as a far-far, near-near suture, based on its entry and exit points; the needle is first inserted far from the incised wound edge and then again exits far from the wound edge on the contralateral side. It is then reinserted near the wound edge on the ipsilateral side and exits near the wound edge on the contralateral side.

Note that the second throw is placed superficial to the first, deeper far-far suture, leading to a nested placement of the suture material. This leads to both wound eversion and wound-edge approximation.

The Allgöwer technique involves performing a half-buried vertical mattress suture: (1) The needle is passed from the far entrance point to the interior of the wound. (2) A buried vertical mattress bite is then taken on the contralateral side, by entering the underside of the dermis and exiting at the incised wound edge. The needle then passes back to the original side, entering near the incised wound edge so that one-half of the wound is closed with a standard vertical mattress suture and the other is closed with a buried vertical mattress.

Drawbacks and Cautions

This technique does not typically permit the same degree of wound-edge apposition as can be accomplished with other transepidermal sutures. In the event that deeper sutures were carefully placed, this may not be a significant drawback, since the wound edges may be well aligned from the placement of these deeper sutures. If not, or if there is a need for improved wound-edge apposition even after placing the vertical mattress suture, additional interrupted sutures may be helpful.

The placement of a vertical mattress suture can sometimes lead to what has been termed the sandwich phenomenon, where the tight dermal wound approximation leads to hyper-eversion of the wound edges and to a raised ridge with epidermal gaping at the center of the wound. If this occurs, placing a simple interrupted suture (see Chapter 5.1) directly over the offending vertical mattress suture can solve this problem.

Suture removal with this technique may be more involved than with simple interrupted sutures, particularly if sutures are left in situ for an extended period of time and some of the suture material has been overgrown by the healing epidermis. To address this problem, some have suggested suturing a length of silicon tubing (such as used in IV lines) along the length of the suture line and incorporating this into the stitch so that the suture can be cut directly over the tubing (or scissors may be inserted into the tubing directly to cut the suture).

As with any suturing technique, knowledge of the relevant anatomy is critical. When placing a vertical mattress suture, it is important to recall that the structures deep to the epidermis may be compromised by the passage of the needle and suture material or that constriction may take place. That said, the vertical orientation of this approach helps minimize this risk.

This technique may elicit an increased risk of track marks, necrosis, and other complications when compared with techniques that do not entail suture material traversing the scar line, such as buried or subcuticular approaches. Therefore, sutures should be removed as early as possible to minimize these complications, and consideration should be given to adopting other closure techniques in the event that sutures will not be able to be removed in a timely fashion.

References

Blattner CM, Markus B, Lear W. Correction of "sandwiching phenomenon" following horizontal mattress suture. *J Am Acad Dermatol.* 2018;78(4):e87-88.

Bolster M, Schipper C, Van Sterkenburg S, Ruettermann M, Reijnen M. Single interrupted sutures compared with Donati sutures after open carpal tunnel release: a prospective randomised trial. *J Plast Surg Hand Surg.* 2013;47(4):289-291.

Dietz UA, Kuhfuss I, Debus ES, Thiede A. Mario Donati and the vertical mattress suture of the skin. *World J Surg.* 2006;30(2):141-148.

Trimbos JB, Mouw R, Ranke G, Trimbos KB, Zwinderman K. The Donati stitch revisited: favorable cosmetic results in a randomized clinical trial. *J Surg Res.* 2002;107(1):131-134.

Zuber TJ. The mattress sutures: vertical, horizontal, and corner stitch. *Am Fam Physician.* 2002;66(12):2231-2236.

Zucchi A, Rovesti M, Satolli F et al. Simplified removal of the Donati stitch. *Dermatol Surg.* 2020;46(2):281-282.

The Shorthand Vertical Mattress Suture

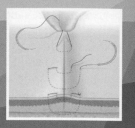

Synonym

Donati suture

Video 5-18. Shorthand vertical mattress suture
Access to video can be found via
mhprofessional.com/atlasofsuturingtechniques2e

Application

This is a modification of the vertical mattress suture, a frequently used everting technique used for closure and epidermal approximation. As with many interrupted techniques, it may be used alone for wounds under minimal tension, such as those formed by either a small punch biopsy or a traumatic laceration. Like its horizontal counterpart, it is also frequently used as a secondary layer to aid in everting the wound edges when the dermis has been closed using a deep suturing technique.

Suture Material Choice

With all techniques, it is best to use the thinnest suture possible in order to minimize the risk of track marks and foreign-body reactions. Suture choice will depend largely on anatomic location and the goal of suture placement.

On the face, a 6-0 or 7-0 monofilament suture may be used, though fast-absorbing gut may be used on the eyelids and ears to obviate the need for suture removal. When the goal of the shorthand vertical mattress suture placement is solely to encourage wound-edge eversion,

fine-gauge suture material may be used on the extremities as well. Otherwise, 5-0 monofilament suture material may be used if there is minimal tension, and 4-0 monofilament suture is useful in areas under moderate tension where the goal of suture placement is relieving tension as well as epidermal approximation. In select high-tension areas, 3-0 monofilament suture may be utilized as well.

Technique

1. The needle is inserted perpendicular to the epidermis, approximately 3 mm distant from the wound edge.
2. With a fluid motion of the wrist, the needle is rotated superficially through the dermis, and the needle tip exits the skin on the contralateral side.
3. The needle body is grasped with surgical forceps in the left hand and pulled upward with the surgical forceps as the body of the needle is released from the needle driver.
4. The needle is then reloaded in a backhand fashion and inserted 6 mm distant from the incised wound edge in line with the exit point on the ipsilateral side.
5. While gently pulling upward on the suture material in order to closely approximate the wound edges, the needle is rotated deep through its arc, exiting on the contralateral side of the wound 6 mm from the incised wound edge.

6. The suture material is then tied off gently, with care being taken to minimize tension across the epidermis and avoid overly constricting the wound edges (Figures 5-18A through 5-18E).

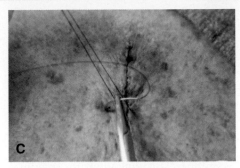

Figure 5-18C. The suture material is grasped with the nondominant hand and gently pulled upward, bringing the wound edges upward, as the needle is reinserted far from the incised wound edge.

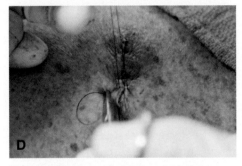

Figure 5-18D. The needle follows a course deep through the dermis, exiting far from the wound edge on the contralateral side.

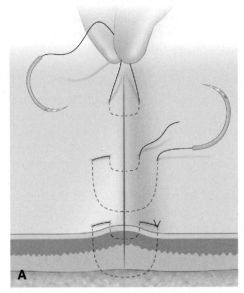

Figure 5-18A. Overview of the shorthand vertical mattress suture.

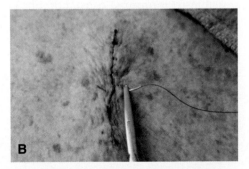

Figure 5-18B. The needle is inserted near the incision line perpendicularly through the epidermis and passes superficially through the dermis, exiting on the contralateral side near the incision line.

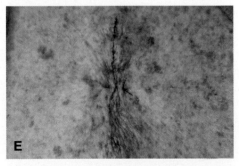

Figure 5-18E. Immediate postoperative appearance after placing a single shorthand vertical mattress suture.

Tips and Pearls

This represents a variation of the standard vertical mattress suture and has been advocated as a faster placement approach for what is functionally the same technique.

As with most transepidermal techniques, it is important to enter the epidermis at 90 degrees when utilizing this technique. This will allow for maximal wound eversion and accurate wound-edge approximation.

The shorthand vertical mattress technique has been termed the near-near, far-far technique, since the suture material enters near the wound edge and exits near the wound edge, and then reenters far from the wound edge and finally exits far from the wound edge. This is in contrast to the standard vertical mattress technique, which is a far-far, near-near technique, since the first bite of suture enters and exits far from the incised wound edge and the second, nested bite of suture enters and exits near the wound edge.

Drawbacks and Cautions

As with the simple interrupted suture, care should be taken to avoid skimming the needle superficially beneath the epidermis. This results from failing to enter the skin at a perpendicular angle and failing to follow the curvature of the needle. This problem may be particularly pronounced with the shorthand vertical mattress suture in novice hands, as the initial, superficially placed throw of suture material may be placed too superficially, resulting in suture material tear-through.

Since the second, deeper loop of suture is placed blindly when using the shorthand technique, care should be taken when working in areas with underlying vessels or nerves that could be pierced or strangulated by the deeper loop of suture. This is less of a problem when using the standard vertical mattress technique, since the deep loop is placed first, permitting full visualization of the underlying structures.

The shorthand vertical mattress technique does not typically permit the same degree of wound-edge apposition as can be accomplished with other transepidermal sutures, since the everting effect of the suture technique may even be associated with a small degree of gaping at the center of the vertical mattress suture.

As with the standard vertical mattress suture, suture removal with this technique may be more involved than with simple interrupted sutures, particularly if sutures are left in situ for an extended period of time and some of the suture material has been overgrown by the healing epidermis.

This technique may elicit an increased risk of track marks, necrosis, and other complications when compared with techniques that do not entail suture material traversing the scar line, such as buried or subcuticular approaches. Therefore, sutures should be removed as early as possible to minimize these complications, and consideration should be given to adopting other closure techniques in the event that sutures will not be able to be removed in a timely fashion.

References

Jones JS, Gartner M, Drew G, Pack S. The shorthand vertical mattress stitch: evaluation of a new suture technique. *Am J Emerg Med.* 1993;11(5):483-485.

Snow SN, Goodman MM, Lemke BN. The shorthand vertical mattress stitch—a rapid skin everting suture technique. *J Dermatol Surg Oncol.* 1989;15(4):379-381.

The Locking Vertical Mattress Suture

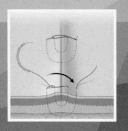

Synonym

Loop mattress suture

Video 5-19. Locking vertical mattress suture
Access to video can be found via
mhprofessional.com/atlasofsuturingtechniques2e

Application

This technique, also known as the loop mattress suture, is a locking variation of the vertical mattress suture that may be used for closure and epidermal approximation. Unlike the standard vertical mattress suture, it adds a section of suture crossing over the top of the incised wound edge, which may be useful to aid in wound-edge apposition. As with many interrupted techniques, it may be used alone for wounds under modest tension, such as those formed by either a small punch biopsy or a traumatic laceration.

Suture Material Choice

With all techniques, it is best to use the thinnest suture possible in order to minimize the risk of track marks and foreign-body reactions. Suture choice will depend largely on anatomic location and the goal of suture placement.

On the face, a 6-0 or 7-0 monofilament suture may be used, though fast-absorbing gut may be used on the eyelids and ears to obviate the need for suture removal. When the goal of the locking vertical mattress suture placement is solely to encourage wound-edge eversion, fine-gauge suture material may be used on the extremities as well. Otherwise, 5-0 monofilament suture material may be used if there is minimal tension, and 4-0 monofilament suture is useful in areas under moderate tension where the goal of suture placement is relieving tension as well as epidermal approximation. In select high-tension areas, 3-0 monofilament suture may be utilized as well.

Technique

1. The needle is inserted perpendicular to the epidermis, approximately 6 mm distant from the wound edge.
2. With a fluid motion of the wrist, the needle is rotated deep through the dermis, and the needle tip exits the skin on the contralateral side. If the needle radius is too small to complete this arc in one movement, this first step may be divided into two, with the needle first exiting between the incised wound edges and then reloaded and reinserted to exit on the contralateral side.
3. The needle body is grasped with surgical forceps in the left hand, with care being taken to avoid grasping the needle tip, which can be easily dulled by repetitive friction against the surgical forceps. It is gently grasped and pulled upward with the surgical forceps as the body of the needle is released from the needle driver. Alternatively, the needle may be

released from the needle driver, and the needle driver itself may be used to grasp the needle from the contralateral side of the wound to complete its rotation through its arc, obviating the need for surgical forceps.

4. The needle is then reloaded in a backhand fashion and inserted at 90 degrees perpendicular to the epidermis approximately 3 mm from the wound edge on the same side of the incision line as the exit point.

5. The needle is rotated superficially through its arc, exiting on the contralateral side of the wound 3 mm from the incised wound edge. Suture material is not pulled tight, however, and a loop of suture, formed by the exit of the suture material laterally and its reentry medially, is left in place.

6. In order to lock the suture over the top of the wound, the needle is passed through the loop formed by the exit and entry of suture material on the contralateral side.

7. The suture material is then tied off gently, with care being taken to

minimize tension across the epidermis and avoid overly constricting the wound edges (Figures 5-19A through 5-19F).

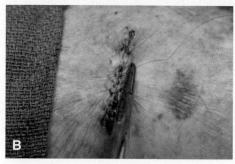

Figure 5-19B. The needle is inserted at 90 degrees to the skin and follows the curvature of the needle, exiting at the contralateral side.

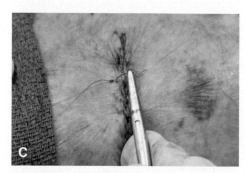

Figure 5-19C. The needle is then reloaded in a backhand fashion and inserted just medial to its exit point.

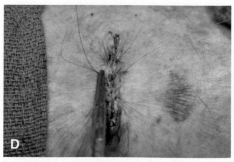

Figure 5-19D. The needle follows a shallow course and exits on the contralateral side, medial to the original insertion point.

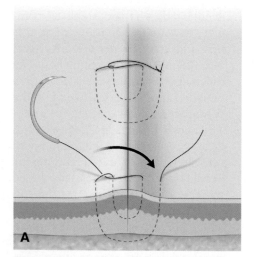

Figure 5-19A. Overview of the locking vertical mattress suture.

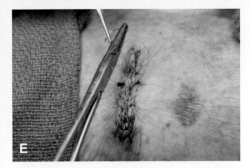

Figure 5-19E. The needle is then passed through the loop created by its exit and subsequent reentry on the contralateral side.

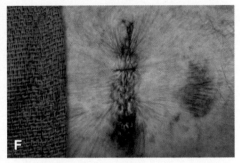

Figure 5-19F. Immediate postoperative appearance, showing the locking portion of the suture traversing the incised wound edge.

Tips and Pearls

This approach may be conceptualized as a hybrid between a vertical mattress suture, a simple interrupted suture, and a pulley suture. Like the vertical mattress suture, this technique leads to pronounced wound-edge eversion. Like the simple interrupted suture, this approach affords excellent wound-edge approximation. And like the pulley suture, the multiple loops lead to a reduction in needed tension across the suture material.

As with most transepidermal techniques, it is important to enter the epidermis at 90 degrees, following the curvature of the needle when utilizing this technique. This will allow for

maximal wound eversion and accurate wound-edge approximation.

As with the simple interrupted suture, care should be taken to avoid skimming the needle superficially beneath the epidermis. This results from failing to enter the skin at a perpendicular angle and to follow the curvature of the needle. This may result in wound inversion as the tension vector of the shallow bite pulls the wound edges outward and down.

Note that the second throw is placed superficial to the first, deeper far-far suture, leading to a nested placement of the suture material. This leads to both wound eversion and wound-edge approximation, and the final loop of suture material traversing the incised wound edge permits the wound edges to be precisely matched.

Before forming the final locking loop, it is helpful to pull through the bulk of the suture material, leaving only a modest tail and a small residual loop. This will help reduce the risk of the suture material tangling during pull through.

Drawbacks and Cautions

This technique ideally results in an everted wound with excellent wound-edge apposition due to the presence of the locking loop over the surface of the incised wound edge. In practice, the locking step may lead to wound-edge inversion, and therefore, this approach should be used selectively.

With any suturing technique, knowledge of the relevant anatomy is critical. When placing a vertical mattress suture, it is important to recall that the structures deep to the epidermis may be compromised by the passage of the needle and suture material or that constriction may take place. That said, the vertical orientation of this approach helps minimize this risk.

This technique may elicit an increased risk of track marks, necrosis, and other complications when compared with techniques that do not entail suture material traversing the scar line, such as buried or subcuticular approaches. Therefore, sutures should be removed as early as possible to minimize these complications, and consideration should be given to adopting other closure techniques in the event that sutures will not be able to be removed in a timely fashion.

Reference

Gault DT, Brain A, Sommerlad BC, Ferguson DJ. Loop mattress suture. *Br J Surg.* 1987;74(9):820-821.

The Running Vertical Mattress Suture

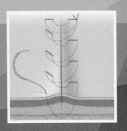

Video 5-20. Running vertical mattress suture
Access to video can be found via
mhprofessional.com/atlasofsuturingtechniques2e

Application

This is a running everting technique used for closure and epidermal approximation. Like any running technique, it may be used alone for wounds under minimal tension, such as wounds on the genitalia or traumatic lacerations. As with its interrupted counterpart, it is most frequently used as a secondary layer to aid in everting the wound edges when the dermis has been closed using a deep suturing technique.

Suture Material Choice

With all techniques, it is best to use the thinnest suture possible in order to minimize the risk of track marks and foreign-body reactions. Suture choice will depend largely on anatomic location and the goal of suture placement.

On the face, a 6-0 or 7-0 monofilament suture may be used, though fast-absorbing gut may be used on the eyelids and ears to obviate the need for suture removal. When the goal of the running vertical mattress suture placement is solely to encourage wound-edge eversion, fine-gauge suture material may be used on the extremities as well. Otherwise, 5-0 monofilament suture material is used if there is minimal tension, and 4-0 monofilament suture is useful in areas under moderate tension where the goal of suture placement is relieving tension as well as epidermal approximation. Occasionally, 3-0 monofilament suture may be utilized as well.

Technique

1. The needle is inserted perpendicular to the epidermis, approximately 6 mm distant to the wound edge.
2. With a fluid motion of the wrist, the needle is rotated through the dermis, taking the bite wider at the deep margin than at the surface, and the needle tip exits the skin on the contralateral side. If the needle radius is too small to complete this arc in one movement, this first step may be divided into two, with the needle first exiting between the incised wound edges and then reloaded and reinserted to exit on the contralateral side.
3. The needle body is grasped with surgical forceps in the left hand, with care being taken to avoid grasping the needle tip, which can be easily dulled by repetitive friction against the surgical forceps. It is gently grasped and pulled upward with the surgical forceps as the body of the needle is released from the needle driver. Alternatively, the needle may be released from the needle driver, and the needle driver itself may be used to grasp the needle from the contralateral side of

271

the wound to complete its rotation through its arc, obviating the need for surgical forceps.

4. The needle is then reloaded in a backhand fashion and inserted at 90 degrees perpendicular to the epidermis approximately 3 mm from the wound edge on the same side of the incision line as the exit point.

5. The needle is rotated superficially through its arc, exiting on the contralateral side of the wound 3 mm from the incised wound edge.

6. The suture material is then tied off gently, with care being taken to minimize tension across the epidermis and avoid overly constricting the wound edges.

7. Only the loose end of suture is trimmed.

8. The needle is then reinserted as in step (1), now just proximal (relative to the surgeon) and lateral (relative to the incised wound edge) to its exit point. This new entry point is therefore in line with the first entry point.

9. Steps (1) through (5) are then repeated sequentially, and after each set of steps, the new entry point—proximal and lateral to the exit point—permits a running placement of sutures.

10. Once the end of the wound is reached, the suture material is gently tied off (Figures 5-20A through 5-20G).

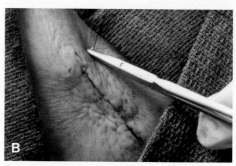

Figure 5-20B. Starting at the distal wound apex, the needle is inserted through the skin far from the incised wound edge at 90 degrees, exiting on the contralateral side far from the incised wound edge.

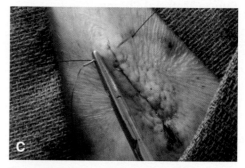

Figure 5-20C. The needle is then reloaded in a backhand fashion and inserted near the wound edge, following a superficial arc, and exits on the contralateral side, medial to the original entry point. The suture material is then tied, forming an anchoring vertical mattress suture.

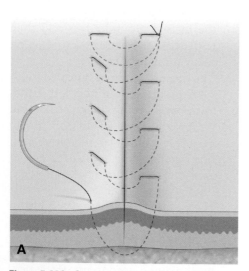

Figure 5-20A. Overview of the running vertical mattress suture.

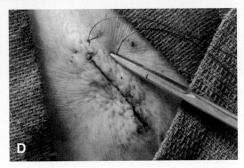

Figure 5-20D. The needle is then advanced along the length of the wound and inserted far from the incised wound edge, again exiting on the contralateral side of the wound far from the incised wound edge.

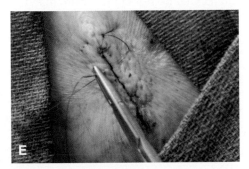

Figure 5-20E. The needle is then reloaded in a backhand fashion and inserted near to the incised wound edge following a shallow course and exiting on the contralateral side of the wound.

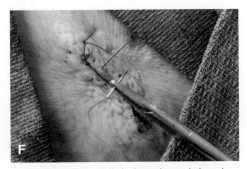

Figure 5-20F. The needle is then advanced along the wound and inserted, again far from the incised wound edge, and the pattern is repeated.

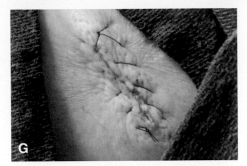

Figure 5-20G. Immediate postoperative appearance.

Tips and Pearls

This approach permits relatively rapid placement of an everting layer of suture material and was proposed as an even faster technique for vertical mattress suture placement than the shorthand (near-near, far-far) technique.

Like the interrupted vertical mattress technique, this approach should be avoided either when inversion is desired or when exaggerated eversion has already been accomplished with a buried suture.

As with most transepidermal techniques, it is important to enter the epidermis at 90 degrees, allowing the needle to travel slightly laterally away from the wound edge before fully following the curvature of the needle when utilizing this technique. This will allow for maximal wound eversion and accurate wound-edge approximation.

An advantage of this approach is that no suture material traverses the incised wound edge and that the suture similarly does not cross the surface of the wound. While this may be less than desirable when attempting to fine-tune epidermal apposition, it is helpful in minimizing the risk of unsightly track marks.

As with the interrupted vertical mattress approach, the second throw is placed superficial to the first, deeper far-far suture, leading to a nested placement of the suture material. This leads to both wound eversion and wound-edge approximation.

Drawbacks and Cautions

As a running technique, the integrity of the entire suture line rests on the security of the two anchoring knots. Since this approach is not relied on for tension relief, suture material breakage or knot failure, while undesirable, does not generally lead to catastrophic wound dehiscence. Indeed, the traction across the suture material itself affords a small degree of security, which may be sufficient to maintain eversion even in the face of knot breakage.

As with the interrupted vertical mattress approach, this technique does not typically permit the same degree of wound-edge apposition as can be accomplished with other transepidermal sutures, since the everting effect of the suture technique may even be associated with a small degree of gaping at the center of the running vertical mattress suture. In the event that deeper sutures were carefully placed, this may not be a significant drawback, since the wound edges may be well aligned from the placement of these deeper sutures.

Suture removal with this technique may be more involved than with simple interrupted sutures, particularly if sutures are left in situ for an extended period of time and some of the suture material has been overgrown by the healing epidermis.

As with any suturing technique, knowledge of the relevant anatomy is critical. When placing a vertical mattress suture, it is important to recall that the structures deep to the epidermis may be compromised by the passage of the needle and suture material or that constriction may take place. That said, the vertical orientation of this approach helps minimize this risk.

This technique may elicit an increased risk of track marks, necrosis, and other complications when compared with techniques that do not entail suture material traversing the scar line, such as buried or subcuticular approaches. Therefore, sutures should be removed as early as possible to minimize these complications, and consideration should be given to adopting other closure techniques in the event that the sutures will not be able to be removed in a timely fashion.

References

Kolbusz RV, Bielinski KB. Running vertical mattress suture. *J Dermatol Surg Oncol.* 1992;18(6):500-502.

Stiff MA, Snow SN. Running vertical mattress suturing technique. *J Dermatol Surg Oncol.* 1992;18(10):916-917.

The Running Alternating Simple and Vertical Mattress Suture

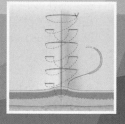

Synonym

Running combined simple and vertical mattress suture

Video 5-21. Running alternating simple and vertical mattress suture

Access to video can be found via mhprofessional.com/atlasofsuturingtechniques2e

Application

This is a hybrid running everting technique used for closure and epidermal approximation. Like any running technique, it may be used alone for wounds under minimal tension, such as wounds on the genitalia or traumatic lacerations. It is most frequently used as a secondary layer to aid in everting the wound edges when the dermis has been closed using a deep suturing technique, where the vertical mattress component helps with eversion and the simple running component aids with wound-edge approximation.

Suture Material Choice

With all techniques, it is best to use the thinnest suture possible in order to minimize the risk of track marks and foreign-body reactions. Suture choice will depend largely on anatomic location and the goal of suture placement.

On the face, a 6-0 or 7-0 monofilament suture maybe used, though fast-absorbing gut may be used on the eyelids and ears to obviate the need for suture removal. When the goal of the running alternating simple and vertical mattress suture placement is solely to encourage wound-edge eversion, fine-gauge suture material may be used on the extremities as well. Otherwise, 5-0 monofilament suture material is used if there is minimal tension, and 4-0 monofilament suture is useful in areas under moderate tension where the goal of suture placement is relieving tension as well as epidermal approximation. In select high-tension areas, 3-0 monofilament suture may be utilized as well.

Technique

A simple interrupted anchoring suture is placed as follows:
1. The needle is inserted perpendicular to the epidermis, approximately one-half the radius of the needle distant to the wound edge. This will allow the needle to exit the wound on the contralateral side at an equal distance from the wound edge by simply following the curvature of the needle.
2. With a fluid motion of the wrist, the needle is rotated through the dermis, taking the bite wider at the deep margin than at the surface, and the needle tip exits the skin on the contralateral side.
3. The needle body is grasped with surgical forceps in the left hand, with care being taken to avoid grasping the needle tip, which can be easily dulled by repetitive friction against the surgical forceps. It is gently grasped and pulled

upward with the surgical forceps as the body of the needle is released from the needle driver. Alternatively, the needle may be released from the needle driver and the needle driver itself may be used to grasp the needle from the contralateral side of the wound to complete its rotation through its arc, obviating the need for surgical forceps.

4. The suture material is then tied off gently, with care being taken to minimize tension across the epidermis and avoid overly constricting the wound edges.

5. The loose end of the suture material is then trimmed.

6. The needle is reinserted perpendicular to the epidermis, approximately 6 mm distant from the wound edge, just proximal relative to the surgeon from its exit point.

7. With a fluid motion of the wrist, the needle is rotated through the dermis at a 45-degree angle toward the surgeon (and away from the prior stitch), and the needle tip exits the skin on the contralateral side, equidistant from the incised wound edge and proximal, relative to the surgeon, from its entry point.

8. The needle is then reloaded in a backhand fashion and inserted at 90 degrees perpendicular to the epidermis approximately 3 mm from the wound edge on the same side of the incision line as the exit point.

9. The needle is rotated superficially through its arc, exiting on the contralateral side of the wound 3 mm from the incised wound edge.

10. The needle is then reloaded in a standard fashion and reinserted on the ipsilateral side of the wound edge but now approximately 6 mm from the incised wound edge, yet still in line with its exit point.

11. The needle is then reinserted as in step (1), now just proximal (relative to the surgeon) and lateral (relative to the incised wound edge) to its exit point. This new entry point is therefore in line with the first entry point.

12. The needle is again passed at a 45-degree angle toward the surgeon (and away from the prior stitch), and the needle tip exits the skin on the contralateral side, equidistant from the incised wound edge and proximal, relative to the surgeon, from its entry point.

13. The needle is then inserted on the contralateral side of the incised wound edge, equidistant from the incised edge and further proximal relative to the surgeon.

14. Steps (6) through (13) are then repeated sequentially, until the end of the wound is reached.

15. Once the end of the wound is reached, the suture material is gently tied off (Figures 5-21A through 5-21I).

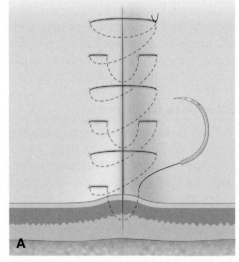

Figure 5-21A. Overview of the running alternating simple and vertical mattress technique.

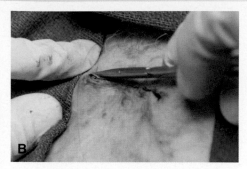

Figure 5-21B. Placement of the anchoring suture. Note the entry and exit of the suture at 90 degrees.

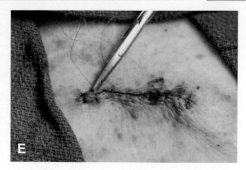

Figure 5-21E. The running component continues, with the needle entering the skin lateral to its exit point and continuing along a diagonal path across the wound edge.

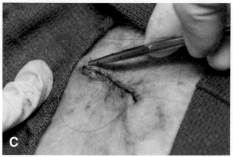

Figure 5-21C. The simple running component begins. Note that the path of suture follows a diagonal relative to the wound edge.

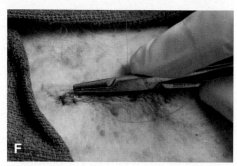

Figure 5-21F. The intermittent simple loop is placed directly across the wound edge.

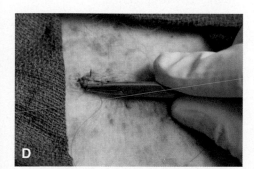

Figure 5-21D. The vertical mattress component—the needle is inserted medial to its exit point and follows a superficial path, exiting on the contralateral wound edge.

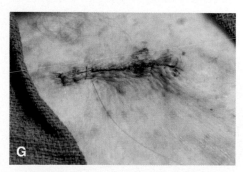

Figure 5-21G. Appearance after the placement of the first set of running and vertical mattress sutures.

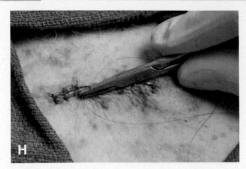

Figure 5-21H. The vertical mattress component continues.

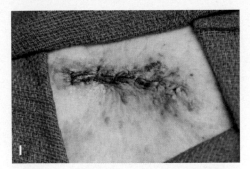

Figure 5-21I. Immediate postoperative appearance, prior to cleaning the wound. Note that the wound-edge approximation is better where the simple loops are present, although wound edges are well everted overall.

Tips and Pearls

This approach permits relatively rapid placement of an everting layer of vertical mattress sutures, and the incorporation of the simple loops means that it is even faster to place than the running vertical mattress suture, since the simple loops require only a single forehand throw of suture material versus the two throws needed for each vertical mattress suture.

The presence of the simple loops also affords easier suture removal, as the loops of interrupted suture may be easily grasped and cut at the time the sutures are removed.

Of course, like the interrupted vertical mattress technique, this approach should be avoided when either inversion

is desired or when exaggerated eversion has already been accomplished with a buried suture.

As with the interrupted vertical mattress approach, the second throw of the vertical mattress component is placed superficial to the first, deeper far-far suture, leading to a nested placement of the suture material. This leads to both wound eversion and wound-edge approximation. Similarly, each of the simple sutures should be placed by taking a larger bite of tissue at their deep portion in order to better evert the wound edges.

Drawbacks and Cautions

Unlike many other running techniques, this approach relies on the suture material traversing the wound at a 45-degree angle in order to permit the individual vertical mattress components to remain perpendicular to the incised wound edge and simultaneously allow the running nature of this technique to progress along the length of the wound. While this results in a neat postoperative appearance, with visible suture material sitting perpendicular to the incised wound edge, it also means that the tension vector of the sutures is at an angle to the underlying tension across the incised wound edge.

As a running technique, the integrity of the entire suture line rests on the security of the two anchoring knots. Since this approach is not relied on for tension relief, suture material breakage or knot failure, while undesirable, does not generally lead to catastrophic wound dehiscence. Indeed, the weaving of the suture material itself affords a small degree of security that may be sufficient to maintain eversion even in the face of knot breakage.

With any suturing technique, knowledge of the relevant anatomy is critical. When placing a vertical mattress suture, it is important to recall that the structures deep to the epidermis may be compromised by the passage of the needle and suture material or that constriction may take place. That said, the vertical orientation of this approach helps minimize this risk.

This technique may elicit an increased risk of track marks, necrosis, and other complications when compared with techniques that do not entail suture material traversing the scar line, such as buried or subcuticular approaches. Therefore, sutures should be removed as early as possible to minimize these complications, and consideration should be given to adopting other closure techniques in the event that sutures will not be able to be removed in a timely fashion.

Reference

Krunic AL, Weitzul S, Taylor RS. Running combined simple and vertical mattress suture: a rapid skin-everting stitch. *Dermatol Surg.* 2005;31(10):1325-1329.

The Hybrid Mattress Suture

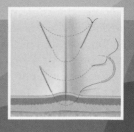

 Video 5-22. Hybrid mattress suture
Access to video can be found via
mhprofessional.com/atlasofsuturingtechniques2e

Application

This is a niche everting technique used for closure and epidermal approximation. It represents a cross between the vertical mattress and horizontal mattress techniques. As with many interrupted techniques, it may be used alone for wounds under minimal tension, such as those formed by either a small punch biopsy or a traumatic laceration.

Suture Material Choice

With all techniques, it is best to use the thinnest suture possible in order to minimize the risk of track marks and foreign-body reactions. Suture choice will depend largely on anatomic location and the goal of suture placement.

On the face, a 6-0 or 7-0 monofilament suture is used, though fast-absorbing gut may be used on the eyelids and ears to obviate the need for suture removal. When the goal of the hybrid mattress suture placement is solely to encourage wound-edge eversion, fine-gauge suture material may be used on the extremities as well. Otherwise, 5-0 monofilament suture material is used if there is minimal tension, and 4-0 monofilament suture is useful in areas under moderate tension where the goal of suture placement is relieving tension as well as epidermal approximation. Occasionally, 3-0 monofilament suture may be utilized as well.

Technique

1. The needle is inserted perpendicular to the epidermis, approximately 6 mm distant to the wound edge.
2. With a fluid motion of the wrist, the needle is rotated through the dermis, taking the bite wider at the deep margin than at the surface, and the needle tip exits the skin on the contralateral side. If the needle radius is too small to complete this arc in one movement, this first step may be divided into two, with the needle first exiting between the incised wound edges and then reloaded and reinserted to exit on the contralateral side.
3. The needle body is grasped with surgical forceps in the left hand, with care being taken to avoid grasping the needle tip, which can be easily dulled by repetitive friction against the surgical forceps. It is gently grasped and pulled upward with the surgical forceps as the body of the needle is released from the needle driver.
4. The needle is then reloaded in a backhand fashion and inserted at 90 degrees perpendicular to the epidermis approximately 3 mm from the wound edge on the same side of the incision line as the exit point, proximal from the exit point relative to the surgeon.

5. The needle is rotated through its arc, exiting on the contralateral side of the wound 3 mm from the incised wound edge.

6. The suture material is then tied off gently, with care being taken to minimize tension across the epidermis and avoid overly constricting the wound edges (Figures 5-22A through 5-22E).

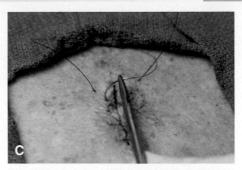

Figure 5-22C. The needle is reloaded in a backhand fashion and inserted "near" the incised wound edge.

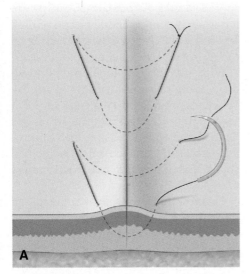

Figure 5-22A. Overview of the hybrid mattress suture technique.

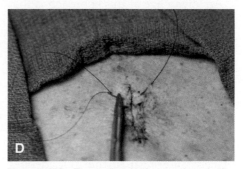

Figure 5-22D. The needle exits the contralateral side of the wound, again "near" the wound edge.

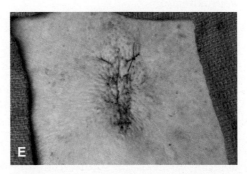

Figure 5-22E. Immediate postoperative appearance. Note the subtle trapezoidal configuration and pronounced wound eversion.

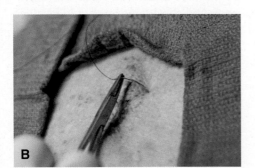

Figure 5-22B. The needle is inserted at 90 degrees, "far" from the incised wound edge, exiting on the contralateral wound edge, again relatively far from the edge.

Tips and Pearls

This technique has been advocated as a cross between a vertical and horizontal mattress suture, affording the benefits of both a vertical and horizontal mattress suture.

As with most transepidermal techniques, it is important to enter the epidermis at 90 degrees, allowing the needle to travel slightly laterally away from the wound edge before fully following the curvature of the needle when utilizing this technique.

An advantage of this approach is that no suture material traverses the incised wound edge and that the suture similarly does not cross the surface of the wound. While this may be less than desirable when attempting to fine-tune epidermal apposition, it is helpful in minimizing the risk of unsightly track marks.

As with the vertical mattress technique, note that the second throw is placed superficial to the first, deeper far-far suture, leading to a nested placement of the suture material. This leads to both wound eversion and wound-edge approximation.

Drawbacks and Cautions

In practice, this technique does not typically afford significant benefits over a horizontal mattress suture, and like other mattress approaches, it does not typically permit the same degree of wound-edge apposition as can be accomplished with other transepidermal sutures, since the everting effect of the suture technique may even be associated with a small degree of gaping at the center of the vertical mattress suture. In the event that deeper sutures were carefully placed, this may not be a significant drawback, since the wound edges may be well aligned from the placement of these deeper sutures. If not, or if there is a need for improved wound-edge apposition even after placing the vertical mattress suture, additional interrupted sutures may be helpful.

As with other mattress techniques, suture removal with this technique may be more involved than with simple interrupted sutures, particularly if sutures are left in situ for an extended period of time and some of the suture material has been overgrown by the healing epidermis.

With any suturing technique, knowledge of the relevant anatomy is critical. When placing a hybrid mattress suture, it is important to recall that the structures deep to the epidermis may be compromised by the passage of the needle and suture material or that constriction may take place.

This technique may elicit an increased risk of track marks, necrosis, and other complications when compared with techniques that do not entail suture material traversing the scar line, such as buried or subcuticular approaches. Therefore, sutures should be removed as early as possible to minimize these complications, and consideration should be given to adopting other closure techniques in the event that sutures will not be able to be removed in a timely fashion.

References

Hoffman MD, Bielinski KB. Surgical pearl: the hybrid mattress suture. *J Am Acad Dermatol.* 1997;36(5 pt 1):773-774.

Makkar S, Sharma R, Nanda V. Hybrid mattress suture. *Plast Reconstr Surg.* 2004;114(7): 1971-1973.

The Tip Stitch

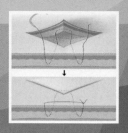

Synonym

Half-buried horizontal mattress suture

Video 5-23. Tip stitch
Access to video can be found via
mhprofessional.com/atlasofsuturingtechniques2e

Application

This technique is designed to bring three ends of tissue together and is often used in the context of a flap, where it permits the tip of tissue to be inset. It is also utilized to repair V-shaped lacerations. This approach may be conceptualized as a half-buried horizontal mattress suture. Since it is used only when attempting to approximate three segments of skin, it is a niche technique.

Suture Material Choice

Suture choice is dependent in large part on location, though as always, the smallest gauge suture material appropriate for the anatomic location should be utilized. On the face, where this technique may be used for flap repairs, a 6-0 or 7-0 monofilament nonabsorbable suture is appropriate. On the trunk, extremities, and scalp, a 3-0 or 4-0 nonabsorbable suture material may be used. Fast-absorbing gut may also be used, obviating the need for suture removal but increasing the risk of tissue reactivity.

Technique

1. The flap is brought into place using buried sutures, allowing the tip to rest with only minimal tension in its desired position.
2. The needle is inserted into the distal edge of the distal nonflap section of skin at 90 degrees with a trajectory running toward the planned entry point in the tip.
3. The needle is then grasped with the surgical pickups and simultaneously released by the hand holding the needle driver. As the needle is freed from the tissue with the pickups, the needle is grasped again by the needle driver in an appropriate position to place the next throw.
4. The needle is inserted into the distal portion of the tip at the level of the superficial dermis, which should be the same depth at which it exited in the prior step. Keeping the needle running horizontally, parallel with the skin surface, it is rotated through the dermis of the tip, exiting on the proximal side of the tip at the same depth.
5. The needle is then reloaded in a backhand fashion and inserted into the dermis of the proximal nontip section of skin, exiting parallel to its initial entry point.

6. The suture material is then gently tied utilizing an instrument tie. Care should be taken to minimize tension on this suture to mitigate the risk of flap tip necrosis (Figures 5-23A through 5-23G).

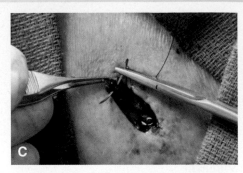

Figure 5-23C. The needle is then inserted through the mid-dermis of the tip.

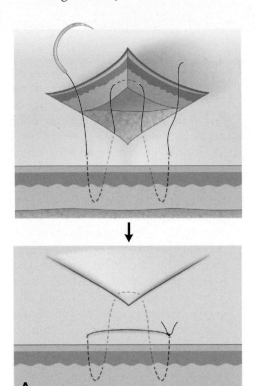

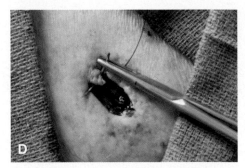

Figure 5-23D. View of the needle passing through the tip. Note that the needle does not pierce the epidermis of the tip.

Figure 5-23A. Overview of the tip stitch.

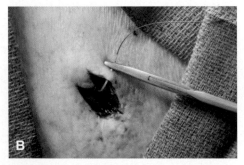

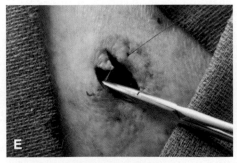

Figure 5-23B. The needle is inserted through the epidermis at 90 degrees on the nontip skin, exiting the mid-dermis.

Figure 5-23E. The needle is then inserted from the deep dermis through to the outside of the skin on the contralateral nontip wound edge.

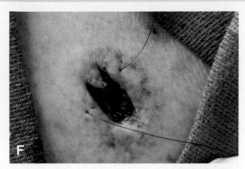

Figure 5-23F. Appearance of the suture prior to tying.

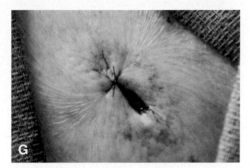

Figure 5-23G. Immediate postoperative appearance immediately after suture tying. Note that the tip is brought into place in close alignment with the other wound edges.

Tips and Pearls

The tip stitch is very useful when bringing the tip of a flap into place and is used frequently in this situation. Importantly, this technique is designed to gently approximate the tissues so that the flap is properly inset in the surrounding skin. While it bears a technical resemblance to the half-buried horizontal mattress, it is important to appreciate that the tip stitch is not designed to work under significant tension, as tension across the suture may lead to necrosis of the delicate and lightly vascularized tip of the flap.

Placing set-back dermal sutures, imbrication sutures, or suspension sutures prior to placement of the tip stitch will ensure that the tip itself is not under tension when it is approximated with the surrounding skin.

Drawbacks and Cautions

Flap tip necrosis is the greatest risk with this technique, since suture material traverses the dermis containing the tip's vascular supply. This risk may be mitigated by tying the suture relatively loosely so that the tip is not overly constricted when the knot is tied. Additionally, if the bites of dermis are sufficiently set back from the wound edge, a small bite comprising less than half of the dermis in the tip could be taken. This would allow blood supply to the tip even in the context of a relatively tight loop running through the distal flap.

There is sometimes a tendency for the tip to sit deeper than the surrounding tissues. This may be related to the relative upward pull on the nontip sections of skin by the transepidermal sutures.

Finally, while flap tip necrosis is a risk, studies have suggested that the tip stitch provides less vascular constriction than other options, such as placing two vertically oriented sutures at the edges of the tip or a suture directly through the tip itself. Vascular compromise and ensuing necrosis of the flap tip are always a risk, even if no sutures are placed through the tip itself, and therefore, the tip stitch approach likely provides a reasonable balance between tissue approximation and adequate vascular supply.

References

Bechara FG, Al-Muhammadi R, Sand M, et al. A modified corner stitch for fixation of flap tips. *Dermatol Surg.* 2007;33(10):1277-1279.

Kandel EF, Bennett RG. The effect of stitch type on flap tip blood flow. *J Am Acad Dermatol.* 2001;44(2):265-272.

McQuown SA, Cook TA, Brummett RE, Trachy RE. Gillies' corner stitch revisited. *Arch Otolaryngol.* 1984;110(7):450-453.

The Vertical Mattress Tip Stitch

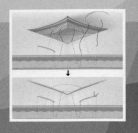

Synonym

Modified corner stitch

Video 5-24. Vertical mattress tip stitch
Access to video can be found via
mhprofessional.com/atlasofsuturingtechniques2e

Application

This technique, also described as the modified corner stitch, is designed to bring three ends of tissue together and is used in the context of a flap, where it permits the tip of tissue to be inset. This can be conceptualized as a vertical mattress variation of the tip stitch, permitting circumferential tissue advancement while concomitantly encouraging wound eversion and mitigating the risk that the tip is set deeper than the surrounding wound edges. Since it is used only when attempting to approximate three segments of skin, this is a niche technique.

Suture Material Choice

Suture choice is dependent in large part on location, though as always, the smallest gauge suture material appropriate for the anatomic location should be utilized. On the face, where this technique may be used for flap repairs, a 6-0 suture is appropriate. On the trunk, extremities, and scalp, a 3-0 or 4-0 suture material may be used. Monofilament nonabsorbable suture material is generally appropriate when utilizing this technique.

Technique

1. The flap is brought into place using buried sutures, allowing the tip to rest with only minimal tension in its desired position.
2. The needle is inserted through the epidermis at 90 degrees starting at the far right edge of the distal nonflap section of skin, with a trajectory running toward the tip. This entry point through the epidermis should be approximately 3 mm set back from the epidermal edge, depending on the thickness of the dermis and the anticipated degree of tension across the tip. The needle, and therefore the suture, should exit in the mid-dermis on the same portion of nonflap skin. Bite size is dependent on needle size.
3. The needle is then grasped with the surgical pickups and simultaneously released by the hand holding the needle driver. As the needle is freed from the tissue with the pickups, the needle is grasped again by the needle driver in an appropriate position to place a suture through the dermis on the flap tip to the left of the previously placed suture.
4. A small amount of suture material is pulled through, and the needle is inserted into the dermis in the flap tip, at the same depth as it exited from the nonflap edge, and the needle is passed through the dermis on the flap tip at a uniform

depth following a trajectory tracing an imaginary circle around the point where all three segments of skin will meet. The needle is then grasped with surgical forceps and released from the needle driver.

5. Attention is then shifted to the proximal nonflap edge of skin, where the needle is inserted in the mid-dermis of the incised edge, with the needle exiting through the epidermis in a mirror image of step (2).

6. The needle is reinserted through the epidermis just medial to the exit point, exiting through the dermis at the incised wound edge of the nonflap skin.

7. The needle is then reinserted in the dermis on the flap in a mirror-image of the technique utilized in step (4), running at the same depth of the dermis but distal to the suture material placed in step (4) relative to the flap tip.

8. The needle is then inserted through the dermis at the incised wound edge on the initial edge of nonflap skin, exiting medial and superior to the original entry point.

9. The suture material is then tied utilizing an instrument tie (Figures 5-24A through 5-24H).

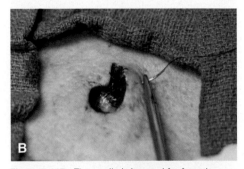

Figure 5-24B. The needle is inserted far from the wound edge, exiting at the level of the deep dermis.

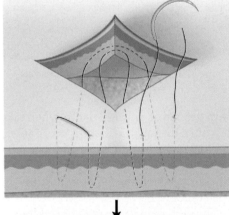

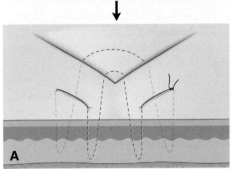

Figure 5-24A. Overview of the vertical mattress tip stitch.

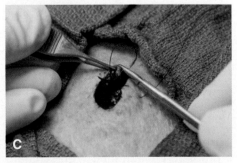

Figure 5-24C. The needle is then inserted through the dermis of the tip, moving laterally along the dermis, without penetrating the epidermis.

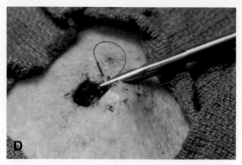

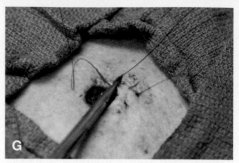

Figure 5-24D. The needle is then inserted through the dermis of the nontip skin, exiting far from the wound edge.

Figure 5-24G. The needle is then inserted through the dermis of the nontip skin, exiting medial to its original entry point. The suture is then tied.

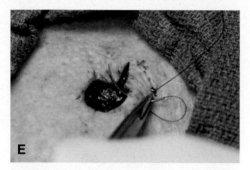

Figure 5-24E. The needle is then inserted closer to the incised wound edge.

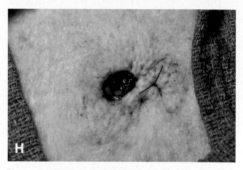

Figure 5-24H. Immediate postoperative appearance.

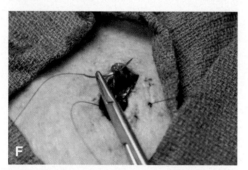

Figure 5-24F. The needle is then inserted through the dermis of the tip, superficial to its prior arc of passage.

Tips and Pearls

This technique was developed to solve a problem encountered with standard tip stitch techniques—the tendency of the flap tip to sit deep relative to the surrounding skin. Some of this problem may be due to lack of attention to the

importance of uniform depth when taking bites through the dermis on all sides, though more likely, it is related to the relative upward pull on the nontip sections of skin by the transepidermal sutures in the standard tip stitch.

The vertical mattress variation of the tip stitch therefore allows better wound eversion and has less of a tendency toward a depressed tip than the standard approach.

The tip stitch is very useful when bringing the tip of a flap into place. Importantly, this technique is designed to gently approximate the tissues so that the flap is properly inset in the surrounding skin. While it bears a technical resemblance to the buried purse-string approach, it is important to appreciate that the tip stitch is not designed to work under significant tension, as tension across the suture may lead to necrosis of the delicate and lightly vascularized tip of the flap.

This is particularly important here, since the vertical mattress tip stitch places two loops of suture material through the tip, increasing the risk of necrosis and tissue strangulation.

Placing set-back dermal sutures, imbrication sutures, or suspension sutures prior to placement of the tip stitch will ensure that the tip itself is not under tension when it is approximated with the surrounding skin.

Yet another variation of this technique entails burying the bite through the second nonflap wound edge so that the only percutaneous sutures are in the first nonflap edge of skin. In this case, steps (5) and (6) are replaced by taking a bite through the dermis alone before beginning the return course of the suture. This approach may slightly lessen the chance of infection and residual dimpling since the suture material on that edge does not traverse the epidermis. This half-buried approach is similar to the Allgöwer variation of the vertical mattress suture.

Drawbacks and Cautions

Flap tip necrosis is the greatest risk with this technique, since two loops of suture material traverse the dermis containing the tip's vascular supply. This risk may be mitigated by tying the suture together relatively loosely so that the tip is not overly constricted when the knot is tied.

Additionally, if the bites of dermis are sufficiently set back from the wound edge, a small bite comprising less than half of the dermis in the tip could be taken. This would allow blood supply to the tip even in the context of a relatively tight loop running through the distal flap.

Since this technique entails the placement of two loops of suture through the flap tip, it may be associated with a higher rate of necrosis than other variations of the tip stitch. Therefore, unless the better wound-edge approximation of the vertical mattress placement is needed, it may be preferable to adopt other variations of the tip stitch that do not require the additional loop of suture through the tip.

Finally, while flap tip necrosis is a risk, studies have suggested that the tip stitch provides less vascular constriction than other options, such as placing two vertically oriented sutures at the edges of the tip or a suture directly through the tip itself. Vascular compromise and ensuing necrosis of the flap tip are always a risk, even if no sutures are placed through the tip itself, and therefore, the tip stitch approach likely provides a reasonable balance between tissue approximation and adequate vascular supply.

References

Bechara FG, Al-Muhammadi R, Sand M, et al. A modified corner stitch for fixation of flap tips. *Dermatol Surg.* 2007;33(10):1277-1279.

Kandel EF, Bennett RG. The effect of stitch type on flap tip blood flow. *J Am Acad Dermatol.* 2001;44(2):265-272.

The Hybrid Mattress Tip Stitch

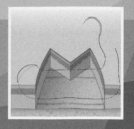

Synonym

Vertical mattress tip stitch

Video 5-25. Hybrid mattress tip stitch

Access to video can be found via
mhprofessional.com/atlasofsuturingtechniques2e

Application

This technique is designed to bring three ends of tissue together and is used in the context of a flap or M-plasty, where it permits the tip of tissue to be inset. This approach may be conceptualized as a hybrid mattress suture that encompasses the dermis of the tip of suture in its near-near step. Since it is used only when attempting to approximate three segments of skin, it is a niche technique.

Suture Material Choice

Suture choice is dependent in large part on location, though as always, the smallest gauge suture material appropriate for the anatomic location should be utilized. On the face, where this technique may be used for flap repairs, a 6-0 or 7-0 monofilament nonabsorbable suture is appropriate. On the trunk, extremities, and scalp, a 3-0 or 4-0 nonabsorbable suture material may be used. Fast-absorbing gut may also be used, obviating the need for suture removal but increasing the risk of tissue reactivity.

Technique

1. The flap is brought into place using buried sutures, allowing the tip to rest with only minimal tension in or close to its desired position.
2. Starting approximately 4 mm distal from the point where the flap tip will be inset, the needle is inserted perpendicular to the epidermis, approximately 6 mm distant to the wound edge.
3. With a fluid motion of the wrist, the needle is rotated through the dermis, taking the bite wider at the deep margin than at the surface, and the needle tip exits the skin on the contralateral side. If the needle radius is too small to complete this arc in one movement, this first step may be divided into two, with the needle first exiting between the incised wound edges and then reloaded and reinserted to exit on the contralateral side.
4. The needle body is grasped with surgical forceps in the left hand, with care being taken to avoid grasping the needle tip, which can be easily dulled by repetitive friction against the surgical forceps.
5. The needle is then reloaded in a backhand fashion and inserted at 90 degrees perpendicular to the epidermis approximately 3 mm from the wound edge on the same side of the incision line as the exit point, distal

from the exit point relative to the surgeon so that it is approximately 2 mm proximal to the flap tip.

6. The needle is rotated superficially through its arc, exiting in the undermined space.

7. The needle is then reloaded, again in a backhand fashion, and a modest bite of the dermis in the flap tip is taken. The needle moves parallel to the skin surface and does not penetrate the epidermis of the tip.

8. The needle is then again reloaded in a backhand fashion and inserted into the superficial dermis on the contralateral side, exiting through the epidermis similarly to steps (5) and (6).

9. The suture material is then tied off gently, with care being taken to minimize tension across the epidermis and avoid overly constricting the wound edges. Care should be taken to minimize tension on this suture to mitigate the risk of flap tip necrosis (Figures 5-25A through 5-25G).

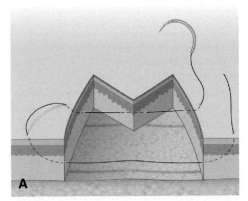

Figure 5-25A. Overview of the hybrid mattress tip stitch.

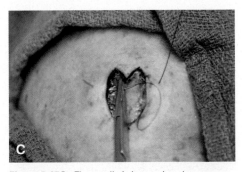

Figure 5-25C. The needle is inserted on the contralateral wound edge, exiting far from the incised wound edge.

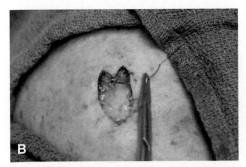

Figure 5-25B. The needle is inserted at 90 degrees to the skin, far from the skin edge and far from the tip, exiting in the open wound space.

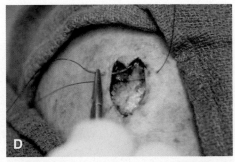

Figure 5-25D. The needle is then inserted closer to the skin edge and closer to the tip, exiting in the undermined space.

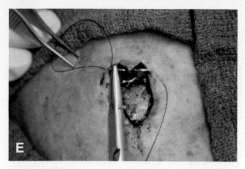

Figure 5-25E. The needle is then passed through the dermis on the tip; it does not penetrate the epidermis of the tip and instead stays at a constant depth in the dermis.

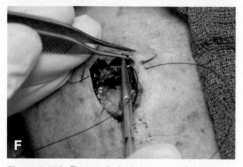

Figure 5-25F. The needle is then inserted from the underside of the dermis, exiting the epidermis close to the wound edge. The suture material is then tied, securing the tip in place.

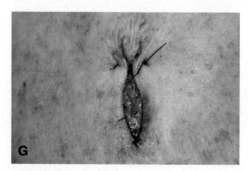

Figure 5-25G. Immediate postoperative view.

Tips and Pearls

The hybrid mattress tip stitch is very useful when bringing the tip of an M-plasty into position. Importantly, as with the standard tip stitch, this technique is designed to gently approximate the tissues so that the flap is properly inset in the surrounding skin. While it bears a technical resemblance to the hybrid mattress, it is important to appreciate that the hybrid mattress tip stitch is not designed to work under significant tension, as tension across the suture may lead to necrosis of the delicate and lightly vascularized tip of the flap.

As with the tip stitch, placing set-back dermal sutures, imbrication sutures, or suspension sutures prior to placement of the tip stitch will ensure that the tip itself is not under tension when it is approximated with the surrounding skin.

Note that the near-near step incorporating the flap tip bite is taken just proximal to the tip of the flap, while the initial far-far bite is taken distal to the flap tip. The sling-like effect of this approach forces the tip into place, securing it in its desired position.

The vertical mattress component of this approach helps mitigate the risk of flap tip inversion, an occasional drawback of the standard tip stitch technique.

Drawbacks and Cautions

As with all tip stitch techniques, flap tip necrosis is the greatest risk with this technique, since suture material traverses the dermis containing the tip's vascular supply. This risk may be mitigated by tying the suture relatively loosely so that the tip is not overly constricted when the knot is tied. Additionally, if the bites of dermis are sufficiently set back from the wound edge, a small bite comprising less than half of the dermis in the tip could be taken. This would allow blood supply to the tip even in the context of a relatively tight loop running through the distal flap.

Finally, while flap tip necrosis is a risk, studies have suggested that the tip stitch provides less vascular constriction than other options, such as placing two vertically oriented sutures at the edges of the tip or a suture directly through the tip itself. Vascular compromise and ensuing necrosis of the flap tip are always a risk, even if no sutures are placed through the tip itself, and therefore, the tip stitch approach likely provides a reasonable balance between tissue approximation and adequate vascular supply.

References

Kandel EF, Bennett RG. The effect of stitch type on flap tip blood flow. *J Am Acad Dermatol.* 2001;44(2):265-272.

Starr J. Surgical pearl: the vertical mattress tip stitch. *J Am Acad Dermatol.* 2001;44(3):523-524.

The Percutaneous Tip Stitch

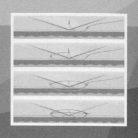

Synonym

Three-dimensional continuous suturing technique

Video 5-26. Percutaneous tip stitch

Access to video can be found via mhprofessional.com/atlasofsuturingtechniques2e

Application

This technique is designed to bring three ends of tissue together and is generally used in the context of a flap or cleft lip repair, where it permits the tip of tissue to be inset. It is also utilized to repair V-shaped lacerations. This approach may be conceptualized as a percutaneous variation of the traditional tip stitch. Since it is used only when attempting to approximate three segments of skin, it is a niche technique.

Suture Material Choice

Suture choice is dependent in large part on location, though as always, the smallest gauge suture material appropriate for the anatomic location should be utilized. On the face, where this technique may be used for flap repairs, a 6-0 or 7-0 monofilament nonabsorbable suture is appropriate. On the trunk, extremities, and scalp, a 3-0 or 4-0 nonabsorbable suture material may be used. Fast-absorbing absorbable sutures may also be used, obviating the need for suture removal but increasing the risk of tissue reactivity.

Technique

1. The flap is brought into place using buried sutures, allowing the tip to rest with only minimal tension in its desired position.
2. The needle is inserted into the distal nonflap section of skin at 90 degrees with a trajectory running toward the planned entry point in the center of the triangular section of skin (the tip).
3. The needle is inserted through the undersurface in the center of the triangular section of skin, following its curvature and exiting. As the needle is freed from the tissue with the pickups, the needle is grasped again by the needle driver in an appropriate position to place the next throw.
4. The needle is then inserted into the proximal nonflap portion of skin at 90 degrees with a trajectory running toward the planned entry point in the center of the triangular section of skin (the tip), directly adjacent to its exit point.
5. The needle is inserted through the undersurface in the center of the triangular section of skin, following its curvature and exiting. As the needle is freed from the tissue with the pickups, the needle is grasped again by the needle driver in an appropriate position to place the next throw.
6. The needle is then inserted into the distal nonflap section of skin at 90 degrees adjacent to its original entry

point, now with a trajectory running toward the proximal edge of the nonflap section of skin.

7. The needle exits at the proximal nonflap section adjacent to its prior exit point.

8. The suture material is then gently tied utilizing an instrument tie. Care should be taken to minimize tension on this suture to mitigate the risk of flap tip necrosis (Figures 5-26A through 5-26G).

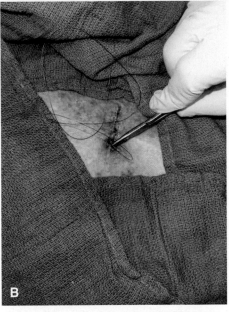

Figure 5-26B. The needle is inserted into the distal section of skin at 90 degrees with a trajectory running toward the planned entry point in the center of the triangular section of skin (the tip).

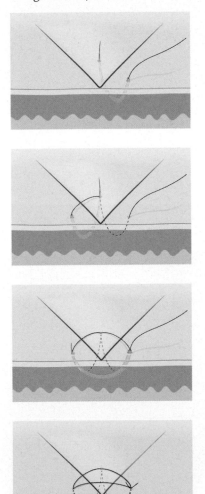

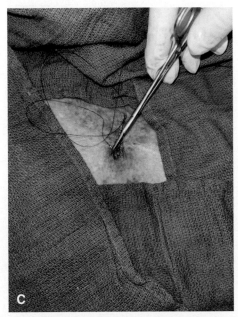

Figure 5-26C. The needle is passed through the tip and reloaded.

Figure 5-26A. Overview of the percutaneous tip stitch.

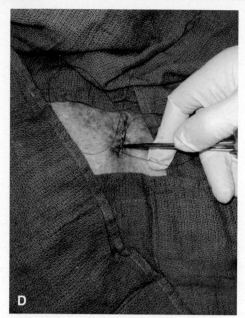

D

Figure 5-26D. The needle is then inserted into the proximal portion of skin at 90 degrees with a trajectory running toward the planned entry point in the center of the triangular section of skin (the tip), directly adjacent to its exit point.

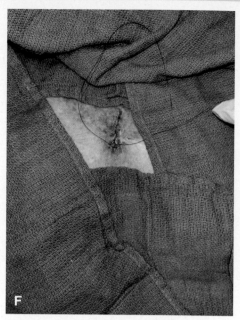

F

Figure 5-26F. Appearance after needle exit.

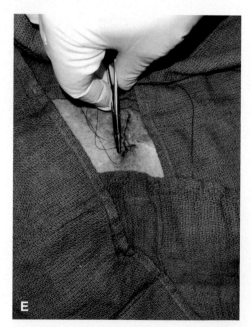

E

Figure 5-26E. The needle is then inserted into the distal section of skin at 90 degrees adjacent to its original entry point, now with a trajectory running toward the proximal edge of the section of skin.

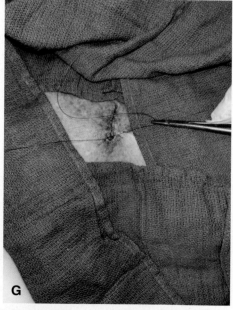

G

Figure 5-26G. Appearance after tying the suture. Note that the tip is now held snug.

Tips and Pearls

The percutaneous tip stitch is useful when bringing the tip of a flap into place. Importantly, this technique is designed to gently approximate the tissues so that the flap is properly inset in the surrounding skin. The percutaneous tip stitch is not designed to work under significant tension, as tension across the suture may lead to necrosis of the delicate and lightly vascularized tip of the flap or residual suture track marks.

Placing set-back dermal sutures, imbrication sutures, or suspension sutures prior to placement of the tip stitch will ensure that the tip itself is not under tension when it is approximated with the surrounding skin.

Drawbacks and Cautions

Flap tip necrosis is the greatest risk with this technique, since suture material traverses the dermis containing the tip's vascular supply. This risk may be mitigated by tying the suture relatively loosely so that the tip is not overly constricted when the knot is tied.

Vascular compromise and ensuing necrosis of the flap tip are always a risk, even if no sutures are placed through the tip itself, and therefore, the percutaneous tip stitch approach likely provides a reasonable balance between tissue approximation and adequate vascular supply.

Reference

Wang X, Fang W, Zhao W, et al. Clinical application of 3-dimensional continuous suturing technique for triangular wounds. *Ann Plast Surg.* 2018;81(3):316-321.

The Pulley Suture

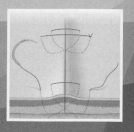

Application

The pulley suture technique relies on the pulley effect of multiple loops of suture to permit the closure of wounds under even significant tension. Since this approach may lead to marked tension across the wound surface, it is typically used in scalp reduction surgery or other areas where the final cosmesis is less critical. This approach may also be used as a temporary technique to better approximate wound edges and allow deep sutures to be placed expeditiously, after which the pulley sutures may be removed.

Suture Material Choice

Suture choice is dependent in large part on location, though because this technique is expressly designed for wounds under marked tension, a 3-0 nonabsorbable suture works well on the scalp and back. However, when the area is under particularly marked tension, a 2-0 nonabsorbable suture may be helpful.

Technique

1. The needle is inserted perpendicular to the epidermis, approximately 8-12 mm distant to the wound edge.

2. With a fluid motion of the wrist, the needle is rotated through the dermis, and the needle tip exits between the incised wound edges.

3. The needle is then reloaded and reinserted from the underside of the dermis on the contralateral wound edge, exiting approximately 4 mm from the wound edge. The exit point is just distal (relative to the surgeon) from the entry point on the original side.

4. The needle is then reloaded and inserted at 90 degrees perpendicular to the epidermis approximately 4 mm from the wound edge on the contralateral side of the incision line (the original entry side).

5. With a fluid motion of the wrist, the needle is rotated through the dermis, and the needle tip exits between the incised wound edges.

6. The needle is then reloaded and reinserted from the underside of the dermis on the contralateral wound edge, exiting approximately 8-12 mm from the wound edge. The exit point is just proximal (relative to the surgeon) from the entry point.

7. The suture material is then tied off (Figures 5-27A through 5-27G).

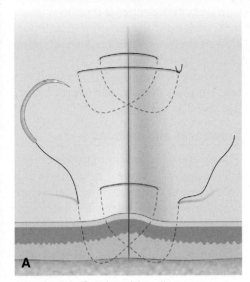

Figure 5-27A. Overview of the pulley suture.

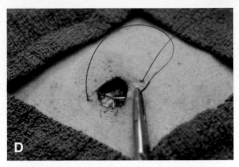

Figure 5-27D. The needle is then inserted directly across from its exit point, again near to the wound edge.

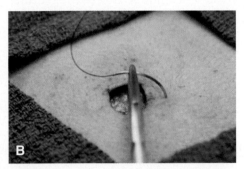

Figure 5-27B. The needle is inserted through the skin, far from the wound edge, exiting the underside of the dermis in the undermined wound space.

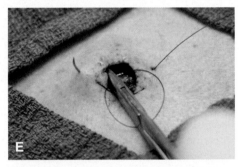

Figure 5-27E. The needle is then inserted again from the underside of the dermis, exiting far from the wound edge directly across from its original entry point.

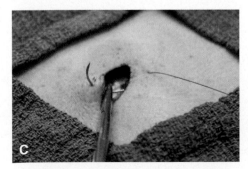

Figure 5-27C. The needle is then inserted on the contralateral wound edge, distal to its exit point along the length of the wound, exiting near to the incised wound edge.

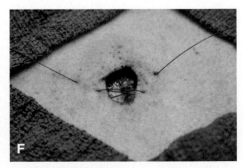

Figure 5-27F. Appearance after placement of the pulley suture prior to tying.

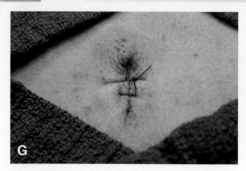

Figure 5-27G. Postoperative appearance after tying the knot.

Tips and Pearls

This is a useful technique for select wounds, as it permits the wound edges to come together even under marked tension. Since the sutures are transepidermal, however, they may also be associated with significant cross-hatching or residual suture track marks if they are left in place for any amount of time. Therefore, one frequently used approach is to use pulley sutures on a temporary basis intraoperatively to permit placement of other sutures; once the other sutures have been placed, the pulley sutures may be removed before the end of the procedure.

If pulley sutures are left in place, they should probably be removed in a timely fashion and certainly should not be left in place for longer than 1 week.

The two loops of suture are slightly offset from each other, as the suture traverses the incised wound edge on an oblique angle, which helps lessen the risk of tissue necrosis and tear-through.

This technique may be used to prepare the wound for placement of a buried pulley suture, such as the pulley set-back dermal suture. As long as undermining has been carried out effectively, utilizing a pulley technique with a thicker gauge suture material should allow for effective closure of all but the tightest wounds.

In areas under extreme tension, a three-loop variation of this approach is possible as well, allowing for an even more dramatic pulley effect.

A double variation of this approach, the tandem pulley stitch, has been recently described as well.

Drawbacks and Cautions

The greatest drawbacks of this approach are the possible residual track marks and wound spread that may be seen when wounds under marked tension are closed. This technique may elicit an increased risk of track marks, necrosis, and other complications when compared with techniques that do not entail suture material traversing the scar line, such as buried pulley techniques. Therefore, sutures should be removed as early as possible (ideally intraoperatively) to minimize these complications, and consideration should be given to adopting other closure techniques in the event that sutures will not be removed in a timely fashion.

Suture removal with this technique may be more involved than with simple interrupted sutures; the inner loop is generally easier to cut at the time of suture removal, though if sutures are left in place for an extended period of time, they may have a tendency to be overgrown by the surrounding epidermis.

References

Field LM. Closure of wounds under tension with the pulley suture. *J Dermatol Surg Oncol.* 1993;19(2):173-174.

Hitzig GS, Sadick NS. The pulley suture. Utilization in scalp reduction surgery. *J Dermatol Surg Oncol.* 1992;18(3):220-222.

Lee CH, Wang T. A novel suture technique for high-tension wound closure: the tandem pulley stitch. *Dermatol Surg.* 2015;41:975-976.

Snow NS. Closure of wounds under tension with the pulley suture. *J Dermatol Surg Oncol.* 1993;19(2):174.

The Purse-String Suture

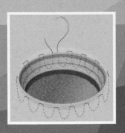

Application

This technique is designed to either shrink the size of a defect or obviate it entirely, depending on the degree of tension and the size of the defect. It is a niche technique, since the purse-string effect tends to lead to a slight puckering in the surrounding skin, a feature that may be acceptable (and will likely resolve with time) on areas such as the forearms and back but is less desirable in cosmetically sensitive locations such as the face. The running nature of the technique means that compromise at any point in the course of suture placement may result in wound dehiscence, though for this reason, a larger gauge suture material is generally utilized.

Suture Material Choice

Suture choice is dependent in large part on location, though as always, the smallest gauge suture material appropriate for the anatomic location should be utilized. On the back and shoulders, 2-0 or 3-0 nonabsorbable suture material is effective, and on the extremities and scalp, a 3-0 or 4-0 absorbable suture material may be used. Since the technique requires easy pull through of suture material, monofilament nonabsorbable suture is generally preferable.

Technique

1. The wound edges are broadly undermined.
2. With the tail of the suture material resting between the surgeon and the far end of the wound, the needle is inserted through the epidermis on the far edge of the wound with a trajectory running parallel to the incision. The entry point in the epidermis should be approximately 3-6 mm set back from the epidermal edge, depending on the thickness of the dermis and the anticipated degree of tension across the closure. The needle, and therefore the suture, should pass through the deep dermis into the undermined space at a uniform depth.
3. The needle is then grasped with the surgical pickups and simultaneously released by the hand holding the needle driver. As the needle is freed from the tissue with the pickups, the needle is grasped again by the needle driver in an appropriate position to repeat the previous step to the left of the previously placed suture.
4. A small amount of suture material is pulled through and the needle is inserted into the dermis to the left of the previously placed suture, and the same movement is repeated.
5. The same technique is repeated moving stepwise around the entire wound until the needle exits close to

the original entry point at the far end of the wound. Once the point closest to the surgeon is reached, it may be more comfortable to shift to a back-hand technique.

6. Once the desired number of throws has been placed, the suture material is then pulled taut, leading to complete or partial closure of the wound, and tied utilizing an instrument tie. Alternatively, a hand tie may be used if desired (Figures 5-28A through 5-28G).

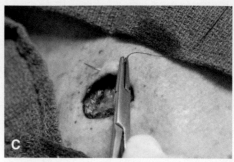

Figure 5-28C. Completion of the first throw of the purse-string suture. Note that the suture continues to follow the curvature of the wound edge.

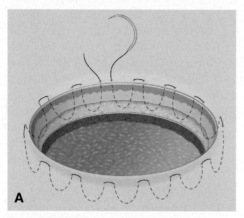

Figure 5-28A. Overview of the purse-string suture technique.

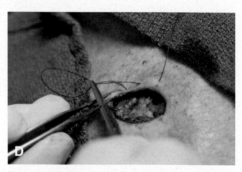

Figure 5-28D. Beginning of the second throw of the purse-string suture. Again, the suture continues to follow the curvature of the wound edge.

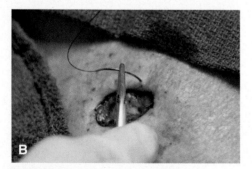

Figure 5-28B. Initiation of the purse-string suture technique. Note the needle enters at 90 degrees and follows a course parallel to the wound.

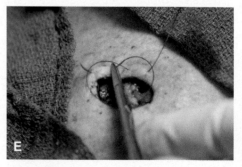

Figure 5-28E. Completion of the second throw.

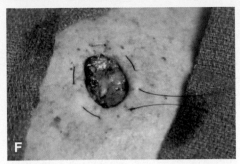

Figure 5-28F. The purse-string suture now encircles the entire wound. Note the intentionally large bites taken for demonstration purposes.

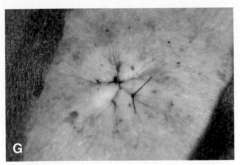

Figure 5-28G. The completed purse-string closure. Note the stellate appearance of the wound, which is more pronounced when repairing areas with a thicker dermis or when taking larger bites.

Tips and Pearls

This technique is designed as an efficient method of wound area reduction. In many cases, placing a purse-string suture can effect complete wound closure, and therefore, it represents an alternative to a layered repair of a fusiform incision. Despite reports of the technique's usefulness as an alternative to linear closure, a randomized controlled trial demonstrated that purse-string closures do not result in appreciably improved scarring compared with secondary intention healing.

It has been suggested that some defects on the back and extremities, particularly in elderly patients with loose skin, are better closed with a purse-string approach than with a traditional linear closure, since linear closures often heal with a residual scar and require a significantly longer excision line, while the puckering that may be present immediately postoperatively with purse-string closures is likely to resolve with time. That said, in the right hands, linear closures on the trunk and extremities often heal with subtle scarring, even when wounds are closed under tension.

On a pragmatic level, this approach is generally utilized either when a patient is unwilling to undergo a traditional linear closure or when a patient's comorbidities make the additional length of the incision for a linear closure an unrealistic option.

As with linear running dermal techniques, this technique may be used as a modified winch or pulley suture, since the multiple loops help minimize the tension across any one loop and permit closure of wounds under marked tension. Because each throw is not tied off, however, it is important to adequately secure the knot.

A monofilament suture is generally used to permit easy pull through as well as straightforward suture removal. Some have also advocated oversewing a defect closed with a purse-string closure with a simple running suture to reduce residual bunching.

The purse-string technique may also be used to effect hemostasis in the case of an oozing wound. For wounds in highly vascular areas, such as the scalp, a purse-string suture may be performed distant from the wound edge; small vessels will be captured within the ring of the purse-string suture and compressed when the suture material is tightened, leading to improved hemostasis. A double ring of purse-string sutures may be used as well to take even better advantage of this hemostatic effect.

Tying a purse-string closure under significant tension may be challenging, as suture material tends to slip after the first knot throw. Utilizing hemostats to secure the suture ends in position during suture lockdown may help mitigate this problem.

Drawbacks and Cautions

As with other transepidermal approaches, this technique may leave suture marks, and since this suture is generally tied under marked tension and is left in place for an extended period of time to permit the wound edges to firmly realign, this problem may be more pronounced with this technique than with other transepidermal approaches. Therefore, if the purse-string approach is to be utilized at all, it may be preferable to adopt the buried approach.

The pucker effect of this closure sometimes resolves rapidly in atrophic skin, though it can persist in other areas; patients should realize that some degree of residual puckering toward the center of the wound is to be expected. As with the buried purse-string approach, this technique may be used to help recreate the nipple-areola complex if full reconstruction is not desired and the nipple is lost to a local tumor.

Since the entire closure is held by a single knot, this approach may be associated with a higher rate of wound dehiscence, as knot failure or failure in the suture material at any point leads to an immediate loss of tension on the closure. Given the concern regarding knot breakage, it may be helpful to attempt to better secure the knot. This may be done by paying particularly close attention to knot tying, tying an extra full knot, adding extra throws, or leaving a longer tail than would traditionally be executed.

This approach provides less wound eversion than vertically oriented approaches such as the set-back dermal or buried vertical mattress sutures. Therefore, consideration should be given to adding additional superficially placed everting sutures, such as the vertical mattress suture, in order to mitigate this problem. Since this approach is generally adopted when the surgeon has accepted that the cosmetic outcome may be less than ideal, it may be reasonable to use this approach as a solitary closure.

References

Cohen PR, Martinelli PT, Schulze KE, Nelson BR. The cuticular purse string suture: a modified purse string suture for the partial closure of round postoperative wounds. *Int J Dermatol.* 2007;46(7):746-753.

Cohen PR, Martinelli PT, Schulze KE, Nelson BR. The purse-string suture revisited: a useful technique for the closure of cutaneous surgical wounds. *Int J Dermatol.* 2007;46(4):341-347.

Field LM. Inadvertent and undesirable sequelae of the stellate purse-string closure. *Dermatol Surg.* 2000;26(10):982.

Greenbaum SS, Radonich M. Closing skin defects with purse-string suture. *Plast Reconstr Surg.* 1998;101(6):1749-1751.

Harrington AC, Montemarano A, Welch M, Farley M. Variations of the pursestring suture in skin cancer reconstruction. *Dermatol Surg.* 1999;25(4):277-281.

Hoffman A, Lander J, Lee PK. Modification of the purse-string closure for large defects of the extremities. *Dermatol Surg.* 2008;34(2):243-245.

Joo J, Custis T, Armstrong AW, et al. Purse-string suture vs second intention healing: results of a randomized, blind clinical trial. *JAMA Dermatol.* 2015;151:265-270.

Ku BS, Kwon OE, Kim DC, et al. A case of erosive adenomatosis of nipple treated with total excision using purse-string suture. *Dermatol Surg.* 2006;32(8):1093-1096.

Maher IA, Fosko S, Alam M. Experience vs experiments with the purse-string closure: unexpected results. *JAMA Dermatol.* 2015;151:259-260.

Marquart JD, Lawrence N. The purse-string lockdown. *Dermatol Surg.* 2009;35:853-855.

Patel KK, Telfer MR, Southee R. A "round block" purse-string suture in facial reconstruction after operations for skin cancer surgery. *Br J Oral Maxillofac Surg.* 2003;41(3):151-156.

Peled IJ, Zagher U, Wexler MR. Purse-string suture for reduction and closure of skin defects. *Ann Plast Surg.* 1985;14(5):465-469.

Randle HW. Modified purse string suture closure. *Dermatol Surg.* 2004;30(2 pt 1):237.

Romiti R, Randle HW. Complete closure by purse-string suture after Mohs micrographic surgery on thin, sun-damaged skin. *Dermatol Surg.* 2002;28(11):1070-1072.

Spencer JM, Malerich SA, Moon SD. A regional survey of purse-string sutures for partial and complete closure of Mohs surgical defects. *Dermatol Surg.* 2014;40(6):679-685.

Teitelbaum S. The purse-string suture. *Plast Reconstr Surg.* 1998;101(6):1748-1749.

Zhu JW, Wu XJ, Lu ZF, Cai SQ, Zheng M. Purse-string suture for round and oval defects: a useful technique in dermatologic surgery. *J Cutan Med Surg.* 2012;16(1):11-17.

The Winch Stitch

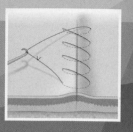

Video 5-29. Winch stitch
Access to video can be found via
AtlasofSuturingTechiniques2e.com.

Application

This is a niche intraoperative tissue expansion approach. When closing wounds under marked tension, buried or transepidermal pulley sutures may be insufficient to permit closure. Placing a temporary winch stitch, in order to take advantage of mechanical tissue creep, aids in closing these select defects. The suture is removed intraoperatively, after other tension-relieving sutures have been placed.

Suture Material Choice

Since this is a temporary suture, choice of suture material is guided more by resilience and resistance to breakage than by any concern regarding permanent track marks. Therefore, a 2-0 or 3-0 monofilament nonabsorbable suture is generally appropriate in most areas where this technique would be used, such as the trunk and scalp.

Technique

1. The needle is inserted perpendicular to the epidermis, approximately one-half the radius of the needle distant to the wound edge. This will allow the needle to exit the wound on the contralateral side at an equal distance from the wound edge by simply following the curvature of the needle.
2. With a fluid motion of the wrist, the needle is rotated through the dermis,

and the needle tip exits the skin on the contralateral side.
3. The needle body is grasped with surgical forceps in the left hand, with care being taken to avoid grasping the needle tip, which can be easily dulled by repetitive friction against the surgical forceps.
4. The loose tail of suture material may be secured in place with the aid of a hemostat.
5. Starting proximal to the prior throw relative to the surgeon, steps (1) through (3) are then repeated sequentially until the desired number of throws is placed.
6. The leading edge of suture is then tied to the loose end where the hemostat was placed (Figures 5-29A through 5-29H).

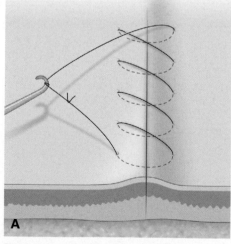

Figure 5-29A. Overview of the winch stitch.

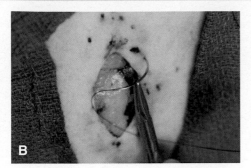

Figure 5-29B. The needle is inserted at 90 degrees through the epidermis close to one pole of the wound.

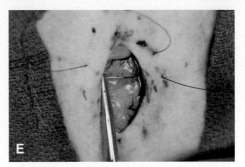

Figure 5-29E. The needle is then inserted on the contralateral wound edge. This pattern continues along the length of the wound.

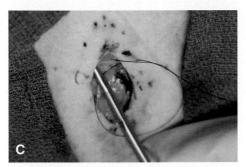

Figure 5-29C. The needle is then inserted on the contralateral side, exiting through the skin.

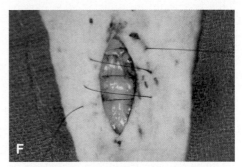

Figure 5-29F. Appearance after placing a series of sutures along the length of the wound.

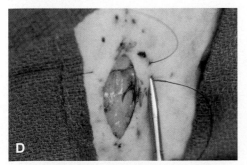

Figure 5-29D. Moving along the wound edge, the needle is again inserted through the skin at 90 degrees.

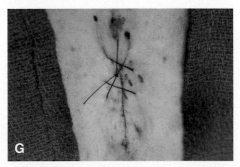

Figure 5-29G. The two ends of the suture are then tied together over the top of the wound.

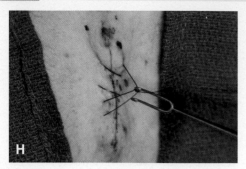

Figure 5-29H. A skin hook may be used to pull up on the tied loop of suture, further tightening the line of sutures.

Tips and Pearls

This is a multiple pulley tissue expansion technique that relies on the multiple throws of suture to minimize tension and secure the wound edges in position. After securing the winch stitch, it may be tightened intermittently by pulling on the suture material with a skin hook, permitting even greater mechanical skin creep.

This technique is not an actual closure technique; that is, the sutures are not left in place to permit tension reduction or wound-edge apposition, but rather to allow placement of the actual tension-relieving sutures that may not be easily placed in extreme high-tension closures.

The individual bites should be large enough to minimize suture material tear-through; otherwise, wounds under extreme tension, especially those with a relatively atrophic dermis, may not support the suture material, which could simply tear through the friable skin, leading to additional defects and associated cosmetic compromise.

Drawbacks and Cautions

Depending on the degree of tension and the thickness and resilience of the dermis, this technique may lead to some epidermal and dermal damage that may not be desirable. Therefore, care should be taken to use this approach only when absolutely needed. The risk of necrosis, while mitigated by the fact that these sutures are only left in place temporarily, is still a possibility, and even in the absence of true tissue necrosis, the trauma of crush injury to the delicate dermal vasculature is a possible risk as well.

Although this approach is designed to take advantage of mechanical tissue creep, it is not a dynamic suture technique, since the ends of the suture material are tied together. Therefore, the suture material may be pulled with a skin hook every few minutes intraoperatively to take advantage of tissue creep but is not secured in the new position, since the suture was tied after its initial placement.

As with any suturing technique, knowledge of the relevant anatomy is critical, and it is important to recall that the structures deep to the epidermis may be compromised by the passage of the needle and suture material. For example, the needle may pierce a vessel, leading to increased bleeding.

Given the possible problems associated with this approach, a double or pulley buried suture is preferable for effecting closure in high-tension areas when feasible. This technique remains a useful adjunct, however, in cases of extreme tension where mechanical tissue creep may be relied on to add laxity to a very tight closure.

Reference

Casparian JM, Monheit GD. Surgical pearl: the winch stitch-a multiple pulley suture. *J Am Acad Dermatol.* 2001;44(1):114-116.

The Dynamic Winch Stitch

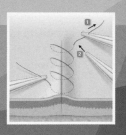

Synonym

Modified winch stitch

 Video 5-30. Dynamic winch stitch
Access to video can be found via
mhprofessional.com/atlasofsuturingtechniques2e

Application

Like the standard winch stitch, this is a niche intraoperative tissue expansion approach. When closing wounds under marked tension, buried or transepidermal pulley sutures may be insufficient to permit closure. Placing a temporary winch stitch, in order to take advantage of mechanical tissue creep, aids in closing these select defects. The suture is removed intraoperatively, after other tension-relieving sutures have been placed.

Suture Material Choice

Since this is a temporary suture, choice of suture material is guided more by resilience and resistance to breakage than by any concern regarding permanent track marks. Therefore, a 2-0 or 3-0 monofilament nonabsorbable suture is generally appropriate in most areas where this technique would be used, such as the trunk and scalp.

Technique

1. The needle is inserted perpendicular to the epidermis, approximately one-half the radius of the needle distant to the wound edge. This will allow the needle to exit the wound on the contralateral side at an equal distance from the wound edge by simply following the curvature of the needle.
2. With a fluid motion of the wrist, the needle is rotated through the dermis, and the needle tip exits the skin on the contralateral side.
3. The needle body is grasped with surgical forceps in the left hand, with care being taken to avoid grasping the needle tip, which can be easily dulled by repetitive friction against the surgical forceps.
4. The loose tail of suture material is secured in place with the aid of a hemostat.
5. Starting proximal to the prior throw relative to the surgeon, steps (1) through (3) are then repeated sequentially until the desired number of throws is placed.
6. The leading edge of suture is then pulled taut and secured in place with a hemostat.
7. After allowing time for tissue creep to occur, one hemostat is gently pulled, increasing tension across the sutures and bringing the wound edges closer together. At maximal pull, an additional hemostat is then placed at the junction of the skin and the suture material, securing the suture material in position. The hemostat that was pulled is then removed. This step is repeated until the desired degree of tension relief has been accomplished.

8. Once permanent sutures are placed, the hemostats are removed and the suture material is pulled out (Figures 5-30A through 5-30H).

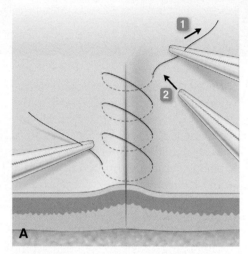

Figure 5-30A. Overview of the dynamic winch technique.

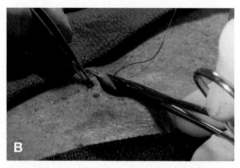

Figure 5-30B. The needle is inserted perpendicular to the skin and exits on the contralateral side.

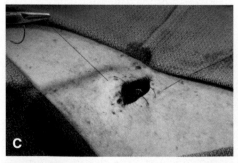

Figure 5-30C. This procedure is repeated sequentially until several large, deep bites are taken, in the fashion of a simple running suture.

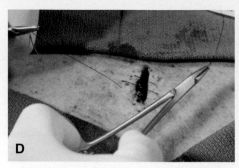

Figure 5-30D. Both the leading and trailing ends of suture are grasped with needle drivers or hemostats, placing tension along the suture material and gently pulling the wound edges together with a pulley technique.

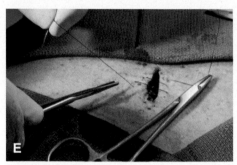

Figure 5-30E. With one end of the suture securely grasped by a needle driver, the other end is pulled taut, and a needle driver or hemostat is placed on the suture where it exits the skin.

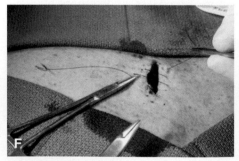

Figure 5-30F. The other needle driver or hemostat is then pulled laterally, tightening the suture.

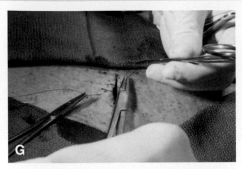

Figure 5-30G. A third needle driver is then placed on the suture at the junction of the suture and the skin, again securing the now tighter suture in place.

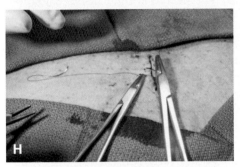

Figure 5-30H. This procedure is then sequentially repeated until all the slack has been removed from the suture material and the wound edges are well approximated. This will allow for placement of a permanent suture across the now temporarily approximated wound edges.

Tips and Pearls

This is a multiple pulley tissue expansion technique that relies on the multiple throws of suture to minimize tension and secure the wound edges in position.

This technique is not an actual closure technique; that is, the sutures are not left in place to permit tension reduction or wound-edge apposition, but rather to allow placement of the actual tension-relieving sutures that may not be easily placed in extreme high-tension closures.

The individual bites should be large enough to minimize suture material

tear-through; otherwise, wounds under extreme tension, especially those with a relatively atrophic dermis, may not support the suture material, which could simply tear through the friable skin, leading to additional defects and associated cosmetic compromise.

Drawbacks and Cautions

Depending on the degree of tension and the thickness and resilience of the dermis, this technique may lead to some epidermal and dermal damage. Therefore, care should be taken to use this approach only when absolutely needed. The risk of necrosis, while mitigated by the fact that these sutures are only left in place temporarily, is still a possibility, and even in the absence of true tissue necrosis, the trauma of crush injury to the delicate dermal vasculature is a possible risk as well.

With any suturing technique, knowledge of the relevant anatomy is critical, and it is important to recall that the structures deep to the epidermis may be compromised by the passage of the needle and suture material. For example, the needle may pierce a vessel, leading to increased bleeding.

Given the possible problems associated with this approach, a double or pulley buried suture is preferable for effecting closure in high-tension areas when feasible. This technique remains a useful adjunct, however, in cases of extreme tension where mechanical tissue creep may be relied on to add laxity to a very tight closure.

Reference

Casparian JM, Rodewald EJ, Monheit GD. The "modified" winch stitch. *Dermatol Surg.* 2001;27(10):891-894.

The Lembert Suture

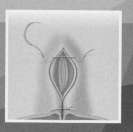

Video 5-31. Lembert suture
Access to video can be found via
mhprofessional.com/atlasofsuturingtechniques2e

Application

This is a niche technique designed to encourage wound-edge inversion and is useful primarily to recreate a natural crease. It may be used to recreate the alar creases as well as to better define the helical rim, and it may also be useful when recreating the mental crease.

Suture Material Choice

With all techniques, it is best to use the thinnest suture possible in order to minimize the risk of track marks and foreign-body reactions. Generally, this suture is used on the face and ears, and therefore, a 6-0 or 7-0 monofilament suture may be best, though fast-absorbing gut may be used to obviate the need for suture removal.

Technique

1. The needle is inserted perpendicular to the epidermis, approximately 8 mm distant to the wound edge.
2. With a fluid motion of the wrist, the needle is rotated superficially through the dermis, and the needle tip exits the skin 2 mm distant from the wound edge on the ipsilateral side.

3. The needle body is grasped with surgical forceps in the left hand and reloaded onto the needle driver.
4. The needle is then inserted perpendicular to the skin on the contralateral side of the wound edge, 2 mm distant from the wound edge.
5. The needle is again rotated superficially through its arc, exiting 8 mm from the incised wound edge.
6. The suture material is then tied off gently, with care being taken to minimize tension across the epidermis and avoid overly constricting the wound edges (Figures 5-31A through 5-31G).

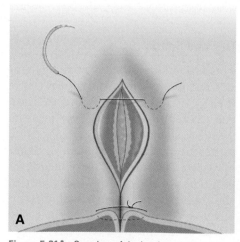

A

Figure 5-31A. Overview of the Lembert suture.

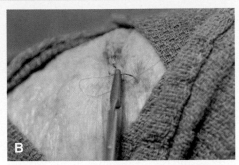

Figure 5-31B. The needle is inserted through the skin far lateral to the wound edge.

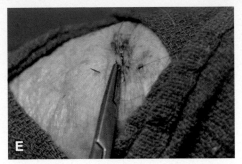

Figure 5-31E. The needle then exits further lateral from the edge of the wound.

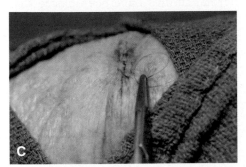

Figure 5-31C. The needle then exits the skin, still lateral to the wound edge.

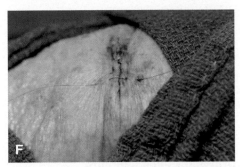

Figure 5-31F. Appearance after suture placement but prior to tying.

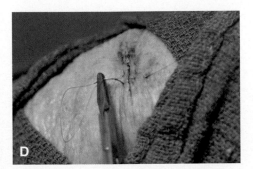

Figure 5-31D. The needle is then inserted through the skin on the contralateral side of the wound, slightly lateral to the edge of the wound.

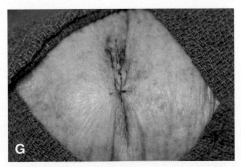

Figure 5-31G. Immediate postoperative appearance. Note the marked wound eversion.

Tips and Pearls

This approach was originally developed for intestinal suturing purposes, where inversion is desirable and indeed necessary.

No suture material traverses the incised wound edges, thus reducing the risk that foreign material could impair effective wound healing. When conceptualizing this technique, the key step is to understand that the suture bites are used only to secure the suture material lateral to the wound and that the actual suture material traverses the top of the wound, leading ultimately to inversion.

This approach is very useful when attempting to recreate a natural crease, especially since traditional everting sutures have a tendency to blunt natural creases. Since the eye is naturally drawn to skin folds and creases, this small change may have a dramatic effect on the ultimate outcome of the repair.

Drawbacks and Cautions

This technique may lead to dramatic wound inversion and, therefore, should only be used when the goal is recreating a natural crease. Moreover, since wound inversion may be associated with inferior cosmesis over the long term, the benefit of accentuated inversion should be weighed against the possibility that the long-term cosmetic outcome of the suture scar may be less than ideal. The overinversion of the wound edges caused by the suturing technique relaxes somewhat after suture removal, allowing the wound edges to meet and heal.

This technique does not contribute at all to epidermal-edge apposition, and therefore, it should ideally be used after dermal sutures have been placed that have effectively aligned the wound edges to permit improved healing.

As with any transepidermal technique, this approach may result in residual track marks; removing sutures in a timely fashion helps mitigate this risk, and utilizing fast-absorbing sutures may also be a reasonable option.

Reference

Antoine Lembert 1802-1851. Study on intestinal suture with a description of a new procedure for performing this surgical operation. 1826. *Dis Colon Rectum.* 1988;31(6):489-494.

The Combined Horizontal Mattress and Simple Interrupted Suture

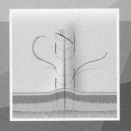

Synonym

Rousso stitch

Video 5-32. Combined horizontal mattress and simple interrupted suture
Access to video can be found via mhprofessional.com/atlasofsuturingtechniques2e

Application

This is an everting technique used for closure and epidermal approximation and is a variation on the horizontal mattress technique. As with many interrupted techniques, it may be used alone for wounds under minimal tension, such as those formed by either a small punch biopsy or a traumatic laceration, or as a secondary layer. Like other mattress sutures, this technique may also be used in the context of atrophic skin, as the broader anchoring bites may help limit tissue tear-through that may be seen with a simple interrupted suture.

Suture Material Choice

With all techniques, it is best to use the thinnest suture possible in order to minimize the risk of track marks and foreign-body reactions. Suture choice will depend largely on anatomic location and the goal of suture placement.

A 5-0 monofilament suture material is appropriate if there is minimal tension across the wound, while 4-0 monofilament suture is used in areas under moderate tension where the goal of suture placement is relieving tension as well as

epidermal approximation. In select high-tension areas, 3-0 monofilament suture may be utilized as well. Though rarely used in these locations, on the face and eyelids, a 6-0 or 7-0 monofilament suture is appropriate, though fast-absorbing gut may be used on the eyelids and ears to obviate the need for suture removal.

Technique

1. The needle is inserted perpendicular to the epidermis, approximately one-half the radius of the needle distant to the wound edge. This will allow the needle to exit the wound on the contralateral side at an equal distance from the wound edge by simply following the curvature of the needle.

2. With a fluid motion of the wrist, the needle is rotated through the dermis, taking the bite wider at the deep margin than at the surface, and the needle tip exits the skin on the contralateral side.

3. The needle body is grasped with surgical forceps in the left hand, with care being taken to avoid grasping the needle tip, which can be easily dulled by repetitive friction against the surgical forceps. It is gently grasped and pulled upward with the surgical forceps as the body of the needle is released from the needle driver.

4. The needle is then reloaded in a backhand fashion and inserted at 90 degrees perpendicular to the

315

epidermis proximal (relative to the surgeon) to its exit point on the same side of the incision line as the exit point.

5. The needle is rotated through its arc, exiting on the right side of the wound (relative to the surgeon) in a mirror image of steps (2) and (3).

6. The needle is then reloaded in standard fashion and inserted on the ipsilateral wound edge distal to the original entry point.

7. With a fluid motion of the wrist, the needle is rotated through the dermis, taking the bite wider at the deep margin than at the surface, and the needle tip exits the skin on the contralateral side.

8. The suture material is then tied off gently, with care being taken to minimize tension across the epidermis and avoid overly constricting the wound edges (Figures 5-32A through 5-32G).

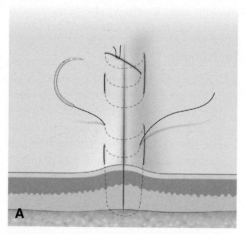

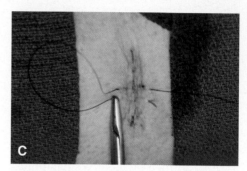

Figure 5-32C. The needle is then reloaded in a backhand fashion and inserted through the epidermis proximal to its exit point along the length of the wound on the ipsilateral side, in a mirror image of the prior step.

Figure 5-32A. Overview of the combined horizontal mattress and simple interrupted suture.

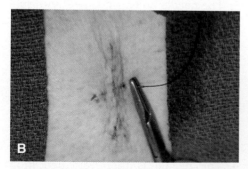

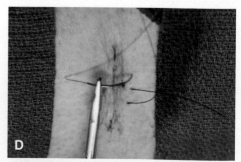

Figure 5-32B. The needle is inserted through the epidermis at a 90-degree angle, exiting on the contralateral wound edge.

Figure 5-32D. The needle is then reinserted through the ipsilateral side, now distal to its original entry point along the length of the wound.

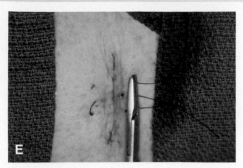

Figure 5-32E. The needle follows its arc through the dermis, exiting on the contralateral side.

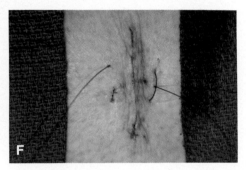

Figure 5-32F. Appearance after placing all of the above sutures.

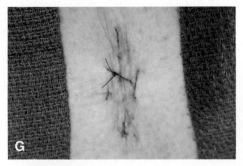

Figure 5-32G. Immediate postoperative appearance. Note the wound-edge eversion.

Tips and Pearls

This approach may be conceptualized as a combined horizontal mattress and simple interrupted suture. Like the locking mattress sutures, this approach makes suture removal more straightforward by

including a portion of suture material traversing over the incised wound edge.

It is important to enter the epidermis at 90 degrees, allowing the needle to travel slightly laterally away from the wound edge before fully following the curvature of the needle when utilizing this technique. This will allow for maximal wound eversion and accurate wound-edge approximation.

As with the simple interrupted suture, care should be taken to avoid skimming the needle superficially beneath the epidermis. This results from failing to enter the skin at a perpendicular angle and failing to follow the curvature of the needle. This may result in wound inversion as the tension vector of the shallow bite pulls the wound edges outward and down.

Since a wide bite of dermis and epidermis is included in the suture arc, it is particularly important to avoid tying the suture material too tightly, as this could lead to wound-edge necrosis.

This approach may reduce the risk of the so-called sandwich phenomenon that occurs occasionally with mattress sutures, since the placement of the simple interrupted portion of the suture helps approximate the wound edges.

Drawbacks and Cautions

With any suturing technique, knowledge of the relevant anatomy is critical. When placing this suture, it is important to recall that the structures deep to the epidermis may be compromised by the passage of the needle and suture material.

Similarly, if the knot is tied relatively tightly, structures deep to the defect may be constricted. This can lead to necrosis due to vascular compromise or even, theoretically, superficial nerve damage. These concerns are more acute with the combined horizontal mattress and simple interrupted suture and other variants of the horizontal mattress suture than with the simple interrupted suture, since the wide arc of the suture material and its horizontal component incorporate more skin and underlying structures, thus increasing the risk of strangulation.

This technique may elicit an increased risk of track marks, necrosis, and other complications when compared with techniques that do not entail suture material traversing the scar line, such as buried or subcuticular approaches. Therefore, sutures should be removed as early as possible to minimize these complications, and consideration should be given to adopting other closure techniques in the event that sutures will not be able to be removed in a timely fashion.

Reference

Kinmon KJ, Rosen RG, Perler AD, London E, Nyska N. The Rousso stitch: a new everting skin closure technique. *J Foot Ankle Surg.* 2003;42(4):244-246.

The Lattice Stitch

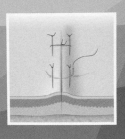

Application

This is a niche technique designed for wounds with an atrophic dermis or under significant tension, where traditional suturing techniques do not allow for adequate tissue recruitment and wound-edge apposition or tension relief. The fundamental principle is to place several interrupted sutures parallel to the wound edge and then tie the interrupted sutures over the wound edge by incorporating the lattice, increasing the stability of the repair and broadly distributing its force.

Suture Material Choice

With all techniques, it is best to use the thinnest suture possible in order to minimize the risk of track marks and foreign-body reactions. A 5-0 monofilament suture material may be used if there is minimal tension, and a 4-0 monofilament suture may be used in areas under moderate tension. In select high-tension areas, a 3-0 monofilament suture may be utilized as well.

Technique

1. Simple interrupted sutures are placed parallel to the incision line, forming the anchoring framework: the needle is inserted perpendicular to the epidermis, approximately 8 mm distant from the wound edge.
2. With a fluid motion of the wrist, the needle is rotated through the dermis, running parallel to the incision line.
3. The suture material is then tied off loosely, leaving a gap between the suture material and the skin.
4. Steps (1) through (3) are then repeated on the contralateral wound edge, forming the contralateral anchoring framework.
5. A simple interrupted suture is then placed, incorporating the suture material from the anchoring framework. The needle is inserted around the anchoring suture on the far end perpendicular to the epidermis.
6. With a fluid motion of the wrist, the needle is rotated through the dermis, taking the bite wider at the deep margin than at the surface, and the needle tip exits the skin on the contralateral side, on the outside of the anchoring framework.
7. The suture material is then tied off gently, with care being taken to minimize tension across the epidermis and avoid overly constricting the wound edges (Figures 5-33A through 5-33H).

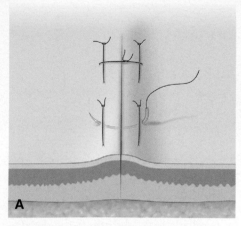

Figure 5-33A. Overview of the lattice suture technique.

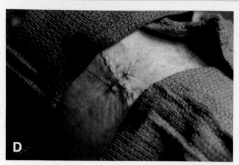

Figure 5-33D. This is repeated on the contralateral wound edge, forming a lattice framework.

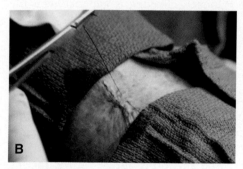

Figure 5-33B. The needle is inserted through the epidermis, parallel to the wound edge.

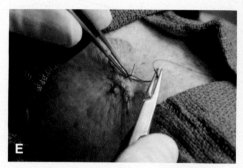

Figure 5-33E. The needle is inserted beneath the interrupted suture on the far side.

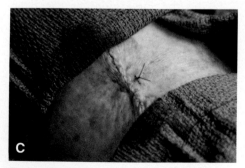

Figure 5-33C. The suture material is tied and trimmed, forming a simple interrupted suture parallel to the incised wound edge.

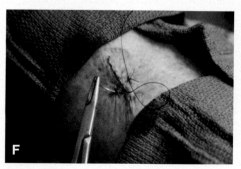

Figure 5-33F. The procedure is repeated on the contralateral side.

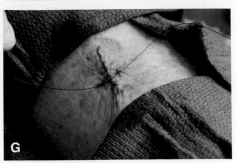

Figure 5-33G. The suture material traversing the wound is now supported by the lattice framework.

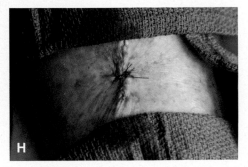

Figure 5-33H. Immediate postoperative appearance.

Tips and Pearls

This technique was developed for closing wounds with an atrophic dermis or where tissue tear-through is a major problem, such as on the lower legs and forearms in patients with extensive actinic damage.

The anchoring sutures are designed to broadly spread the tension across the wound edge, mitigating the risk of tissue tear-through and helping to distribute tension evenly across the wound. The physics of this closure has been explored separately.

This technique has also been described incorporating multiple other approaches, such as a crossed lattice stitch, where the suture running across the wound stretches obliquely from one anchoring suture to the next; the double lattice suture, where two sutures are placed across each set of anchoring sutures; and the stacked (near-far) lattice stitch, where adjacent anchor sutures are placed at variable distances from the wound edge with some overlap.

Drawbacks and Cautions

The greatest drawbacks of this approach are time, suture material use, tear-through, and the risk of oversewing and subsequent tissue necrosis, particularly with multiple closely spaced anchoring sutures. Since each suture crossing the incision requires two anchoring sutures, this technique may take significantly longer to execute than other approaches. Moreover, the excess suture material that needs to be used to incorporate this approach means that on longer closures additional packages of suture material may be needed.

Finally, placing multiple anchoring sutures parallel to the incision line may lead to impaired vascularization and an increased risk of wound-edge necrosis, since a significant proportion of the skin surrounding the wound is encompassed by suture material that has the potential to constrict the underlying vessels.

With any suturing technique, knowledge of the relevant anatomy is critical. When placing these sutures, it is important to recall that the structures deep to the epidermis may be compromised by the passage of the needle and suture material.

This technique may elicit an increased risk of track marks, tear-through, necrosis, and other complications when compared with techniques that do not entail suture material traversing the scar line, such as buried or subcuticular approaches. Therefore, sutures should be removed as early as possible to minimize these complications, and consideration should be given to adopting other closure techniques in the event that sutures will not be able to be removed in a timely fashion. Some studies have also demonstrated an increased rate of dehiscence when utilizing interrupted sutures alone without underlying dermal tension-relieving sutures, highlighting that this technique should be used either for wounds under minimal tension or in concert with deeper tension-relieving sutures.

Reference

Knoell KA. The lattice stitch technique. *Arch Dermatol.* 2011;147(1):17-20.

CHAPTER 5.34

The Adhesive Strip Bolster Technique

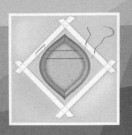

 Video 5-34. Adhesive strip bolster technique
Access to video can be found via mhprofessional.com/atlasofsuturingtechniques2e

Application

This is a niche technique designed for wounds with an atrophic dermis, where standard suturing techniques result in significant tissue tear-through due to atrophic skin. By placing adhesive strips on the skin surrounding the wound, the skin's resistance to tear-through is increased substantially, permitting closures on even very atrophic lower leg and forearm skin.

Suture Material Choice

With this technique, sterile adhesive strips are included on the surgical tray. Other forms of sterile tape or adhesive dressings may be used as well.

On the forearms, a 4-0 monofilament nonabsorbable suture may be used, whereas on the lower legs, a 3-0 monofilament suture may be more effective.

Technique

1. The adhesive strips are placed on the skin surrounding the wound. They should be placed immediately adjacent to the wound margin on dry skin to facilitate adhesiveness.
2. Horizontal mattress sutures are then placed, passing through both the skin and adhesive strips. The needle is inserted perpendicular to the adhesive strip and epidermis, approximately one-half the radius of the needle distant to the wound edge. This will allow the needle to exit the wound on the contralateral side at an equal distance from the wound edge by simply following the curvature of the needle.
3. With a fluid motion of the wrist, the needle is rotated through the dermis, taking the bite wider at the deep margin than at the surface, and the needle tip exits the skin on the contralateral side, piercing the skin and adhesive strip.
4. The needle is then reloaded in a backhand fashion and inserted at 90 degrees perpendicular to the epidermis and adhesive strip proximal (relative to the surgeon) to its exit point on the same side of the incision line as the exit point.
5. The needle is rotated through its arc, exiting on the right side of the wound (relative to the surgeon) in a mirror image of steps (2) and (3).
6. The suture material is then tied off gently, with care being taken to minimize tension across the epidermis and avoid overly constricting the wound edges (Figures 5-34A through 5-34G).

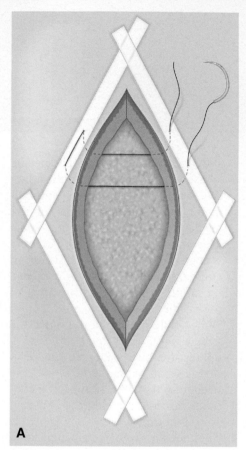

Figure 5-34A. Overview of the adhesive strip bolster technique.

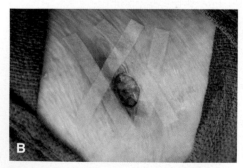

Figure 5-34B. Adhesive strips fixed to the area surrounding the operative wound.

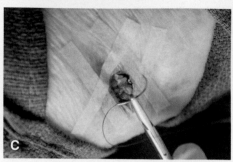

Figure 5-34C. The needle is passed at 90 degrees through the center of the adhesive strip. Note that the area of overlap between two strips provides the greatest bolster effect.

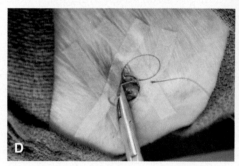

Figure 5-34D. The needle exits on the contralateral side.*

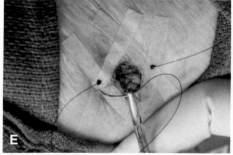

Figure 5-34E. The needle is reinserted on the ipsilateral side, continuing the horizontal mattress suture placement.

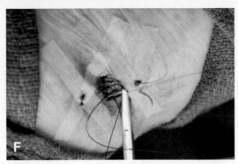

Figure 5-34F. The needle then exits on the contralateral side.

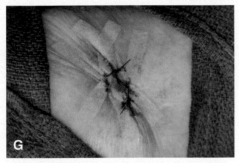

Figure 5-34G. Immediate postoperative appearance after placement of a central horizontal mattress suture and two simple interrupted sutures at the poles.

Tips and Pearls

This technique was developed for closing wounds with an atrophic dermis or where tissue tear-through is a major problem, such as on the lower legs and forearms in patients with extensive actinic damage. It is much faster than other approaches, such as the lattice stitch, and concomitantly does not share some of the lattice stitch's drawbacks that are rooted in oversewing the wound.

One variation of this technique has been described using a hydrocolloid dressing as a bolster, while another variation has focused on utilizing cyanoacrylate glue to bolster the atrophic dermis. The glue is allowed to harden on the skin, adding strength to the atrophic epidermis in a similar fashion to the adhesive strips. While providing a benefit in terms of elegance and ease of wound care, the additional cost of the individually packaged glue for this technique may make it less readily adopted. Regardless of the particular bolster material used, the principle of this approach remains the same—an externally applied material is used to adhere to and strengthen an otherwise atrophic surgical site, permitting placement of sutures when the suture material would otherwise have found little purchase in the thin skin.

In order to recruit maximal dermis, the horizontal mattress technique, as described previously, is often used with this approach, though other techniques, such as simple interrupted sutures or vertical mattress sutures, may be utilized as appropriate.

Care should be taken to avoid skimming the needle superficially beneath the epidermis. This results from failing to enter the skin at a perpendicular angle and failing to follow the curvature of the needle. This may result in wound inversion as the tension vector of the shallow bite pulls the wound edges outward and down.

It is possible to utilize absorbable sutures with this approach as well by incorporating percutaneous approaches, such as the percutaneous set-back dermal suture, so that the percutaneous bites of suture material also capture part of the adhesive strip in order to increase their security. In this case, however, the adhesive strips should be carefully removed approximately 2 weeks postoperatively.

An important advantage of this approach over the lattice technique is that no additional sutures are needed, thus saving time and, more importantly, avoiding the risk that the anchoring sutures themselves could tear through the atrophic skin leading to a more extensive wound.

Drawbacks and Cautions

Patients should be cautioned to expect that the adhesive strips will appear somewhat crusted; generally, these strips serve as a dressing, and when they are removed approximately 10-14 days postoperatively, the underlying wound is found to be clean, dry, and intact. Still, their presence may represent a nidus for bacterial growth.

With any suturing technique, knowledge of the relevant anatomy is critical. When placing these sutures, it is important to recall that the structures deep to the epidermis may be compromised by the passage of the needle and suture material.

This technique may elicit an increased risk of track marks, necrosis, and other complications when compared with techniques that do not entail suture material traversing the scar line, such as buried or subcuticular approaches. Therefore, sutures should be removed as early as possible to minimize these complications. That said, this approach is specifically utilized when the dermis is atrophic, and as such, buried techniques often are not particularly effective in these situations.

References

Mazzurco JD, Krach KJ. Use of a hydrocolloid dressing to aid in the closure of surgical wounds in patients with fragile skin. *J Am Acad Dermatol*. 2012;66(2):335-336.

Tayebi B, Kaniszewska M, Mahoney AM, Tung R. A novel closure method for surgical defects in atrophic skin using cyanoacrylate adhesive and suture. *Dermatol Surg*. 2015;41(1):177-180.

The Frost Suture

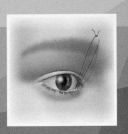

Synonym

Temporary eyelid suspension suture

Application

This is a niche approach that is used to secure the lower eyelid margin in place to help prevent postoperative ectropion. It is useful when there is concern that postoperative edema could result in a downward pull on the lower eyelid during the postoperative period. However, it is not to be used to correct ectropion that is apparent intraoperatively.

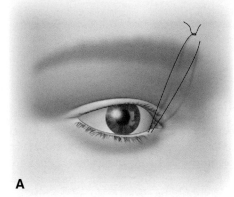

Figure 5-35A. Overview of the Frost suture.

Suture Material Choice

Usually, a 4-0 nonabsorbable monofilament suture is adequate for Frost suture placement.

Technique

1. After the closure has been completed, the needle is inserted through the tarsus or just inferior to it.
2. With a fluid motion of the wrist, the needle is rotated, taking a 3-mm bite.
3. The needle is then reloaded and passed through the skin above the medial eyebrow, keeping the angle and placement of the lower lid in its anatomic position.
4. The suture material is then tied off gently, forming a sling. Alternatively, the positioning above the medial eyebrow may be secured using adhesive strips (Figures 5-35A through 5-35D).

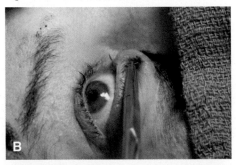

Figure 5-35B. The needle is inserted through the tarsal plate, lateral to the punctum.

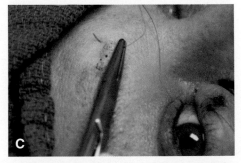

Figure 5-35C. The needle is then inserted through the skin of the medial eyebrow, performing a simple interrupted suture.

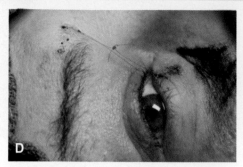

Figure 5-35D. Appearance immediately after suture placement. The eyelid is now suspended in anatomic position, minimizing the risk of developing edema-induced ectropion in the first few postoperative days.

Tips and Pearls

Knowledge of eyelid anatomy is critical before embarking on this oculoplastic technique. The suture should penetrate the tarsus or directly inferior to it, but care should be taken to avoid the inferior lateral punctum or canaliculus.

This technique is designed to prevent the eyelid from developing an ectropion in the postoperative period. However, it is not able to correct an ectropion that is already apparent intraoperatively. Sutures may be removed approximately 3 days

postoperatively but may be left in place longer if a large amount of postoperative edema or bleeding is present.

The superior anchor point may be secured with adhesive strips and liquid adhesive if desired, which also permits adjustment of the tension across the suture in the postoperative period based on the degree of edema.

Drawbacks and Cautions

As noted previously, suture placement in the medial lower eyelid should only be undertaken by those with a thorough familiarity and comfort with eyelid anatomy.

Since the sling of suture projects in front of the eye, patients should be educated regarding postoperative care and may consider using an eye patch in order to protect the area from inadvertent tugging on the suture.

Reference

Desciak EB, Eliezri YD. Surgical pearl: temporary suspension suture (Frost suture) to help prevent ectropion after infraorbital reconstruction. *J Am Acad Dermatol.* 2003;49(6):1107-1108.

The Running Pleated Suture

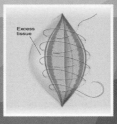

 Video 5-36. Running pleated suture
Access to video can be found via
mhprofessional.com/atlasofsuturingtechniques2e

Application

This technique is designed to correct an imbalance in tissue length on two sides of a wound, as is commonly encountered in flap repairs. When performing advancement and rotation flaps, Burrow's triangles are often taken at the poles of the flap in order to account for the discrepancy in tissue quantity between the two edges of the wound. This technique is designed to take advantage of forming multiple small pleats in the tissue that may be thought of as tiny Burrow's triangles all along the wound length, leading ultimately to a shorter scar.

Suture Material Choice

With all techniques, it is best to use the thinnest suture possible in order to minimize the risk of track marks and foreign-body reactions. Generally, this technique is used on the face, where 6-0 or 7-0 monofilament nonabsorbable suture is appropriate. On flaps on other body sites, 5-0 suture may be appropriate as well.

Technique

1. The needle is inserted perpendicular to the epidermis, approximately one-half the radius of the needle distant to the wound edge. This will allow the needle to exit the wound on the contralateral side at an equal distance from the wound edge by simply following the curvature of the needle.

2. With a fluid motion of the wrist, the needle is rotated through the dermis, taking the bite wider at the deep margin than at the surface, and the needle tip exits the skin on the contralateral side.

3. The suture material is then tied off gently, with care being taken to minimize tension across the epidermis and avoid overly constricting the wound edges. This forms the first anchoring knot for the running line of pleated sutures. The loose tail is trimmed, and the needle is reloaded.

4. Starting proximal to the prior knot relative to the surgeon, the needle is inserted perpendicular to the epidermis on the side without tissue excess, approximately one-half the radius of the needle distant to the wound edge.

5. With a fluid motion of the wrist, the needle is rotated through the dermis, and the needle tip exits into the undermined space.

6. The needle is then reloaded and inserted through the superficial dermis on the contralateral wound edge, taking a more superficial bite on this side of the wound.

7. Steps (4) through (6) are then sequentially repeated until the end of the wound is reached, so that

there is more space between bites on the wound side with excess.

8. For the final throw at the inferior apex of the wound, the needle is loaded with a backhand technique and inserted into the skin at a 90-degree angle in a mirror image of the other throws, entering just proximal to the exit point relative to the surgeon on the same side of the incision line and exiting on the contralateral side.

9. The suture material is only partly pulled through, leaving a loop of suture material on the side of the incision opposite to the needle.

10. The suture material is then tied to the loop using an instrument tie (Figures 5-36A through 5-36H).

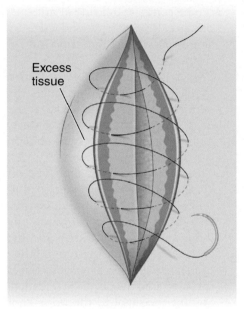

Excess tissue

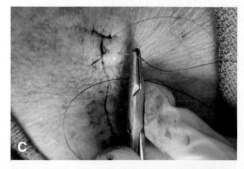

Figure 5-36B. The anchoring suture is tied. Note the presence of excess tissue on the side of the wound where the anchoring suture's knot has been placed.

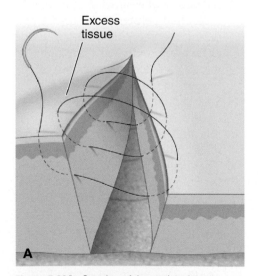

Excess tissue

A

Figure 5-36A. Overview of the running pleated suture.

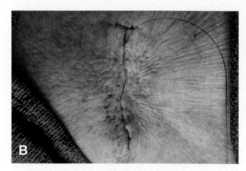

C

Figure 5-36C. The needle is inserted superficially through the dermis on the side of excess, a moderate distance from the anchoring suture.

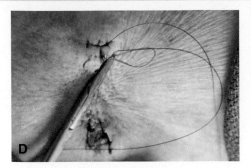

Figure 5-36D. The needle is then inserted deep on the contralateral side, closer to the anchoring suture.

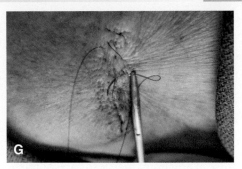

Figure 5-36G. This pattern continues along the course of the wound.

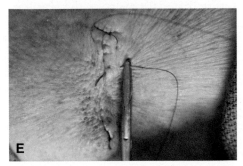

Figure 5-36E. Another superficial bite is taken on the side of excess, again moderately distant from the prior suture.

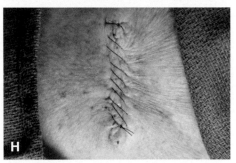

Figure 5-36H. Immediate postoperative appearance. Note that the wound edges now demonstrate less pronounced excess.

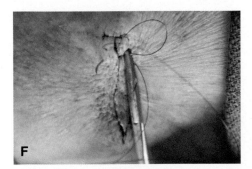

Figure 5-36F. A deep bite is taken, exiting close to the prior suture, on the side without excess.

Tips and Pearls

While originally described for flap repairs, this technique may be used in any situation where there is a differential in tissue quantity between the two sides of a wound. Taking widely spaced superficial bites on the side with excess and narrowly spaced deep bites on the side without excess has the effect of pleating down the wound edge with excess tissue and tacking it into place against the contralateral wound edge.

A deeper layer of sutures should be placed to relieve tension across the wound edges before placing the running pleated suture.

Drawbacks and Cautions

Some visible pleating, particularly on the side with excess, is expected in the immediate postoperative period. In most areas, this will resolve with time as the wound heals.

As with all running techniques, the integrity of the entire suture line rests on two knots, and suture material compromise at any point may lead to a complete loss of the integrity of the line of sutures. Since this technique is designed for low-tension environments, however, even in the face of suture material breakage, the remaining throws of suture may permit some residual epidermal approximation and wound-edge length equalization.

Since all loops of suture are placed in succession, this technique does not permit the same degree of fine-tuning of the epidermal approximation as a simple interrupted suture.

As with any suturing technique, knowledge of the relevant anatomy is critical. When placing running pleated sutures, it is important to recall that the structures deep to the epidermis may be compromised by the passage of the needle and suture material.

Similarly, if the knot is tied relatively tightly, structures deep to the defect may be constricted. This can lead to necrosis due to vascular compromise or even, theoretically, superficial nerve damage; again, this risk may be mitigated by maintaining some laxity in the suture throws.

This technique may elicit an increased risk of track marks, necrosis, inflammation, and other complications when compared with techniques that do not entail suture material traversing the scar line, such as buried or subcuticular approaches. Therefore, sutures should be removed as early as possible to minimize these complications.

Reference

Kouba DJ, Miller SJ. "Running pleated" suture technique opposes wound edges of unequal lengths. *Dermatol Surg.* 2006;32(3):411-414.

The Running Bolster Suture

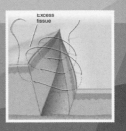

Excess tissue

Synonym

Lilliputian bolster dressing

Video 5-37. Running bolster suture

Access to video can be found via
mhprofessional.com/atlasofsuturingtechniques2e

Application

This is a niche technique used for securing bolsters over the top of skin grafts. It represents a running suture approach for tying over a bolster dressing, which was traditionally performed with multiple interrupted sutures tying down a bolster dressing.

Suture Material Choice

With all techniques, it is best to use the thinnest suture possible in order to minimize the risk of track marks and foreign-body reactions. Generally, a 5-0 or 6-0 nonabsorbable monofilament suture is appropriate, as the suture is not designed to bear significant tension.

Technique

1. After securing the graft in place, the needle is inserted at the 3 o'clock position, 5 mm lateral to the graft edge perpendicular to the epidermis and tangential to the angle of the graft.
2. With a fluid motion of the wrist, the needle is rotated through the dermis, and the needle tip exits 2-3 mm distant from the entry point.
3. The free end of the suture may be secured with a hemostat, or a knot may be tied to secure the suture in place, leaving a long tail.
4. The suture is then passed over the bolster and similarly inserted at the 9 o'clock position relative to the graft, following steps (1) and (2). Note that multiple passes can be performed so that the angle changes by only 30 degrees between each pass.
5. The suture is then similarly inserted at the 12 o'clock position relative to the graft, following steps (1) and (2).
6. The suture is then similarly inserted at the 6 o'clock position relative to the graft, following steps (1) and (2).
7. The needle is passed around the suture material segment between the 9 o'clock and 12 o'clock positions.
8. Nonadherent dressing and gauze are then cut to size and slipped over the top of the graft in the desired position by passing them through the approximately 5 o'clock position.
9. The ends of the suture material may be pulled toward the 3 and 9 o'clock positions to tighten. The suture material is then tied off gently over the top of the bolster, securing the bolster in place (Figure 5-37A).

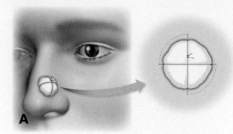

Figure 5-37A. Overview of the running bolster technique.

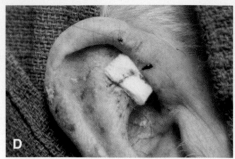

Figure 5-37D. Appearance after placing the sutures, before securing the bolster.

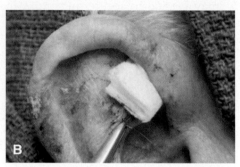

Figure 5-37B. After placing the bolster in place, the needle is inserted parallel to the bolster edge, exiting distally at an equivalent distance from the edge of the bolster.

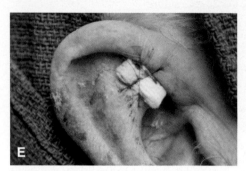

Figure 5-37E. Immediate appearance after suture placement.

Tips and Pearls

This is a niche technique and represents an alternative to the standard tie-over approach for securing full-thickness skin grafts. Since it is a running technique, only one knot is needed, increasing the speed with which the bolster may be placed.

Full-thickness skin grafts benefit from being secured in place to maintain direct contact between the donor and recipient sites and minimize lateral movement. Moreover, a bolster dressing may help decrease the risk of hematoma formation by maintaining constant even pressure across the surface of the graft, though recent studies have suggested that a pressure dressing may be adequate in most cases.

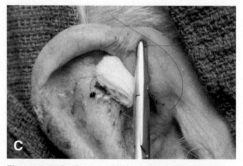

Figure 5-37C. The needle is then inserted through the skin directly across the bolster from its exit point, and the needle travels so that it exits directly across from the original entry point on the contralateral wound edge.

An alternate technique has been described, where each pass of the running bolster suture crosses over the center of the bolster, obviating the need to lock the last loop of suture. Another variation (the Lilliputian approach) notes that the initial suture can be tied and that the angle of each pass can be changed by as little as 30 degrees or less.

A simplified version of this approach (as shown in Figures 5-37B through 5-37E) has also been described for small grafts, where the initial suture enters at 6 o'clock and exits at 9 o'clock and then, after passing over the bolster, enters at 3 o'clock and exits at 12 o'clock. When the suture material is tied, the running bolster is secured.

Drawbacks and Cautions

The central drawback of this approach is that the integrity of the entire suture rests on one knot. Moreover, suture material compromise at any point may lead to a complete loss of the integrity of the running bolster.

Suturing a bolster in place results in additional suture material traversing the skin; this both takes additional time to execute and potentially increases the risk of infection or track marks. Therefore, in many cases, an external pressure dressing may suffice to secure the graft in place and reduce the risk of hematoma formation.

References

Adams DC, Ramsey ML, Marks VJ. The running bolster suture for full-thickness skin grafts. *Dermatol Surg.* 2004;30(1):92-94.

Davenport M, Daly J, Harvey I, Griffiths RW. The bolus tie-over "pressure" dressing in the management of full thickness skin grafts: is it necessary? *Br J Plast Surg.* 1988;41(1):28-32.

De Gado F, Chiummariello S, Monarca C, et al. Skin grafting: comparative evaluation of two dressing techniques in selected body areas. *In Vivo.* 2008;22:503-508.

Jeong HS, Kim KS, Lee HK. Hydrocolloid dressings in skin grafting or immobilization and compression. *Dermatol Surg.* 2011;37:320-324.

Langtry JA, Kirkham P, Martin IC, Fordyce A. Tie-over bolster dressings may not be necessary to secure small full thickness skin grafts. *Dermatol Surg.* 1998;24(12):1350-1353.

Shimizu I, MacFarlane DF. Full-thickness skin grafts may not need tie-over bolster dressings. *Dermatol Surg.* 2013;39(5):726-728.

Skouge JW. The running bolster suture for full thickness skin grafts. *Dermatol Surg.* 2004;30(8):1180-1181.

Srivastava D, Kouba DJ. A "Lilliputian" technique for rapid and efficient securing of bolster dressings over full-thickness skin grafts. *Dermatol Surg.* 2009;35(8):1280-1281.

The Combined Vertical Mattress-Dermal Suture

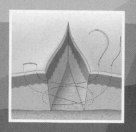

Synonym

Subcutaneous loop suture

Video 5-38. Combined vertical mattress-dermal suture
Access to video can be found via
mhprofessional.com/atlasofsuturingtechniques2e

Application

This is a combination suture that may be conceptualized as a hybrid between a vertical mattress suture and a dermal suture. It was designed to permit closure of deep defects and simultaneously permit wound eversion with a single suture, obviating the need for bilayered closures.

Suture Material Choice

With all techniques, it is best to use the thinnest suture possible in order to minimize the risk of track marks and foreign-body reactions. Suture choice will depend largely on anatomic location and the goal of suture placement.

Typically, 5-0 monofilament nonabsorbable suture material is appropriate if there is minimal tension, and 4-0 monofilament suture may be used in areas under moderate tension. In high-tension areas, 3-0 monofilament suture may be utilized as well.

Technique

1. The needle is inserted perpendicular to the epidermis, approximately 6 mm distant to the wound edge.

2. With a fluid motion of the wrist, the needle is rotated through the dermis, taking the bite wider at the deep margin than at the surface, and the needle tip exits between the incised wound edges.

3. The needle is then reloaded and inserted through the deep dermis on the contralateral wound edge.

4. The needle is then reloaded again in a backhand fashion and inserted through the deep dermis on the original wound edge.

5. The needle is then reloaded, entering from beneath the dermis on the contralateral wound edge and exiting approximately 6 mm from the wound edge.

6. The needle is then reloaded in a backhand fashion and inserted at 90 degrees perpendicular to the epidermis approximately 3 mm from the wound edge on the same side of the incision line as the exit point.

7. The needle is rotated superficially through its arc, exiting on the contralateral side of the wound 3 mm from the incised wound edge.

8. The suture material is then tied off gently, with care being taken to minimize tension across the epidermis and avoid overly constricting the wound edges (Figures 5-38A through 5-38H).

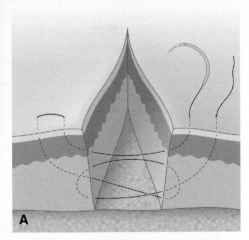

A

Figure 5-38A. Overview of the combined vertical mattress-dermal suture.

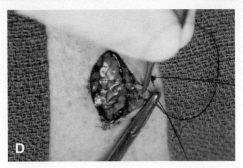

D

Figure 5-38D. The needle is then inserted through the deep dermis on the original side of entry.

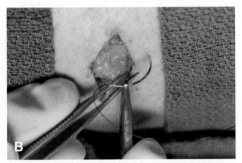

B

Figure 5-38B. The needle is inserted perpendicular to the skin far from the wound edge, exiting in the open wound space.

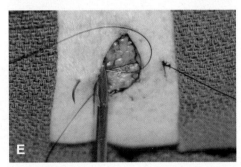

E

Figure 5-38E. The needle is then inserted from the underside of the dermis up through the skin on the contralateral side, far from the wound edge.

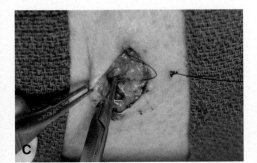

C

Figure 5-38C. The needle is inserted in the deep dermis on the contralateral side.

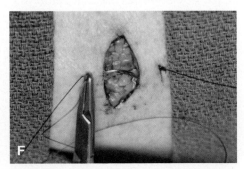

F

Figure 5-38F. The needle is then inserted near the wound edge on the ipsilateral side, exiting in the undermined wound space, following a superficial course.

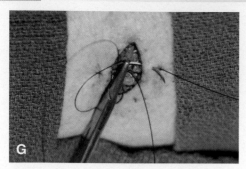

Figure 5-38G. The needle then enters the contralateral side, running superficially and exiting near the wound edge.

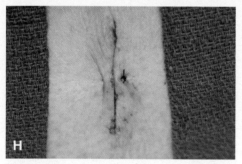

Figure 5-38H. Immediate postoperative appearance. Note the wound-edge eversion.

Tips and Pearls

This technique has been described as a simple approach to closure that permits closure of deeper structures (and dead-space obviation) as well as epidermal approximation and eversion. Perhaps its most useful niche is for the closure of very small defects or punch biopsies, where a single nonabsorbable suture may be used for the entire closure.

Like the standard vertical mattress technique, this technique is generally used for its pronounced effect on wound eversion. Therefore, while it is appropriate for most skin closures, it should be avoided when inversion is desired.

As with most transepidermal techniques, it is important to enter the epidermis at 90 degrees, allowing the needle to travel slightly laterally away from the wound edge before fully following the curvature of the needle when utilizing this technique. This will allow for maximal wound eversion and accurate wound-edge approximation.

An advantage of this approach, as with the vertical mattress technique, is that no suture material traverses the incised wound edge and that the suture similarly does not cross the surface of the wound. While this may be less than desirable when attempting to fine-tune epidermal apposition, it is helpful in minimizing the risk of unsightly track marks.

Drawbacks and Cautions

Since the dermal portion of the suture is executed with the same suture as the vertical mattress portion, if suture removal occurs too early, there is a risk of dehiscence, since no residual absorbable suture material is left in the wound. Similarly, if sutures are left in place for too long, there is a high chance of leaving residual track marks.

As the dermal portion of the suture is performed, it may be challenging to visualize the deep portion of the wound adequately, making placement of the deeper portion of the suture more challenging.

When removing sutures, a greater degree of force may need to be applied to remove the full length of the suture material, since the single length of suture has performed multiple loops in both the dermis and epidermis. Suture material breakage is therefore a possibility, and care should be taken to apply constant gentle traction.

With any suturing technique, knowledge of the relevant anatomy is critical. When placing this suture, it is important to recall that the structures deep to the epidermis may be compromised by the passage of the needle and suture material or that constriction may take place. That said, the vertical orientation of this approach helps minimize this risk.

This technique may elicit an increased risk of track marks, necrosis, and other complications when compared with techniques that do not entail suture material traversing the scar line, such as buried or subcuticular approaches. Therefore, sutures should be removed as early as possible to minimize these complications, and consideration should be given to adopting other closure techniques in the event that sutures will not be able to be removed in a timely fashion.

Reference

Naimer SA, Biton A, Topaz M. The subcutaneous loop: a single suture technique for skin closure after superficial and subcutaneous surgery. *J Drugs Dermatol*. 2006;5(10):966-968.

The Cross Stitch

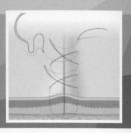

Application

This is a niche technique used for closure, hemostasis, and epidermal approximation of select wounds. It may be conceptualized as a simple running suture that is performed without an anchoring knot and that, when the terminus is reached, travels in the opposite direction toward the original wound apex. While it demonstrates an elegant and symmetrical postoperative appearance, it also entails the placement of a greater number of transepidermal sutures while providing little extra in terms of functional benefit, and therefore, it is used only infrequently.

Suture Material Choice

As with all techniques, it is best to use the thinnest suture possible in order to minimize the risk of track marks and foreign-body reactions. Suture choice will depend largely on anatomic location and the goal of suture placement. The cross stitch may be utilized either to aid in wound-edge approximation or to help with hemostasis. In the latter case, slightly thicker suture material may be utilized.

On the face, a 6-0 or 7-0 monofilament suture may be used for epidermal approximation. Indeed, 5-0 or 6-0 monofilament may be used on the extremities as well, though 4-0 monofilament suture may be utilized in areas under moderate tension

where the goal of suture placement is relieving tension and hemostasis as well as epidermal approximation.

Technique

1. The needle is inserted perpendicular to the epidermis, approximately one-half the radius of the needle distant to the wound edge. This will allow the needle to exit the wound on the contralateral side at an equal distance from the wound edge by simply following the curvature of the needle.

2. With a fluid motion of the wrist, the needle is rotated through the dermis, taking the bite wider at the deep margin than at the surface, and the needle tip exits the skin on the contralateral side.

3. The needle body is grasped with surgical forceps in the left hand and pulled upward with the surgical forceps as the body of the needle is released from the needle driver.

4. A tail of free suture material is then left, and no knot is tied. A hemostat may be used to clamp the tail of the suture to avoid the risk of pulling it through during the subsequent steps.

5. Starting proximal to the prior knot relative to the surgeon, steps (1) through (3) are then repeated sequentially, and the needle is advanced along the course of the wound until the contralateral apex is reached.

6. Once the apex is reached, steps (1) through (3) are then repeated heading

in the contralateral direction, again advancing along the wound, but now with entry and exit points crossing the previously placed line of sutures, forming an X appearance.

7. Once the apex is reached, the leading end of the suture is tied to the tail end of the suture using an instrument tie (Figures 5-39A through 5-39G).

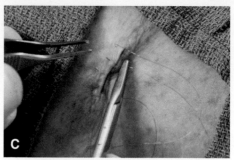

C

Figure 5-39C. Second bite, following the pattern of a simple running suture.

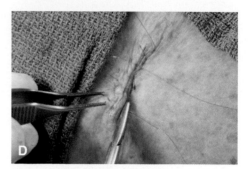

D

Figure 5-39D. The running series continues until the end of the wound is reached.

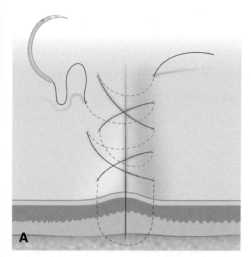

A

Figure 5-39A. Overview of the cross-stitch technique.

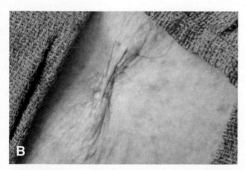

B

Figure 5-39B. Initiation of the suture. Note that a tail is left and there is no traditional anchoring suture to be tied.

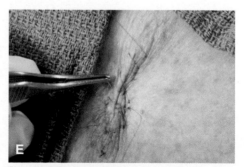

E

Figure 5-39E. After reaching the end of the wound, the suture pattern then reverses direction and moves distally toward the origination point.

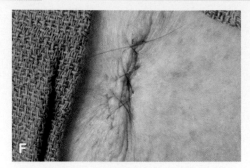

Figure 5-39F. The suture material is then pulled taut, creating a cross-stitch pattern.

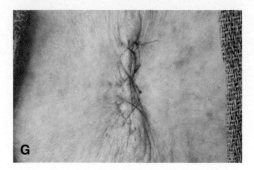

Figure 5-39G. Immediate postoperative appearance.

Tips and Pearls

As with the simple running suture, it is important to enter the epidermis at 90 degrees, allowing the needle to travel slightly laterally away from the wound edge before fully following the curvature of the needle when utilizing this technique. This will allow for maximal wound eversion and accurate wound-edge approximation.

As always, care should be taken to avoid skimming the needle superficially beneath the epidermis. This results from failing to enter the skin at a perpendicular angle and to follow the curvature of the needle. This may result in wound inversion as the tension vector of the shallow bite pulls the wound edges outward and down.

In order to maintain uniformity in the length of the visible running sutures and to allow all of the suture loops to remain parallel, it is important to take uniform bites with each throw. Therefore, each subsequent loop should begin at the same point lateral to the incised wound edge and at a uniform distance closer to the surgeon than the preceding entry point.

Sutures should not be tied too tightly, and it is helpful to permit sufficient laxity between the epidermis and the suture material when using this technique. This approach will help minimize the risk of track marks that may be associated with postoperative edema.

Drawbacks and Cautions

This technique has two main drawbacks. First, the integrity of the entire suture line rests on the integrity of a single knot. When this technique is used only to fine-tune epidermal approximation, knot failure is unlikely to lead to dehiscence, but if there is significant tension across the wound, this may be more problematic. Second, the additional row of simple interrupted sutures used in this technique does little to aid in wound-edge approximation or wound security, while concomitantly increasing the risk of track mark formation. Therefore, unless this approach is being utilized for its hemostatic effects, it may not be the ideal technique in most circumstances.

As with all running techniques, since each loop of the running suture material is designed to hold an equal amount of tension, it follows that areas of the wound under greater tension, such as its central portion, may tend to gape or potentially exist under greater tension, leading to an increased risk of track marks.

As with any suturing technique, knowledge of the relevant anatomy is critical. When placing the cross stitch, it is important to recall that the structures deep to the epidermis may be compromised by the passage of the needle and suture material. Thus, the needle may pierce a vessel, leading to increased bleeding, while a tightly placed suture may lead to necrosis due to vascular compromise or even, theoretically, superficial nerve damage.

This technique may elicit an increased risk of track marks, necrosis, inflammation, and other complications when compared with techniques that do not entail suture material traversing the scar line, such as buried or subcuticular approaches. Therefore, sutures should be removed as early as possible to minimize these complications, and consideration should be given to adopting other closure techniques in the event that sutures will not be able to be removed in a timely fashion.

Reference

Johnson TM, Bichakjian CK, Wang TS. Surgical pearl: the cross-stitch. *J Am Acad Dermatol.* 2001;44(4):673-674.

The Basting Suture

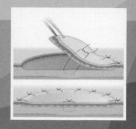

Synonym

Tacking suture

Video 5-40. The basting suture
Access to video can be found via
mhprofessional.com/atlasofsuturingtechniques2e

Application

Like the percutaneous suspension suture, this is a niche technique designed to fix the base of a graft to a deeper structure and is typically used when fixing a graft to underlying structures to minimize the risk of dead-space/hematoma formation and maintain close approximation between the underside of the graft and the underlying vascular bed. This may be used as an alternative or adjunct to tie-over bolster dressings for graft fixation, as the literature is equivocal on the relative benefits of basting sutures and bolster dressings.

Suture Material Choice

Depending on location, a 4-0, 5-0, or 6-0 nonabsorbable or fast-absorbing suture may be used.

Technique

1. After one edge of the graft has been fixed—or, at a minimum, a single suture has been placed to fix the graft, ideally on the distal edge relative to the surgeon—the suture needle is inserted at 90 degrees from the outside of the skin overlying the desired tacking point directly through the dermis, exiting on the undersurface of the graft at the point where fixation to the underlying anchoring point is desired. Since only the distal edge has been fixed, the graft can be gently reflected back, and the exit point of the needle can be easily visualized.

2. The needle is then gently pulled through the graft, regrasped, and inserted through the base of the graft bed at the desired point, and the needle's curvature is followed to take a small bite. Gentle tension can be exerted if desired to ensure than an adequate bite was taken.

3. The needle is then reloaded and inserted back through the underside of the reflected graft adjacent to its original exit point so that it exits on the outside of the graft.

4. The suture material is then tied using an instrument tie (Figures 5-40A through 5-40G).

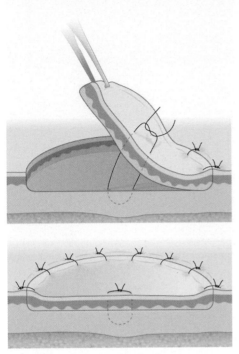

Figure 5-40A. Overview of the basting suture.

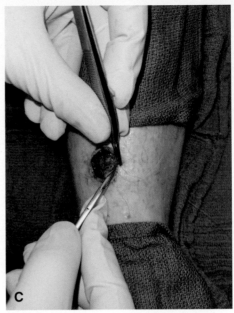

Figure 5-40C. The graft is reflected back, and the needle emerges through the now exposed underside of the graft. It is then reloaded.

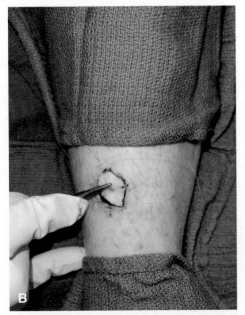

Figure 5-40B. The needle is inserted percutaneously at the desired location, directly through the graft.

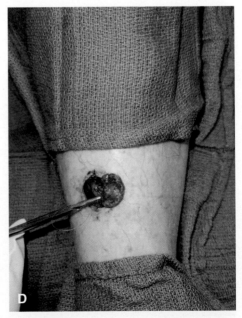

Figure 5-40D. The needle is inserted blindly through the base of the graft recipient site, a small bite is taken, and the needle then exits from the base of the graft.

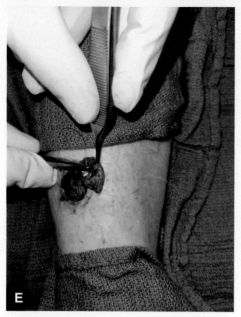

Figure 5-40E. The needle is then reloaded and inserted through the underside of the reflected graft directly adjacent to the original suture.

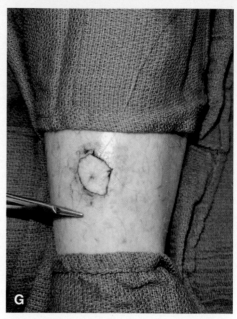

Figure 5-40G. The suture is then tied, and the base of the graft is fixed to the recipient bed. Note that the graft has not yet been trimmed.

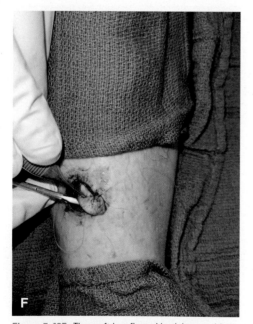

Figure 5-40F. The graft is reflected back into position, and the needle is pulled through.

Tips and Pearls

As with any traditional suspension suture, this technique's use demands familiarity with the underlying anatomy so that no sensitive deeper structures are injured or strangled during the blind placement of the deep anchoring suture. The deep suture should also be placed parallel to the underlying vascular plexus to similarly mitigate this risk.

When working in an area with a natural groove, such as on the nasal ala, or along cosmetic subunit boundaries, placing the basting suture(s) along the groove or boundary with the entry and exit points aligned along the long axis of the groove may help both recreate the natural groove and reduce the risk of graft tenting in the areas where it is most likely to occur.

Drawbacks and Cautions

As with any suspension suture, the anchoring portion of this suture technique carries the risk of damage to an underlying vascular or neural plexus. Familiarity with the underlying bony anatomy is therefore of paramount importance, as it also permits the surgeon to select the best location for suspension suture placement.

Care should be taken to avoid tying the suture too tightly, as this could result in long-term dimpling of the graft.

References

Adnot J, Salasche SJ. Visualized basting sutures in the application of full-thickness skin grafts. *J Dermatol Surg Oncol.* 1987;13(11):1236-1241.

Kromka W, Cameron M, Fathi R. Tie-over bolster dressings vs basting sutures for the closure of full-thickness skin grafts: a review of the literature. *J Cutan Med Surg.* 2018;22(6):602-606.

The Snug Tip Stitch

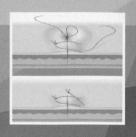

Video 5-41. Snug tip stitch
Access to video can be found via
mhprofessional.com/atlasofsuturingtechniques2e

Application

This is a niche technique used for reducing the appearance of dog ears, or standing cones, at the ends of elliptical excisions or local flaps. While dog-ear minimization is generally accomplished by excising lesions with fusiform incisions, this often extends the length of the wound significantly, which is undesirable. This technique was designed as an approach to mitigate the raised dog-ear appearance of the standing cone while concomitantly avoiding unnecessarily extending the length of the wound.

Suture Material Choice

Suture choice is dependent in large part on location. On the back and extremities, a 2-0, 3-0, or 4-0 nonabsorbable suture material may be used, and on the face and other areas under minimal tension, a 4-0 or 5-0 nonabsorbable suture is adequate. Alternatively, fast-absorbing sutures may be used as well.

Technique

1. The needle is inserted near the base of the dog ear in line with the long axis of the defect.
2. The needle courses deep to the dog ear, exiting where the incision line meets the dog ear.

3. The needle is then reinserted moving in the same direction 3-6 mm further along the wound edge.
4. The needle exits by passing through the epidermis just lateral to the incision line.
5. The suture is then tied with an instrument tie, securing the dog ear snug to the surrounding skin (Figures 5-41A through 5-41D).

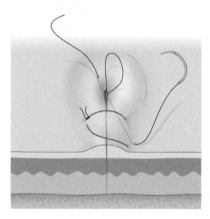

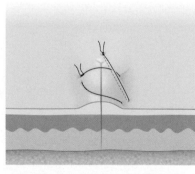

Figure 5-41A. Overview of the snug tip stitch.

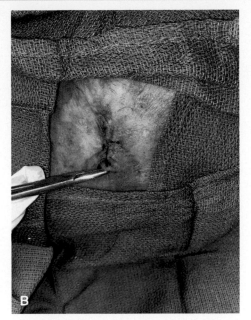

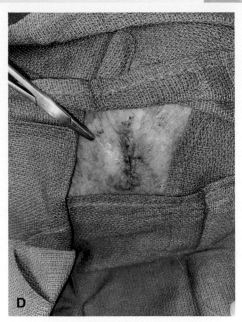

Figure 5-41B. The needle is inserted near the base of the dog ear in line with the long axis of the defect and courses deep to the dog ear, exiting where the incision line meets the dog ear.

Figure 5-41D. The suture is then tied with an instrument tie, securing the dog ear snug to the surrounding skin.

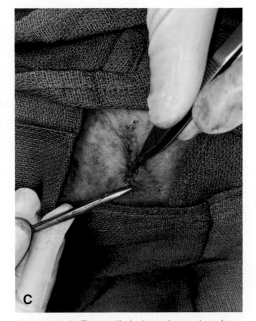

Figure 5-41C. The needle is then reinserted moving in the same direction 3-6 mm further along the wound edge and exits by passing through the epidermis just lateral to the incision line.

Tips and Pearls

This technique works best for small standing cones in lax skin, where all that is needed is for the suture to temporarily tamp down the dog ear. In some locations, such as convexities over the forehead, even defects repaired with a 4:1 ellipse may still display residual standing cones at the apices; therefore, this approach may be used as an adjunct in such cases as well.

Since no additional tissue is excised, this technique will occasionally lead to a rippling effect in the areas where it is utilized, though this is generally preferable to the dramatic bump that would otherwise be present when dog ears are left behind.

Some experience is helpful in deciding what degree of residual standing cone appearance is acceptable. Wounds on the lower legs, for example, often heal well, and residual standing cones may smooth out spontaneously, likely due to the tension over bony prominences. Conversely, standing cones over cheeks and other areas with abundant soft tissue often resolve only minimally over time, and therefore, leaving significant dog ears in these locations should be assiduously avoided if possible, and suturing techniques that mitigate their immediate appearance, such as the snug tip stitch, may be insufficient.

This approach, when used in concert with a technique such as the fascial plication suture, which causes a round or oval defect to appear more fusiform, may permit closure of wounds with significantly less standing cone removal, leading to shorter—and therefore more cosmetically appealing—scars.

Drawbacks and Cautions

The residual focal rippling of the epidermis caused by tissue redundancy will generally resolve with time, though in areas with significant actinic damage and solar elastosis, the lack of underlying elasticity may lead to residual textural changes that do not resolve. In these unusual cases, surgical revision may be useful to excise the residual area, as would be done for a dog-ear removal, thus leading to a more acceptable cosmetic outcome.

This technique is designed to address small standing cones that do not represent significant tissue bulk. In cases where bulky dog ears are present, oversewing them using the snug tip stitch approach may not be sufficient, and residual standing cones may remain.

Reference

Cronin MM, Li Y, Cronin TA, Cronin, TA. The snug tip stitch: a tissue-sparing technique for the correction of small dog ears. *Dermatol Surg.* 2021;47(7):1004-1005.

The Dog-Ear Tip Stitch

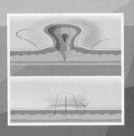

Video 5-42. Dog-ear tip stitch
Access to video can be found via
mhprofessional.com/atlasofsuturingtechniques2e

Application

This is a niche technique used for reducing the appearance of dog ears, or standing cones, at the ends of elliptical excisions or local flaps. While dog-ear minimization is generally accomplished by excising lesions with fusiform incisions, this often extends the length of the wound significantly, which is undesirable. This technique was designed as an approach to mitigate the raised dog-ear appearance of the standing cone while concomitantly avoiding unnecessarily extending the length of the wound.

Suture Material Choice

Suture choice is dependent in large part on location, though as always, the smallest gauge suture material appropriate for the anatomic location should be utilized. On the face, where this technique may be used for flap repairs, a 6-0 or 7-0 monofilament nonabsorbable suture is appropriate. On the trunk, extremities, and scalp, a 3-0 or 4-0 nonabsorbable suture material

may be used. Fast-absorbing absorbable sutures may also be used, obviating the need for suture removal but increasing the risk of tissue reactivity.

Technique

1. The needle is inserted into the proximal edge of the incision line adjacent to the dog ear at 90 degrees, with a trajectory running toward the base of the dog ear.
2. The needle is pulled through adjacent to the base of the dog ear, reloaded, and inserted parallel with the base of the dog ear in an almost horizontal orientation, as would be done for a purse-string suture. As the needle is freed from the tissue with the pickups, the needle is grasped again by the needle driver in an appropriate position to place the next throw.
3. The needle is then reinserted into the underside of the distal wound edge and exits on the distal edge of the incision line, parallel to the original entry point.
4. The suture material is then gently tied utilizing an instrument tie (Figures 5-42A through 5-42H).

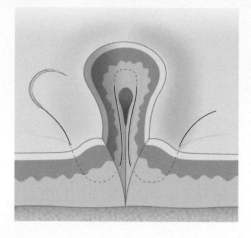

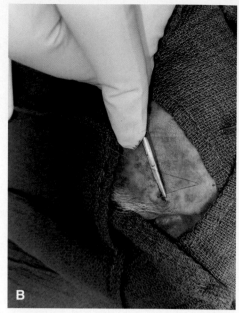

Figure 5-42B. The needle is inserted into the proximal edge of the incision line adjacent to the dog ear at 90 degrees with a trajectory running toward the base of the dog ear.

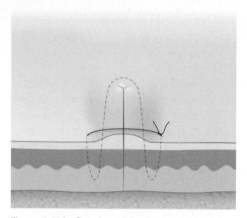

Figure 5-42A. Overview of the dog-ear tip stitch.

Tips and Pearls

This technique works best for small standing cones in lax skin, where all that is needed is for the suture to temporarily tamp down the dog ear. In some locations, such as convexities over the forehead, even defects repaired with a 4:1 ellipse may still display residual standing cones at the apices; therefore, this approach may be used as an adjunct in such cases as well.

Since no additional tissue is excised, this technique will occasionally lead to a rippling effect in the areas where it is

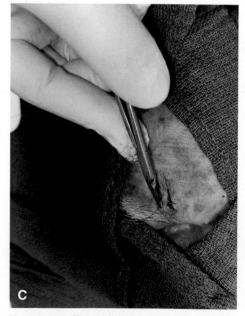

Figure 5-42C. The needle exits adjacent to the base of the dog ear.

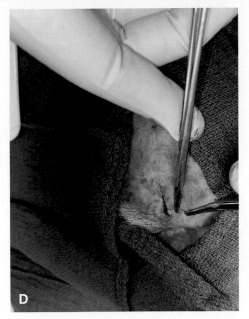

Figure 5-42D. The needle is reloaded.

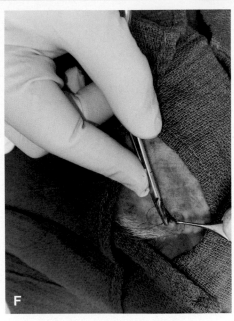

Figure 5-42F. Note the horizontal orientation of the needle.

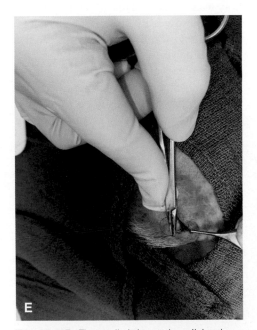

Figure 5-42E. The needle is inserted parallel to the base of the dog ear in an almost horizontal orientation, as would be done for a purse-string suture.

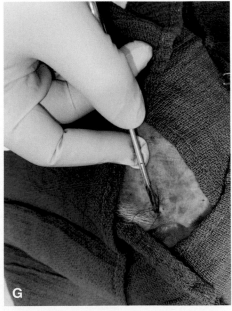

Figure 5-42G. The needle is then reinserted into the underside of the distal wound edge and exits on the distal edge of the incision line, parallel to the original entry point.

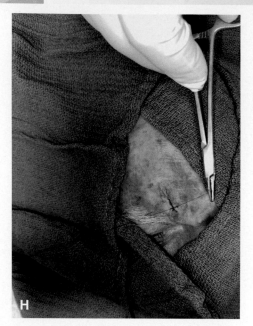

Figure 5-42H. The suture material is then gently tied utilizing an instrument tie.

utilized, though this is generally preferable to the dramatic bump that would otherwise be present when dog ears are left behind.

Some experience is helpful in deciding what degree of residual standing cone appearance is acceptable. Wounds on the lower legs, for example, often heal well, and residual standing cones may smooth out spontaneously, likely due to the tension over bony prominences. Conversely, standing cones over cheeks and other areas with abundant soft tissue often resolve only minimally over time, and therefore, leaving significant dog

ears in these locations should be assiduously avoided if possible, and suturing techniques that mitigate their immediate appearance may be insufficient.

This approach, when used in concert with a technique such as the fascial plication suture, which causes a round or oval defect to appear more fusiform, may permit closure of wounds with significantly less standing cone removal, leading to shorter—and therefore more cosmetically appealing—scars.

This can be thought of as a hybrid between a tip stitch and a purse-string suture in the ways it brings tissue together to reduce the appearance of dog ears.

Drawbacks and Cautions

The residual focal rippling of the epidermis caused by tissue redundancy will generally resolve with time, though in areas with significant actinic damage and solar elastosis, the lack of underlying elasticity may lead to residual textural changes that do not resolve. In these unusual cases, surgical revision may be useful to excise the residual area, as would be done for a dog-ear removal, thus leading to a more acceptable cosmetic outcome.

This technique is designed to address small standing cones that do not represent significant tissue bulk. In cases where bulky dog ears are present, oversewing them using the dog-ear tip stitch approach may not be sufficient, and residual standing cones may remain.

The Percutaneous Dog-Ear Tip Stitch

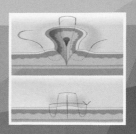

Video 5-43. Percutaneous dog-ear tip stitch
Access to video can be found via
mhprofessional.com/atlasofsuturingtechniques2e

Application

This is a niche technique used for reducing the appearance of dog ears, or standing cones, at the ends of elliptical excisions or local flaps. While dog-ear minimization is generally accomplished by excising lesions with fusiform incisions, this often extends the length of the wound significantly, which is undesirable. This technique was designed as an approach to mitigate the raised dog-ear appearance of the standing cone while concomitantly avoiding unnecessarily extending the length of the wound.

Suture Material Choice

Suture choice is dependent in large part on location, though as always, the smallest gauge suture material appropriate for the anatomic location should be utilized. On the face, where this technique may be used for flap repairs, a 6-0 or 7-0 monofilament nonabsorbable suture is appropriate. On the trunk, extremities, and scalp, a 3-0 or 4-0 nonabsorbable suture material may be used. Fast-absorbing absorbable sutures may also be used, obviating the need for suture removal but increasing the risk of tissue reactivity.

Technique

1. The needle is inserted into the proximal edge of the incision line adjacent to the dog ear at 90 degrees with a trajectory running toward the planned entry point adjacent to the center of the dog ear.
2. The needle is inserted through the undersurface of the dog ear, following its curvature and exiting. As the needle is freed from the tissue with the pickups, the needle is grasped again by the needle driver in an appropriate position to place the next throw.
3. The needle is then reinserted into the dog ear adjacent to its exit point at 90 degrees with a trajectory running toward the planned exit point on the distal edge of the incision line, parallel to the original entry point.
4. The needle exits at the distal exit point.
5. The suture material is then gently tied utilizing an instrument tie (Figures 5-43A through 5-43H).

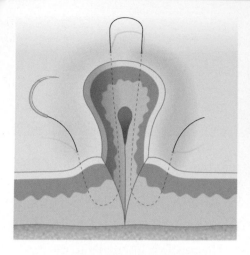

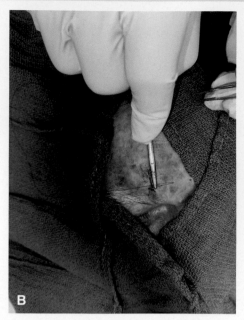

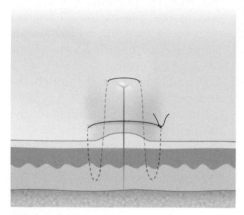

Figure 5-43A. Overview of the percutaneous dog-ear tip stitch.

B

Figure 5-43B. The needle is inserted into the proximal edge of the incision line adjacent to the dog ear at 90 degrees with a trajectory running either toward the incised wound edge or toward the planned entry point adjacent to the center of the dog ear.

Tips and Pearls

This technique works best for small standing cones in lax skin, where all that is needed is for the suture to temporarily tamp down the dog ear. In some locations, such as convexities over the forehead, even defects repaired with a 4:1 ellipse may still display residual standing cones at the apices; therefore, this approach may be used as an adjunct in such cases as well.

Since no additional tissue is excised, this technique will occasionally lead to a rippling effect in the areas where it is

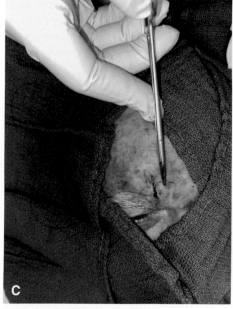

C

Figure 5-43C. The needle is reloaded after exiting in the center of the wound. Alternatively, for smaller dog ears, the needle could be passed directly through the underside of the dog ear, combing this step with the next.

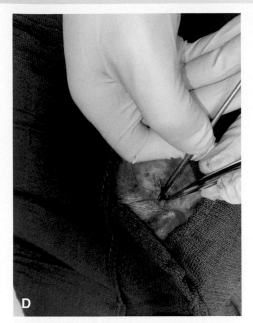

Figure 5-43D. The needle is inserted through the undersurface of the dog ear, following its curvature and exiting.

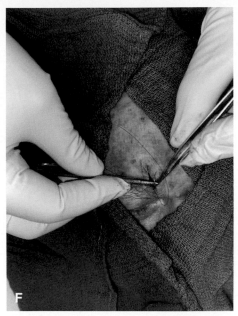

Figure 5-43F. The needle is then reinserted into the dog ear adjacent to its exit point at 90 degrees with a trajectory running toward the planned exit point on the distal edge of the incision line, parallel to the original entry point.

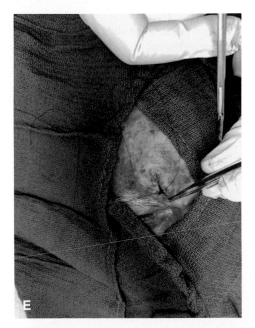

Figure 5-43E. The needle is freed from the tissue with the pickups. It will then be grasped again by the needle driver in an appropriate position to place the next throw.

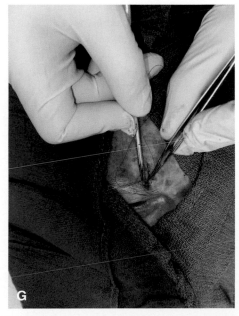

Figure 5-43G. The needle exits at the distal exit point.

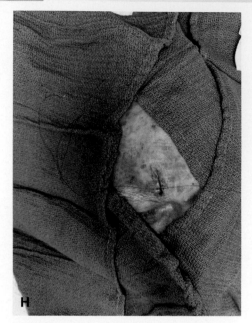

Figure 5-43H. The suture material is then gently tied utilizing an instrument tie.

utilized, though this is generally preferable to the dramatic bump that would otherwise be present when dog ears are left behind.

Some experience is helpful in deciding what degree of residual standing cone appearance is acceptable. Wounds on the lower legs, for example, often heal well, and residual standing cones may smooth out spontaneously, likely due to the tension over bony prominences. Conversely, standing cones over cheeks and other areas with abundant soft tissue often resolve only minimally over time, and therefore, leaving significant dog ears in these locations should be assiduously avoided if possible, and suturing techniques that mitigate their immediate appearance may be insufficient.

This approach, when used in concert with a technique such as the fascial plication suture, which causes a round or oval defect to appear more fusiform, may permit closure of wounds with significantly less standing cone removal, leading to shorter—and therefore more cosmetically appealing—scars.

Drawbacks and Cautions

The residual focal rippling of the epidermis caused by tissue redundancy will generally resolve with time, though in areas with significant actinic damage and solar elastosis, the lack of underlying elasticity may lead to residual textural changes that do not resolve. In these unusual cases, surgical revision may be useful to excise the residual area, as would be done for a dog-ear removal, thus leading to a more acceptable cosmetic outcome.

This technique is designed to address small standing cones that do not represent significant tissue bulk. In cases where bulky dog ears are present, oversewing them using the dog-ear tip stitch approach may not be sufficient, and residual standing cones may remain.

The Three-Dimensional Percutaneous Dog-Ear Tip Stitch

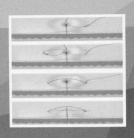

Video 5-44. Three-dimensional percutaneous dog-ear tip stitch
Access to video can be found via
mhprofessional.com/atlasofsuturingtechniques2e

Application

This is a niche technique used for reducing the appearance of dog ears, or standing cones, at the ends of elliptical excisions or local flaps. While dog-ear minimization is generally accomplished by excising lesions with fusiform incisions, this often extends the length of the wound significantly, which is undesirable. This technique was designed as an approach to mitigate the raised dog-ear appearance of the standing cone while concomitantly avoiding unnecessarily extending the length of the wound.

Suture Material Choice

Suture choice is dependent in large part on location, though as always, the smallest gauge suture material appropriate for the anatomic location should be utilized. On the face, where this technique may be used for flap repairs, a 6-0 or 7-0 monofilament nonabsorbable suture is appropriate. On the trunk, extremities, and scalp, a 3-0 or 4-0 nonabsorbable suture material may be used. Fast-absorbing absorbable sutures may also be used, obviating the need for suture

removal but increasing the risk of tissue reactivity.

Technique

1. The needle is inserted into the proximal edge of the incision line adjacent to the dog ear at 90 degrees with a trajectory running toward the planned entry point adjacent to the center of the dog ear.
2. The needle is inserted through the undersurface of the dog ear, following its curvature and exiting. As the needle is freed from the tissue with the pickups, the needle is grasped again by the needle driver in an appropriate position to place the next throw.
3. The needle is then inserted into the distal edge of the skin, directly across from the entry point of the first throw. It follows its curvature, exiting in the center of the dog ear adjacent to its exit point.
4. The needle is then reloaded and enters at the proximal edge of the incision line directly adjacent to its first entry point; it follows a trajectory directly perpendicular to the long axis of the wound, exiting adjacent to the second entry point.
5. The suture material is then gently tied utilizing an instrument tie (Figures 5-44A through 5-44I).

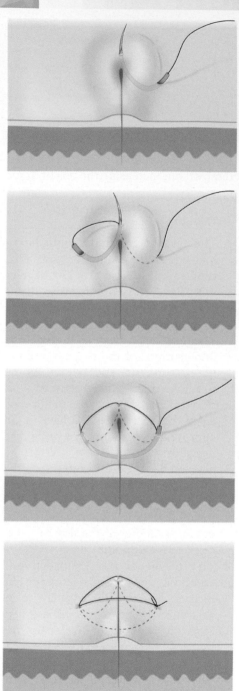

Figure 5-44A. Overview of the three-dimensional percutaneous dog-ear tip stitch.

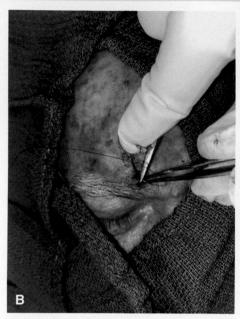

Figure 5-44B. The needle is inserted into the proximal edge of the incision line adjacent to the dog ear at 90 degrees with a trajectory running toward the planned entry point adjacent to the center of the dog ear.

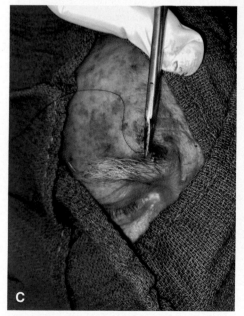

Figure 5-44C. The needle exits through the undersurface of the dog ear, following its curvature and exiting. As the needle is freed from the tissue with the pickups, the needle is grasped again by the needle driver in an appropriate position to place the next throw.

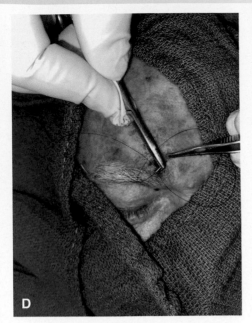

D

Figure 5-44D. The needle is then inserted into the distal edge of the skin, directly across from the entry point of the first throw.

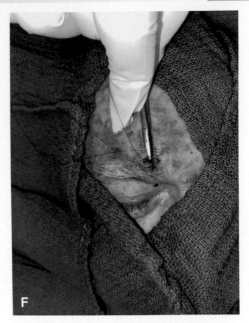

F

Figure 5-44F. The needle is then reloaded and enters at the proximal edge of the incision line directly adjacent to its first entry point and follows a trajectory directly perpendicular to the long axis of the wound.

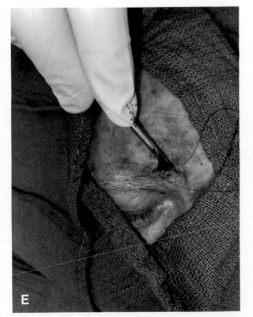

E

Figure 5-44E. The needle follows its curvature, exiting in the center of the dog ear adjacent to its exit point.

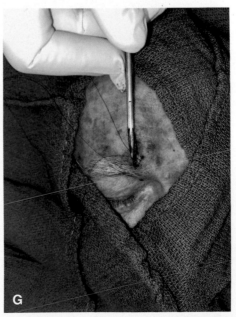

G

Figure 5-44G. The needle exits adjacent to the second entry point.

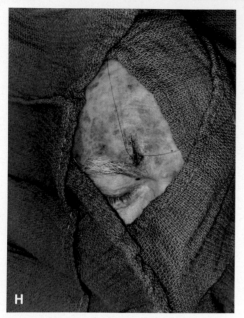

Figure 5-44H. Appearance prior to tying the suture.

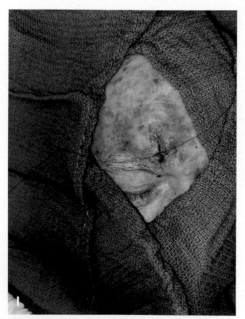

Figure 5-44I. The suture material is then gently tied utilizing an instrument tie.

Tips and Pearls

This technique works best for small standing cones in lax skin, where all that is needed is for the suture to temporarily tamp down the dog ear. In some locations, such as convexities over the forehead, even defects repaired with a 4:1 ellipse may still display residual standing cones at the apices; therefore, this approach may be used as an adjunct in such cases as well.

Since no additional tissue is excised, this technique will occasionally lead to a rippling effect in the areas where it is utilized, though this is generally preferable to the dramatic bump that would otherwise be present when dog ears are left behind.

Some experience is helpful in deciding what degree of residual standing cone appearance is acceptable. Wounds on the lower legs, for example, often heal well, and residual standing cones may smooth out spontaneously, likely due to the tension over bony prominences. Conversely, standing cones over cheeks and other areas with abundant soft tissue often resolve only minimally over time, and therefore, leaving significant dog ears in these locations should be assiduously avoided if possible, and suturing techniques that mitigate their immediate appearance may be insufficient.

This approach, when used in concert with a technique such as the fascial plication suture, which causes a round or oval defect to appear more fusiform, may permit closure of wounds with significantly less standing cone removal, leading to shorter—and therefore more cosmetically appealing—scars.

This approach can be conceptualized as a dog ear–addressing version of the percutaneous tip stitch, as originally described as the three-dimensional continuous suturing technique.

Drawbacks and Cautions

The residual focal rippling of the epidermis caused by tissue redundancy will generally resolve with time, though in areas with significant actinic damage and solar elastosis, the lack of underlying elasticity may lead to residual textural changes that do not resolve. In these unusual cases, surgical revision may be useful to excise the residual area, as would be done for a dog-ear removal, thus leading to a more acceptable cosmetic outcome.

This technique is designed to address small standing cones that do not represent significant tissue bulk. In cases where bulky dog ears are present, oversewing them using the dog-ear tip stitch approach may not be sufficient, and residual standing cones may remain.

This technique involves the placement of numerous percutaneous sutures through a delicately vascularized dog ear, and there is a theoretical risk of necrosis or track marks when using this approach.

CHAPTER 6

Suturing Tips and Approaches by Anatomic Location

The Chest, Back, and Shoulders

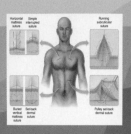

The chest, back, and shoulders are at once among the least challenging areas to repair—given the often ample tissue laxity, low patient expectations for cosmesis, and lack of anatomic danger zones and cosmetic unit boundaries—and among the most challenging, since the rate of hypertrophic scar formation and the tension from repetitive actions of daily living are rather high.

Therefore, reconstruction of these areas affords the flexibility of a potpourri of treatment approaches while demanding a reconstructive technique aimed at assuring that the tension across the wound surface, both at the time of closure and in the perceived future, remains kept to a minimum. Anticipating patient activity levels is of the utmost importance, as wounds in these areas may appear to be under a mild degree of tension at the time of reconstruction, while the patient lays in a restricted position and in a controlled environment; that same patient, however, is likely to be quite active even in the immediate postoperative period, and the tension across the nascent wound may increase exponentially. Therefore, designing a closure with an eye to the future and after gaining a modicum of appreciation of the patient's activity level is absolutely critical, since the same wound may be closed utilizing a variety of suturing techniques depending on the anticipated degree of tension that it will need to withstand.

In general, every effort should be made to close wounds in a linear fashion. This allows for the greatest chance of healing with minimal scarring, obviates the risk of flap or graft necrosis, and is generally the most cost-effective approach.

For the most part, reconstruction of the skin and soft tissues on the trunk does not present any major challenges. Unlike the head and neck, there are few danger zones to avoid, and the relative thickness of the underlying tissue planes makes for a rather forgiving canvas on which to work.

A few areas deserve special mention—the nipple unit and umbilicus may both be thought of as cosmetic subunits of their own. As with facial reconstruction, it is important to appreciate that the eye is drawn to these subunits and that any compromise of their unity leads to a cosmetic impression of imbalance out of proportion to the actual size and nature of the scar. Therefore, every effort should be made to maintain the integrity of these subunit boundaries.

For the nipple and areola, defects in the periareolar zone should be confined to this area. This may be accomplished by the use of rotation flaps in the immediate periareolar area, which may take advantage of the ability to hide incision lines in the outer boundary of the areola. Similarly, transposition flaps, M-plasties, and other approaches to shift the Burow's triangles may also be used to avoid extending the incision onto the areola.

For defects within the areola, every attempt should be made to confine the repair within the boundaries of the areola itself. In the event of complete loss of the nipple or areola, some basic suturing techniques may be useful in reconstructing these anatomic landmarks. For example, the circular appearance of the areola may be evoked by utilizing a purse-string suturing approach, and reconstruction of a lost nipple may be effected by performing an exaggerated purse-string approach leading to bunching of the central skin, creating a rudimentary nipple.

Similarly, the umbilicus should be thought of a unique subunit; defects or wounds in this area should ideally be repaired by either localizing the scar line within the umbilicus or reconstructing a modified umbilicus in cases of larger defects.

Of note, an inverting approach is useful here in order to recreate the natural inversion of the skin at the boundaries of the umbilicus. This may be accomplished with either simple buried dermal sutures or inverting horizontal mattress sutures. The Lembert stitch, or its running variant, the Cushing suture, may also be used to effect dramatic wound inversion.

Meticulous attention to technique remains the fundamental building block of all of these approaches, as even the best-planned flap or most thought-out approach can be waylaid by leaving suture track marks or other residual evidence of past surgical repair.

Suture Material Choice

High-tension areas such as the back, chest, and shoulders should always be closed with the assumption that the patient will have at least a moderate level of activity in the postoperative period. It is far better to use a slightly thicker suture than planned (as long as it is placed in the correct plane) than to err on the side of using too thin a suture for the tension in a given area.

Typically, 2-0 or 3-0 absorbable suture material may be used for fascial and dermal repairs in these areas. While a 0 suture may be used on thicker back dermis, in all but in the rarest of occasions, no suture material thicker than 2-0 should be required, especially if appropriate undermining has been effected.

Needle choice is similarly of critical importance when planning closures in high-tension areas. Smaller needles may easily bend when traversing the thicker dermis of the back; larger, semicircular needles such as the Ethicon CP-2 needle and its equivalents work very well and reliably penetrate even the thickest dermis without losing their curvature.

Not all backs are created equal; some older women, in particular, have relatively thin dermis on the back and attendant laxity; in these cases, a 3-0 suture material is more than adequate.

Suture Technique Choice

Among the most popular technique choices in these areas are the set-back dermal suture and the buried vertical mattress suture techniques. The butterfly suture may be used as well, though it is slightly more challenging to execute than the previously mentioned approaches and does not result in as much eversion as the set-back dermal technique. Because of the high tension in these areas, eversion is particularly critical, and leaving a residual ridge, mainly on the back and shoulders, is desirable as it may result in a more inconspicuous scar as the wound heals and the suture is absorbed.

In cases of particularly high tension, the various pulley suture approaches may be used to allow for better wound-edge approximation even in the face of extreme tension. Buried pulley approaches offer the mechanical advantage of a pulley effect without risking the attendant track marks and necrosis that could be associated with the placement of superficial pulley sutures.

Two easily effected buried pulley approaches for the back include the pulley set-back dermal suture and the pulley buried vertical mattress suture. The former offers significant advantages in terms of eversion and also relegates the suture material to the deeper dermis and avoids placing suture material between the incised wound edges, a significant advantage especially when larger gauge suture material is being used (Figure 6-1).

While the winch stitch or running external pulley suture may be utilized,

it is usually unnecessary in these anatomic locations where a robust dermis allows a great deal of material to be placed in a buried fashion, translating into an easily placed and effective buried pulley suture.

Superficial suture approaches include simple interrupted sutures for added security, as well as for finessing wound-edge approximation. These may also be used toward the edges of an elliptical incision in order to tamp down incipient dog ears, especially when overeverting the bulk of the wound in high-tension areas, as overeversion toward the apices of an elliptical incision may increase the risk of dog-ear formation.

In wounds under extreme tension, a few well-placed interrupted horizontal mattress sutures, using a relatively large-gauge suture material (such as 3-0 nylon),

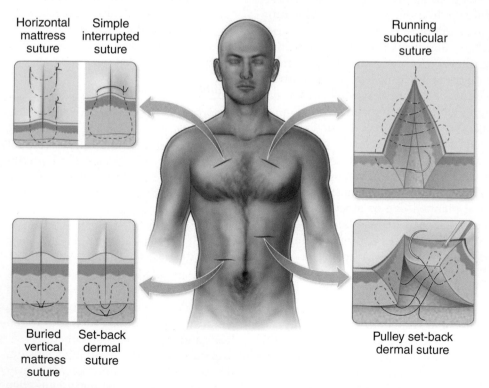

Horizontal mattress suture   Simple interrupted suture   Running subcuticular suture

Buried vertical mattress suture   Set-back dermal suture   Pulley set-back dermal suture

Figure 6-1. Frequently used suturing techniques on the chest and back.

may be useful both for added eversion and for a measure of extra wound security. Care should be taken, however, to remove these sutures early (5-7 days in most cases) in order to reduce the risk of residual track marks. Other mattress approaches, such as the vertical mattress or hybrid mattress, may also be used in high-tension areas.

Running subcuticular sutures may also be used as an outer layer of closure; importantly, this approach adds little if any strength to the wound, though it may be useful in finessing wound-edge approximation. With experience, the need for subcuticular suture material may be largely obviated by meticulous attention to technique in the placement of a sufficient number of buried sutures.

For the back and shoulders, elliptical excisions may be closed with a buried vertical mattress approach toward the apices and a set-back dermal approach toward the center. This allows for sufficient eversion all around with a more dramatic central eversion corresponding to the area that will be under the greatest tension. This also helps reduce the risk of overeverting the apices, as outlined previously.

For the superficial aspect of the closure, if the wound has been effectively closed under minimal tension, a running subcuticular technique may be used to finesse wound-edge approximation. If there is significant tension at the time of the closure or if the patient's activity level is anticipated to be high, placement of a set of simple interrupted sutures may be beneficial. Horizontal mattress sutures may be used toward the center of the wound to allow for additional wound security, though they should be avoided toward the apices to minimize overly dramatic eversion leading to dog-ear formation.

The Arms

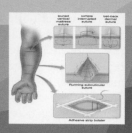

As with the chest and shoulders, the arms are often relatively straightforward to close, as for all but the largest defects, ample tissue is generally available for recruitment. When conceptualizing closure options on the arms, the anatomic location—the upper arm, inner arm, or flexor versus extensor surface—and the degree of atrophy should all be considered.

Classic approaches to closures on the extremities often advocate for attempting closure along the long axis of the extremity. While this approach may be reasonable for large defects, many smaller defects benefit from a closure either perpendicular to the long axis of the arm (ie, horizontally oriented) or on a diagonal. In either event, taking the time preoperatively to assess the degree of skin laxity and its direction is critical in designing the ideal closure. Sometimes, this orientation falls along the relaxed skin tension lines or Langer's lines, but this is not always the case, as closures must consider not only minimizing the tension across the wound but also minimizing the appearance of standing cones or dog ears.

On convex surfaces, such as the outer arms (as well as others, such as the forehead), it may be difficult to ensure a completely flat contour in the immediate postoperative period, though a significant degree of standing cone blunting often occurs in the postoperative period.

Closures along the long axis of the upper arm and forearm similarly may

result in a more profound dog-ear appearance, as the central portions of the closure are tightened relative to the surrounding skin, leading to an exaggerated standing cone appearance at the apices. Therefore, when possible, horizontally oriented closures may be preferable in these anatomic locations.

A major challenge relating particularly to forearm closures is the profound atrophy present in this sun-exposed area. Even closures under minimal tension must contend with the challenges of suture placement in atrophic areas, as the tendency toward suture material tear-through may be a problem even in the absence of marked tension. Percutaneous approaches, horizontally oriented techniques, and the use of tape bolsters may help in effectively closing such atrophic areas.

Suture Material Choice

For modest-tension closures on the upper arms, 3-0 or 4-0 absorbable suture material is generally adequate, while most forearm closures may be accomplished with 4-0 absorbable suture. Rarely, high-tension closures, such as those effected after a large melanoma resection on the muscular upper arm of a young patient, may benefit from 2-0 absorbable suture.

Transepidermal sutures, if used, are usually 5-0 nonabsorbable suture, though 5-0 absorbable monofilament suture may also be used for a subcuticular closure on the upper arm. In atrophic skin, subcuticular approaches are best avoided, as there is little dermis available to grasp and the small volume of surrounding skin means that suture absorption may be delayed.

Suture Technique Choice

The workhorse technique for most arm closures is a vertically oriented buried suture. The set-back dermal suture is highly effective, and the buried vertical mattress suture may be utilized as well.

Wide undermining is very helpful in leading to an effective closure, and undermining at the apices of the ellipse may aid in reducing the appearance of dog ears.

As always, a linear closure is preferable to a flap, and in all but the most extreme cases, most defects on the arms are easily closed in a linear fashion. An S-plasty may be utilized in order to mitigate the appearance of standing cones in select cases (Figure 6-2).

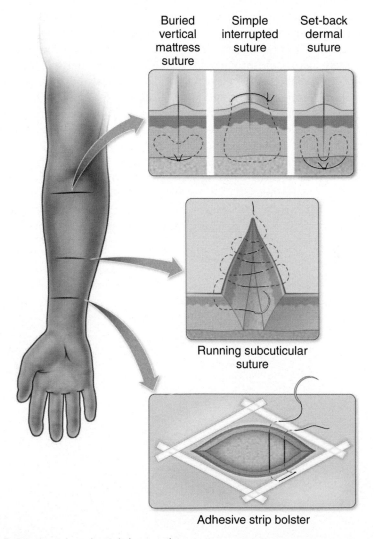

Figure 6-2. Frequently used suturing techniques on the arms.

While buried vertical mattress or set-back dermal sutures are frequently used for the bulk of these closures, other techniques may also be employed. In wounds under marked tension, pulley approaches, such as the pulley set-back dermal suture or pulley buried vertical mattress, may be useful; as always, however, these techniques should only be used if needed as they result in an increased volume of retained suture material when compared with their single-throw equivalents.

In wounds under very mild tension, running buried approaches may be utilized, though in general, interrupted buried sutures are favored whenever possible in order to militate against the problems associated with suture material breakage.

Superficial approaches, if utilized, include the running subcuticular technique, though as noted earlier, this should be avoided on atrophic forearms. Other frequently used approaches include the simple running suture and the running horizontal mattress technique.

On atrophic forearms, patients may benefit from closures using the percutaneous set-back dermal suture, the percutaneous buried vertical mattress suture, or the buried (or percutaneous) horizontal mattress suture. When the degree of atrophy is extreme, an adhesive strip bolster technique may be most appropriate.

As in other anatomic locations, combining the set-back dermal suture for the bulk of wound closure with buried vertical mattress sutures at the wound apices may help effect marked wound eversion while concomitantly avoiding extreme eversion (and thus standing cone formation) at the apices.

In wounds under extreme tension, a pulley set-back dermal suture or pulley buried vertical mattress suture may be placed at the center of the wound, with standard set-back or buried vertical mattress sutures placed over the remainder of the wound.

Similarly, when superficial sutures are used, placing a horizontal mattress suture toward the center of the wound coupled with a simple interrupted suture at the wound apex may be a useful approach.

The Legs

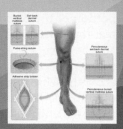

When contemplating wound closures on the lower extremities, clinicians should keep in mind that closures above the knee are fundamentally different from their below-the-knee counterparts. Thigh closures may be conceptualized as similar to closures on the upper arm—the dermis is moderate in thickness, and the area is under often substantial tension. On the shins, however, closures are often significantly more challenging. The presence of impaired circulation and high tension means that closures below the knee may be technically challenging to effect and are concomitantly fraught with an increased risk of infection and dehiscence when compared with closures elsewhere on the body.

An important principle when closing wounds below the knee is to anticipate the high risk of closure failure and therefore minimize the size of the defect. Thus, concerns regarding standing cone formation should be set aside when closing most shin defects. The high tension in these areas also means that as the repair heals over time the tension across the central portion of the wound may lead to blunting of the initial valley created by the closure, and therefore, the appearance of the dog ears will eventually resolve.

As with other highly mobile areas, it is important to plan appropriately when developing an ideal axis of wound closure. Therefore, the leg should be examined preoperatively both flexed and extended, and individual closure approaches should be tailored to each patient so that a patient who spends most of the day seated at a computer or in a wheelchair may have their wound closed on a slightly different axis than a highly active patient.

Suture Material Choice

Most wounds on the thighs are closed with a 3-0 absorbable suture material, though in small wounds under minimal tension, a 4-0 absorbable suture may be used. Similarly, wounds on the shins are often closed with a 3-0 absorbable suture, though when an adhesive strip bolster technique is used, a 3-0 nonabsorbable suture may be used as well.

Suture Technique Choice

The standard approaches to closure include the set-back dermal suture and the buried vertical mattress suture for most leg closures. Generally, these approaches are used on the thighs, though of course with larger defects under marked tension, a pulley variation of the previously mentioned techniques is possible as well. When closing wounds on the shins, however, other specific challenges may emerge. These wounds are often very narrow, and the skin is often fairly inelastic and, therefore, may not permit easy placement of buried vertically oriented sutures. In such cases, placing a percutaneous set-back dermal suture may be an alternative. Other approaches include the percutaneous buried vertical mattress technique (though the shallow portion of the bite may result in tissue tear-through in the thin skin of the shins) and the percutaneous horizontal mattress suture (where the horizontal orientation allows for a broader and more robust bite of dermis). The adhesive strip bolster approach utilized in concert with a horizontal mattress suture is also a mainstay of therapy for closing narrow atrophic wounds on the shins (Figure 6-3).

Superficial closures may be performed utilizing a running subcuticular technique; when absorbable monofilament suture is used with this approach, it affords the benefit of long-lasting wound-edge approximation. Other interrupted sutures may be used as well, with simple interrupted, horizontal mattress, and vertical mattress representing some of the most frequently used techniques for wounds on the thighs.

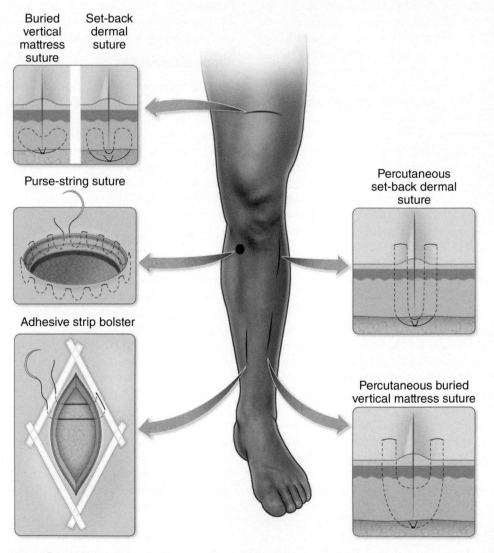

Figure 6-3. Frequently used suturing techniques on the legs.

On the shins, care should be taken not to oversew the area. There is sometimes a temptation to add additional sutures when the wound edges are not precisely approximated. While other anatomic locations, such as the face, are very forgiving when extra sutures are placed, the poor vascular supply to the lower legs means that adding extra suture material, except when necessary, should be avoided.

An additional option when closing the lower legs is to perform a purse-string closure. Since cosmesis on the shins is often subpar and keeping the wound as small as possible is of paramount importance, the purse-string approach may be a useful adjunct. Because the skin on the shins is often atrophic, the percutaneous purse-string technique may generally be the most appropriate in this location.

On the thighs, the usual approach of utilizing set-back dermal sutures except at the apices where buried vertical mattress techniques are used may be the most appropriate. On the knees, adding additional horizontal mattress sutures layered over top of set-back dermal sutures may aid in tension reduction in these high-mobility areas.

The percutaneous purse-string technique may be used on the shins in concert with simple interrupted or horizontal mattress sutures to obtain wound-edge approximation. Partial closure of large defects on the lower leg with purse-string closures may be augmented by allowing the remainder of the wound to close via secondary intention healing.

The Hands and Feet

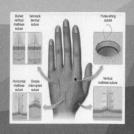

The hands and feet present some novel challenges to wound closure. First, these areas are highly mobile—by their very nature, these locations are under constant stress, so that the dorsal hands are subject to significant stretching when making a fist or grasping an object. Second, these areas are subject to repetitive friction—on the hands when they are put in a pocket or purse and on the feet while wearing shoes. Moreover, since the hands are frequently exposed to bacteria in the course of everyday events and the feet often spend the day occluded and are bathed in a significant bacterial load during showers, these areas also have a theoretically higher risk of postoperative infection.

Due to these considerations, wound repair on the hands and feet is best accomplished by effecting a robust closure with a minimal degree of transepidermal suture placement. As with all anatomic locations, linear closure is generally preferred if at all possible, and the overwhelming majority of defects on the hands and feet may be closed in a linear fashion.

Careful broad undermining is very helpful in these locations where the vasculature is often easily visualized in the subdermal plane. As with all closures, examining patients throughout their range of motion may be helpful in determining the best axis for closure. Generally, longitudinal closures along the long axis of the hand or foot are favored, both in terms of minimizing tension and mitigating the risk of postoperative lymphedema. That said, individual variations and individual propensities must always be taken into account when designing a closure.

Suture Material Choice

On the hands and feet, 3-0 or 4-0 absorbable suture material is often used as the mainstay of closure. Although the skin in these areas is often under marked tension, smaller needles such as the PS-3 or P-3 needle may be most useful since the defects are generally modest in size and the dermis on the hands, while tougher on younger patients, may become markedly atrophic with age and accumulated solar damage.

For superficial closures, 5-0 absorbable suture may be used for a subcuticular closure, while 5-0 nonabsorbable suture may be used for transepidermal closures. On the feet of younger patients, 4-0 or even 3-0 nonabsorbable suture may also be used when placing interrupted transepidermal sutures.

Suture Technique Choice

As in most locations, the set-back dermal suture or buried vertical mattress suture is generally the technique of choice on the hands and feet. Since these wounds are sometimes fairly narrow, percutaneous approaches such as the percutaneous set-back dermal suture, percutaneous buried vertical mattress suture, or buried horizontal mattress suture may be useful as well (Figure 6-4).

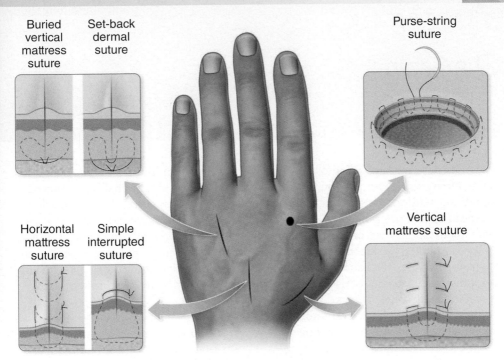

Figure 6-4. Frequently used suturing techniques on the hands and feet.

In wounds under marked tension, the pulley set-back dermal or pulley buried vertical mattress sutures may be useful techniques, particularly when placed toward the center of a wound under tension. The relatively robust dermis on the hands and feet of younger patients means that everting horizontally or obliquely oriented techniques, including the butterfly suture, are viable options as well.

The presence of significantly sized vessels very close to the underside of the dermis means that caution should be exerted when placing transepidermal sutures on the dorsal hands and feet. With wide undermining in the appropriate plane, these larger vessels are easily visualized when placing buried sutures.

Transepidermal sutures could easily perforate a superficial vessel, and therefore, unless they are necessary, it may be best to avoid traditional approaches such as the simple running suture. Instead, utilizing either skin adhesive or a running subcuticular approach may be preferable, especially on the highly vascular dorsal hands. This has the added benefit of minimizing the amount of suture material extruding from the skin that could be caught when placing the hand in a pocket or purse in the postoperative period.

In select cases, purse-string approaches may be useful as well, although the postoperative cosmesis is generally not as appealing as when using linear closures.

The Scalp

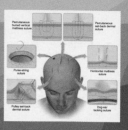

Closures on the scalp, like those on the shins, often involve narrow wounds under significant tension. Most surgical repairs on the scalp take place on the bald scalp of older men, where years of actinic damage have contributed to skin cancer development. In such cases, the skin may be slightly atrophic, and the degree of tissue mobility is variable, with some patients demonstrating a remarkably elastic and redundant tissue reserve and others presenting with a tight scalp with minimal laxity.

Closures on the hair-bearing scalp, such as those effected after a nonmelanoma skin cancer or pilar cyst excision, often occur in areas with a thicker dermis that has not been exposed to the same degree of actinic damage and where the ensuing atrophy has not taken place. In such cases, the benefit of working with a thicker dermis may be mitigated by the complexity of closing a wound in a hair-bearing location.

As with all closures, it is preferable to utilize a linear repair when possible. Smaller defects are easily closed in this fashion, though larger defects on the scalp may necessitate flap or graft closure. Secondary intention healing is also, of course, an option, particularly for thinner defects.

It is also important to recall that there may be significant atrophy in this sun-exposed area. Even closures under minimal tension must contend with the challenges of suture placement in atrophic areas, as the tendency toward suture material tear-through may be a problem even in the absence of marked tension.

The convex nature of the scalp also lends itself to unique challenges, as repairs over a convex surface have a tendency to lead to pronounced dog-ear formation even when utilizing narrow ellipses with a high length-to-width ratio. Specific techniques, including the dog-ear tacking suture, may be helpful in such cases.

Suture Material Choice

Repairs on the scalp under moderate tension may benefit from utilizing a 3-0 absorbable suture, while those under minimal tension, such as defects created by excising a pilar cyst, can be closed with 4-0 absorbable suture. Moderately sized needles, such as the FS-2, are a reasonable choice for most scalp closures. Superficial sutures may include suture material ranging from a 3-0 nonabsorbable suture that may be used for additional tension relief in large closures to a 5-0 nonabsorbable suture that may be used for improving wound-edge approximation.

Suture Technique Choice

As in most locations, either the set-back dermal suture or the buried vertical mattress suture is generally the technique of choice on the scalp. Since scalp wounds are often fairly narrow, approaches such as the percutaneous set-back dermal suture, percutaneous buried vertical mattress, or percutaneous horizontal mattress may be useful (Figure 6-5). The percutaneous set-back dermal technique may be the approach of choice as it is easy to place and has only minimal chance of tissue tear-through. The percutaneous vertical mattress suture, especially when placed on the atrophic skin of the scalp, may lead to tear-through of its superficially placed arms.

In scalp wounds under marked tension, the pulley set-back dermal and pulley buried vertical mattress sutures may be useful techniques, particularly when placed toward the center of a wound under tension. For narrow low- to moderate-tension wounds, a running percutaneous set-back dermal technique

may be effective, as it is easy to place in narrow wounds.

Since the convex surface of the scalp may lead to dog-ear formation, the dog-ear tacking suture may be useful in some scalp wounds. The postoperative appearance of dimpling at the apices of the wound is generally not of major concern to the patient, and as the suture is absorbed, a significant reduction of dimpling gradually occurs. As in all convex areas, care should be taken to avoid overly chasing the dog ears, as they may remain apparent even after extensive dog-ear corrections are undertaken.

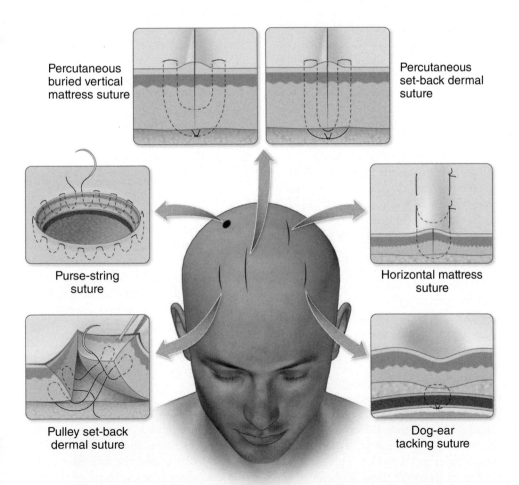

Percutaneous buried vertical mattress suture

Percutaneous set-back dermal suture

Purse-string suture

Horizontal mattress suture

Pulley set-back dermal suture

Dog-ear tacking suture

Figure 6-5. Frequently used suturing techniques on the scalp.

The Forehead

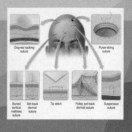

The forehead presents unique challenges and opportunities to the surgeon. The convex surface may increase the tendency toward dog-ear formation, as even ellipses with large length-to-width ratios may result in a residual standing cone appearance.

Additionally, the relatively immobile skin and minimal laxity coupled with the nearby presence of the eyebrows may also translate into a risk of long-standing brow asymmetry in select cases. While this is generally addressed when designing the closure, suture technique may play a role here as well.

The natural furrows and wrinkles present, particularly on the muscular forehead of elderly men, also need to be considered when designing forehead closures and when choosing suture techniques, as blunting a dramatic wrinkle may draw attention toward an otherwise well-designed repair. In such cases, an inverting technique may be preferable. Conversely, patients treated with neurotoxins to mitigate the appearance of forehead wrinkles may benefit from everting techniques that will leave only barely perceptible scars as they heal.

As always, linear closures are preferable to flap and graft techniques whenever possible. Often, such closures are directed transversely across the forehead, so that the suture line remains hidden in the natural lines and wrinkles. This must also be weighed against the risk of causing an asymmetrical brow lift. Suture techniques directed at fixing the lower portion of the repair in place or maximally mobilizing the upper portion of the repair, such as suspension sutures, may be useful in these situations. Occasionally, however, especially with medially located defects, causing a subtle brow lift may be desirable.

For larger defects on the forehead, vertically oriented repairs may be useful as well. As with paramedian forehead flaps, a full-thickness incision and subgaleal undermining may be used to further mobilize tissue and to permit a straightforward linear closure.

Suture Material Choice

For mild- to moderate-tension closures on the forehead, 5-0 absorbable suture is generally sufficient. Using a small needle, such as the P-3 reverse cutting needle, is often adequate. For wounds under greater tension, 4-0 absorbable suture material may be used as well, particularly if a deep incision has been made and the wound is being closed with plication or deep soft tissue sutures. Fine-gauge 6-0 or 7-0 nonabsorbable suture material may be used for transepidermal sutures.

Suture Technique Choice

As with most closures on the face, workhorse techniques such as the set-back dermal suture and the buried vertical mattress suture are the usual approaches of choice (Figure 6-6).

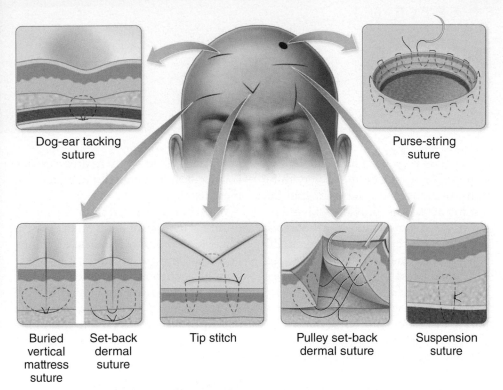

Dog-ear tacking suture

Purse-string suture

Buried vertical mattress suture

Set-back dermal suture

Tip stitch

Pulley set-back dermal suture

Suspension suture

Figure 6-6. Frequently used suturing techniques on the forehead.

As briefly noted earlier, an important exception to this approach would be utilizing inverting techniques when attempting to hide a closure within pronounced skin folds or wrinkles on the forehead. This should be reserved for use in wrinkles that are profound and in cases where the patient has no plans to utilize neurotoxins or other approaches to mitigate the appearance of their wrinkles in the future. Utilizing a simple buried dermal suture technique for the deep sutures combined with an inverting horizontal mattress or Lembert suture for the transepidermal component may aid in promoting wound-edge inversion.

Given the tendency for forehead closures to resist dog-ear correction, the dog-ear tacking suture may be considered in such cases. The immediate postoperative dimpling effect generally resolves with time, permitting closures to remain relatively short while avoiding the exaggerated dog ears that would otherwise be present. When advancement flaps are utilized, the tip stitch, or one of its variants, is frequently utilized.

For larger defects in the upper forehead, occasionally the purse-string technique or one of its modifications may be useful as well; while this does not result in a fine linear scar, it may permit more rapid healing than would be seen with secondary intention healing alone.

The Eyelids

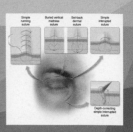

The eyelids present unique challenges to the surgeon—the dermis is very thin, with a near absence of subcutaneous fat in some areas. This provides only minimal tissue volume to aid in absorbable suture material breakdown, potentially increasing the chance of suture spitting or suture abscess formation. Moreover, the highly elastic eyelid skin also means that a disfiguring residual pull is possible, so that ectropion—while something to avoid at all costs—is only the most extreme outcome along a spectrum of lid pull abnormalities.

The unique challenges associated with eyelid repair mean that some of the standard buried suturing techniques may be less useful in these locations, and the lack of significant tension along most eyelid repairs means that running or transepidermal techniques, which should be used sparingly in many locations to minimize the risk of scar spread, may be appropriate. Medial canthal eyelid repairs should sometimes be avoided altogether, as this area tends to heal well by secondary intention.

Suture Material Choice

When absorbable suture material is used in eyelid repairs, 5-0 or 6-0 braided or monofilament suture material may be used. It is important to avoid using thicker suture material on the eyelids, as the large volume of suture material in knots relative to the thickness of the dermis may impede the process of suture

material breakdown by hydrolysis. Fine P-3 needles are generally adequate for these repairs.

When transepidermal sutures are used, 6-0 or 7-0 monofilament is often the best. These locations may also heal well using fast-absorbing gut suture (or the newer rapidly absorbing synthetic sutures), where the disadvantage of higher tissue reactivity should be weighed against the benefit of utilizing a rapidly absorbing suture material that obviates the need for suture removal.

Suture Technique Choice

Despite the often-thin dermis present on the eyelids, standard approaches such as the set-back dermal suture and the buried vertical mattress technique are often utilized. Care should be taken to avoid skimming the needle too superficially, leading to an essentially percutaneous repair (Figure 6-7).

In patients with a very thin dermis or with marked atrophy, placing absorbable sutures may be particularly challenging. In such cases, simple interrupted sutures may be used to easily approximate eyelid skin. Running variations, such as the simple running suture, may be used as well. While overeversion of the eyelid skin should be avoided, transepidermal everting techniques, such as the running horizontal mattress or running diagonal mattress suture, may be used as well. Unlike repairs in anatomic locations under tension, the transepidermal closures may

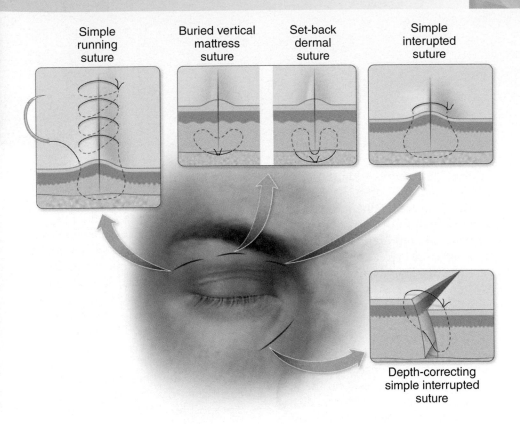

Figure 6-7. Frequently used suturing techniques on the eyelids.

be used as a solitary approach for some eyelid closures under minimal tension.

When working on the lower eyelid at the eyelid-cheek junction, a marked difference in dermal thickness may be appreciated between the thin eyelid skin and the thicker dermis of the upper cheek. In such cases, the depth-correcting simple interrupted suture may be helpful to maintain precise wound-edge apposition.

Finally, the Frost suture may be used to mitigate the risk of developing ectropion due to tissue edema in the immediate postoperative period. It is important to recall that this approach will not help when ectropion is present; rather, it is designed to minimize the chance that the postoperative edema and ecchymosis seen after lower lid surgery will lead to an iatrogenic ectropion. The benefit of placing a Frost suture should be weighed against the risk of the patient traumatizing the suture material, where an accidental pull could lead to a painful and possibly damaging outcome. Therefore, Frost sutures should only be left in place for a minimum period of time and should be covered with a wound dressing to avoid accidental tugging.

The Lips

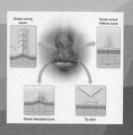

The lips, like the eyelids, represent a special site; they often have only a modest dermal component, necessitating consideration of alternative repair strategies, and represent a free margin, as they are fixed in place only by muscle. Therefore, any lateral tension across the lips often translates into a long-standing residual pull that does not resolve with time.

Accurate reapproximation of the vermilion border is of critical importance in lip repairs and reconstructions. Similarly, any residual dog ears on the lips, and particularly at the vermilion, do not resolve with time. Therefore, adequately extending linear excisions and performing a wedge resection when needed is of paramount importance.

Appreciating the anatomic subtleties and detail regarding the boundaries of the cosmetic subunits of the lip, while beyond the scope of this book, is a critical prerequisite to approaching any repairs in this cosmetically and functionally sensitive area.

While linear closures are, as always, preferred, the lack of any bony attachments means that residual pull will often not resolve on the lip. Therefore, larger defects may benefit from flap closures, where additional suture techniques, such as the tip stitch, buried tip stitch, vertical mattress tip stitch, or hybrid mattress tip stitch, could be useful.

Suture Material Choice

In general, 5-0 or 6-0 absorbable suture material is often used on the lips, as it is elsewhere on the face. Depending on surgeon preference, braided or monofilament suture material may be used.

Since lip repairs are generally approached in a layered fashion, absorbable suture may be used for both muscle and dermal repairs. For full-thickness defects, when the inner mucosal surface needs to be repaired first, fast-absorbing gut may be used first to reapproximate this difficult to reach layer.

For most lip repairs, 6-0 or 7-0 nonabsorbable sutures are generally appropriate. Transepidermal lip repairs often take advantage of the softness of silk suture material; while it is among the most reactive suture materials, its pliability makes it a good choice when repairs on the vermilion and mucosal lip are necessary in order to avoid the poking effect of nylon sutures. Similarly, fast-absorbing gut suture may also be used in these locations and confers the added advantage that suture removal is not necessary.

Suture Technique Choice

Standard buried dermal techniques, such as the set-back dermal and buried vertical mattress approaches, are frequently used on the lips (Figure 6-8). One important exception is around the vermilion border,

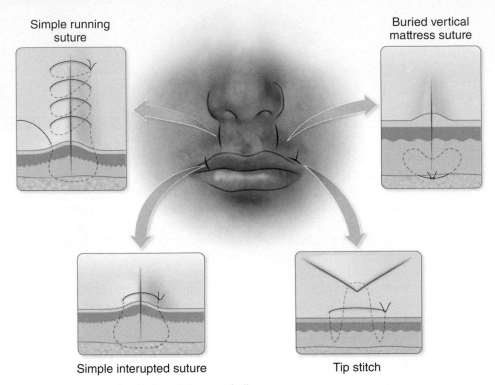

Simple running suture

Buried vertical mattress suture

Simple interupted suture

Tip stitch

Figure 6-8. Frequently used suturing techniques on the lips.

where overeversion should be assiduously avoided in order to preserve the integrity of the white line. In these areas, buried vertical mattress techniques, or even a simple buried dermal approach, may sometimes be more appropriate. As with the eyelids, since the lips represent a free margin, dog ears or marked hyper-eversion may resolve slowly, if at all (Figure 6-8).

Transepidermal approaches should be used with caution on the mucosal lip, and the rich vasculature of the lip should be kept in mind when placing transepidermal sutures that may lead to inadvertent piercing of underlying vessels. Conversely, mild residual oozing may be approached by placing a series of simple interrupted sutures or simple running sutures, as the hemostatic effect of this approach may place indirect pressure on the small leaking vessels, leading to adequate hemostasis. The running locking suture, while expressly advocated for this purpose, is rarely needed on the lip if adequate hemostasis was obtained prior to final closure. When it is used, however, care should be taken to avoid overtightening the individual loops of suture, as this may lead to tissue necrosis.

Simple interrupted sutures and depth-correcting simple interrupted sutures may also be useful when fine-tuning approximation of the lip margin. The ability of these interrupted approaches to guarantee precise wound-edge alignment is of paramount importance on these cosmetically sensitive closures, where a single millimeter of misalignment could have a dramatic effect on overall facial cosmesis.

The Nose

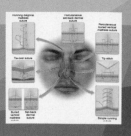

The nose is a frequently encountered surgical site for clinicians who focus on cutaneous reconstruction; the propensity for nonmelanoma skin cancer development in this area and the prominent location of the nose in the central face solidify the importance of appropriate repair approaches in this area.

While understanding and appreciating the importance of cosmetic subunits is an essential prerequisite for all skin and soft tissue reconstruction on the face, nowhere is this more important than on the nose. Understanding that defects must be approached with cosmetic subunit repair in mind and with an attention to restoration of the natural subunit boundaries and contours is perhaps the fundamental theoretical building block of all nasal reconstruction.

The three-dimensional complexity of the nose similarly necessitates particular attention. This is important not only for surface anatomy, where the inversion of the alar groove, for example, must always be recreated if violated, but also for the various layers of tissue that may require individual suturing and reconstruction— from cartilage to muscle to dermis.

All of these fundamental reconstructive and anatomic considerations necessarily translate into a rich array of suturing techniques that may be utilized when approaching nasal defects. Some stem from necessity, as narrow nasal wounds may not easily permit insertion of typical vertically oriented buried sutures, while others come from a need to recreate a natural depression, such as the alar groove or nasofacial sulcus.

Linear repairs on the nose are often possible even for larger defects, as wide undermining and the potential for tissue recruitment may permit midline repairs even when at first blush this does not seem feasible. Careful attention to dog-ear correction is of paramount importance. Local flaps and grafts, of course, may be utilized very frequently on the nose, though larger flaps, such as the paramedian forehead flap, are very useful for reconstructing large defects of the entire nasal tip subunit.

Nasal repairs of all sorts, since they take place on sebaceous skin, may benefit from dermabrasion approximately 3-9 months postoperatively. This may help smooth out any obvious repair lines on the nose, which may appear depressed relative to the surrounding sebaceous skin. It is important to adequately prepare patients for this possible eventuality.

Suture Material Choice

Often, 5-0 absorbable suture is used for the deeper layers of nasal reconstruction, though both thicker and thinner suture material is sometimes useful depending on individual circumstances. The P-3 reverse cutting needle is the most frequently used on the nose, though the narrowness of some nasal wounds means that a smaller semicircular needle, such as the P-2 needle, may be useful as well in order to permit insertion of the needle body into the wound for placement of vertically oriented buried sutures. While less readily available, consideration could also be given to utilizing a small cutting needle (or even a tapered needle), as opposed to a reverse cutting needle, since sometimes the atrophic sebaceous nasal skin has a tendency to tear as the reverse cutting needle moves superficially through the upper dermis.

For transepidermal techniques, 6-0 or 7-0 suture material is generally used on the nose. Since this outside layer of sutures often bears minimal tension, a fast-absorbing gut suture may be used as well, obviating the need for suture removal while potentially increasing the risk of tissue reactivity.

Suture Technique Choice

Standard buried techniques, such as the set-back suture or buried vertical mattress suture, are frequently used on the nose, though for smaller closures, it may be difficult to place these vertically oriented sutures. Utilizing a small P-2 needle may permit easier placement of vertically oriented buried sutures, though the semicircular nature of the needle means that it is more suited to set-back suture placement than buried vertical mattress suturing (Figure 6-9).

Another approach to closing narrow nasal wounds is the use of the percutaneous variations of the vertically oriented approaches, such as the percutaneous set-back suture or percutaneous buried vertical mattress suture. The percutaneous horizontal mattress suture could be used as well, though it provides less precise wound-edge apposition and has a higher theoretical risk of tissue necrosis. If percutaneous approaches are used,

the individual nasal skin type should be addressed, as patients with highly sebaceous skin may have a greater tendency to have trouble with residual dimpling from the percutaneous portions of the sutures.

Hyper-everting the wound edges should be avoided when working in the nasofacial groove, as eversion in this area may not resolve with time and could therefore leave a residual ridge. Similarly, the alar groove and other natural creases may be recreated using inverting techniques such as the simple buried suture, the inverting horizontal mattress suture, or the Lembert suture.

Suspension sutures may be used when recreating the more dramatic skin folds, such as the nasofacial sulcus and nasolabial folds. In addition to standard suspension sutures, the tie-over suture may be utilized, as well as the buried vertical mattress suspension suture, which add the benefit of being able to tack the suture material once the buried dermal suture is placed and the degree of tenting (or lack of inversion) is established.

Suspension sutures may also be used to maintain the patency of the alar valve. Traditionally, cartilage grafts have been placed to bridge open the alar valve, but placing a single superolaterally based suspension suture may quickly accomplish the same goal with only minimal morbidity and no need for a graft harvest.

Quilting sutures may be useful on large flaps in order to maintain the natural contour of the nose and minimize the risk of hematoma formation. These sutures may be conceptualized as an externally placed percutaneous tacking suture, where the epidermis is tacked to the underlying soft tissues.

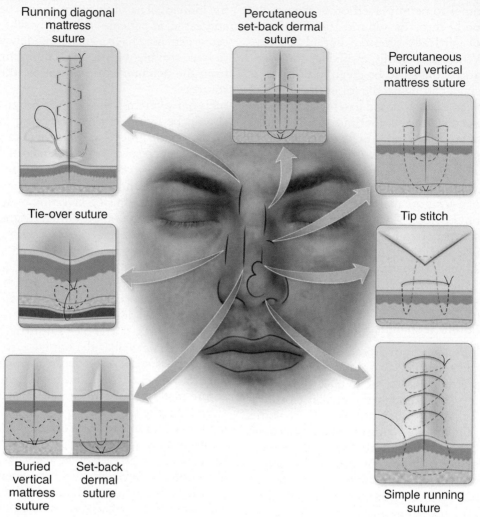

Running diagonal mattress suture

Percutaneous set-back dermal suture

Percutaneous buried vertical mattress suture

Tie-over suture

Tip stitch

Buried vertical mattress suture

Set-back dermal suture

Simple running suture

Figure 6-9. Frequently used suturing techniques on the nose.

The Ears

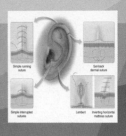

The ears, like the nose, have a complex three-dimensional array of ridges and valleys that must be respected if a reconstruction is to return the appearance of normal. Since the cartilaginous strut of the ear provides its basic structural integrity, the ear represents a type of free margin. Appreciating where the rigidity of the cartilaginous strut will force a dermal repair back toward the appearance of normalcy is an important principle of ear reconstruction and may permit linear closures of larger defects.

Tissue recruitment from the posterior ear, retroauricular sulcus, and mastoid allows for complex flap repairs on the helix and beyond. When the immediate postoperative effect is pinning back the ear, this may resolve with time, and therefore, retroauricular sulcus-based transposition flaps may be an excellent option for many helical repairs.

While as a general rule skin grafts should often be avoided in favor of flap repairs, repairs of the nonmargin areas of the ear, such as the conchal bowl, are readily accomplished with full-thickness skin grafts, where the retroauricular area provides a locus of plentiful donor tissue.

The ears are also unique in that flap repairs can twist in three dimensions so that an advancement or rotation flap may also have a significant twisting component, permitting even greater tissue recruitment and mobility.

These repair considerations are important when approaching suturing techniques, which serve as the fundamental building blocks of effective cosmetically appealing repairs. Many small defects along the helix may be repaired with a small complex linear repair perpendicular to the helical rim, while larger defects may necessitate a single or double advancement flap. Precise suturing techniques help hide scars along the cosmetic subunits of the ear, where eversion is critical to healing, particularly when transversely oriented repairs are used so that the suture line crosses cosmetic subunit boundaries.

Suture Material Choice

Generally, 5-0 absorbable suture is used for the deeper component of most ear repairs, though a heavier suture may be used when securing larger flaps in place in the retroauricular area or when tacking back the ear. Though the P-3 reverse cutting needle is generally used, narrower repairs may benefit from the smaller P-2 needle.

Transepidermal repairs may use 6-0 nonabsorbable suture, though 5-0 or 6-0 fast-absorbing gut may be useful as well and obviate the need for suture removal. For grafts, 5-0 or 6-0 gut or the newer rapid-absorbing synthetic sutures are excellent options as they avoid the need for suture removal, which on a graft site could traumatize the delicate graft and potentially impair healing.

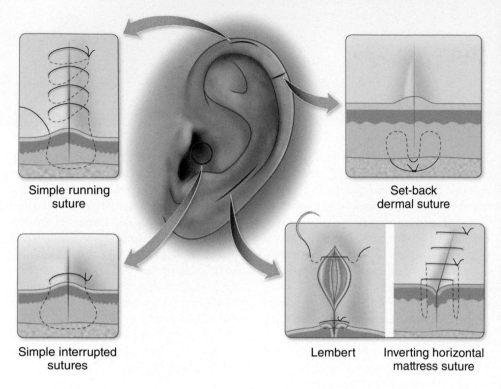

Simple running suture

Set-back dermal suture

Simple interrupted sutures

Lembert   Inverting horizontal mattress suture

Figure 6-10. Frequently used suturing techniques on the ears.

Suture Technique Choice

Everting set-back dermal or buried vertical mattress sutures are useful when closing most ear defects, as they provide excellent wound-edge approximation and eversion. Since some ear defects may be very narrow, percutaneous variations of these approaches may be utilized as well.

Another effective approach for the closure of narrow wounds is the percutaneous horizontal mattress suture. This technique also permits a smaller number of sutures to be placed in total, as each suture incorporates a broader area.

For recreating natural grooves, the inverting horizontal mattress suture and Lembert suture may be utilized. In pronounced cases, suspension sutures may be utilized as well, but care should be taken when tacking sutures to underlying cartilage (Figure 6-10).

When securing a graft, placing a series of simple interrupted sutures is often the best approach. Simple running sutures may also be used; either way, starting the suture from the graft and securing it to the surrounding skin may help minimize graft motion during active suturing. Fast-absorbing gut suture allows for easy suture placement without the need for suture removal. If a bolster is then used to secure the graft, it may be sutured in placed with a running or interrupted bolster suture.

CHAPTER 7

Approach to Technique Selection by Closure Type

Linear Excisions and Repairs

Suturing techniques play a critical role in the efficiency of surgical reconstruction, and technique choice may also affect the design of linear closures.

Historically, most linear closures relied on a bilayered closure approach, with sutures placed in the dermis for tension relief and transepidermally for wound-edge approximation. This paradigm has shifted over the past few years, with the realization that recruiting deeper tissue planes may have a profound effect on wound strength and cosmesis.

Fascial plication is one of the most useful techniques for linear closures, as it confers several advantages simultaneously.[1] First, it leads to significant tension reduction over the wound surface by shifting tension to the deep fascia. Second, it decreases the amount of undermining needed to permit effective closure, theoretically improving vascular supply to the undersurface of the advancing wound edges and reducing the risk of potential space formation that may increase the risk of hematoma formation. Finally, fascial plication has a significant effect on wound geometry, as a single fascial plication suture shifts a wound from a 3:1 fusiform shape to a 6:1 ratio and decreases the apical angles significantly.

Fascial plication sutures need not be used for all linear closures. This technique is most appropriate for areas under significant tension or large excisions where minimizing the postoperative wound length is desirable. On the face, recruiting the superficial musculoaponeurotic system (SMAS) may be very helpful. When designing the closure of a round defect, the fascial plication suture should be placed prior to removing the dog ears. The risks of fascial plication sutures include possible pain, a theoretically increased infection risk (since the fascial envelope has been pierced by suture), and a theoretical risk of vascular compromise through inadvertent pressure-induced ligation of perforating vessels. In practice, these complications are infrequent, though patients may experience transient pain during needle entry and immediately after the fascial plication suture is tied. If pain persists for more than 5 minutes, the suture should be removed.

Buried dermal sutures are the cornerstone of linear repairs. Two central suturing techniques are useful, the buried vertical mattress suture and the set-back dermal suture. The former yields significant wound-edge eversion and epidermal approximation, while the latter is easier to execute, provides even more eversion, and results in better cosmesis. Indeed, a randomized controlled trial has suggested that the set-back suture leads to cosmetically more appealing scarring than the buried vertical mattress suture. Its ease of use is a significant advantage as well, particularly as effective wound-edge eversion is one of the most challenging (and clinically critical) components of the linear excision and closure.

Set-back dermal sutures result in marked wound-edge eversion, though this can be adjusted based on how set back each bite is taken from the incised wound edge.

Though many manuscripts and chapters addressing linear closures advocate the placement of a key suture in the center of the wound followed by closure using the rule of halves, in practice, this may be less desirable than starting at one edge of the wound—typically the edge most distant from the clinician—and moving proximally. The latter technique allows tension to be gradually relieved, minimizing the tension across any single suture. This permits tissue creep to gradually take place over the course of the closure.

The set-back or buried vertical mattress sutures may be placed closer together in the center of the wound, where tensile forces are greatest. After placement of a full row of buried sutures, the wound edges should be well everted and ideally drape together under no tension. With assiduous attention to detail, this layer of sutures may lead to ideal wound-edge approximation, obviating the need for transepidermal sutures.

If transepidermal sutures are placed, they may be performed in a simple interrupted or running fashion. Ideally, there should be no tension across the wound surface after deep suture placement, and therefore, running sutures may be appropriate. Alternatively, some mild depth correction may be needed, and in such cases, depth-correcting simple interrupted sutures can be used. Running horizontal mattress sutures, often with intermittent simple loops, may also be helpful for yielding excellent wound eversion and avoiding suture material crossing over the incised wound edge. Running

subcuticular sutures may be used as well, though in the context of well-placed buried sutures, they often confer only minimal advantage while introducing additional foreign body material across the wound.

Laceration and Surgical Incision Repair

Lacerations and surgical incisions are often under minimal tension, since unlike excisions they do not require the removal of tissue that must then be accommodated by pulling a wound together under tension. Therefore, these circumstances often benefit from straightforward suturing techniques, such as set-back sutures and buried vertical mattress sutures, as workhorse techniques and simple running sutures or running subcuticular sutures as a secondary layer. Note that running subcuticular sutures remain very popular, although with meticulous placement of buried sutures, they may add little to a closure other than time and suture material. Running horizontal mattress sutures, often incorporating simple loops, may also be a useful approach, particularly when additional eversion is desired.

Flaps

Many of the same principles apply when suturing a local flap into place. A key distinction, however, is that well-designed flaps—like laceration repairs and incisional surgical repairs—may be under less tension, and therefore require less wound eversion, than some linear excisions and repairs. Therefore, in all but the most unusual of circumstances, if surgeons find that they are working under extreme tension and require pulley versions of suturing techniques, this may be a sign that their flap design is imperfect. Therefore, as with linear closures, set-back sutures and buried vertical mattress sutures are the fundamental building blocks of flap suturing.

Grafts

As with flaps, graft repairs—or, at least, the graft recipient site—should generally be under very little to no tension. Such closures thus benefit from a combination of simple interrupted, simple running, and depth-correcting simple interrupted sutures at their periphery and basting sutures (or their variants, such as pinpoint pexing sutures) in the center. Fast-absorbing suture material can be very useful in these circumstances as it obviates the need for suture removal, thus saving both a visit and potential discomfort for the patient.

References

Kantor J. The fascial plication suture: an adjunct to layered wound closure. *Arch Dermatol.* 2009;145(12):1454-1456.

Dzubow LM. The use of fascial plication to facilitate wound closure following microscopically controlled surgery. *J Dermatol Surg Oncol.* 1989;15(10):1063-1066.

Wang AS, Kleinerman R, Armstrong AW, et al. Setback versus buried vertical mattress suturing: results of a randomized blinded trial. *J Am Acad Dermatol.* 2015;72(4):674-680.

Alam M, Nodzenski M, Yoo S, Poon E, Bolotin D. Objective structured assessment of technical skills in elliptical excision repair of senior dermatology residents: a multirater, blinded study of operating room video recordings. *JAMA Dermatol.* 2014;150(6):608-612.

Wang SQ, Goldberg LH. Surgical pearl: running horizontal mattress suture with intermittent simple loops. *J Am Acad Dermatol.* 2006;55(5):870-871.

Moody BR, McCarthy JE, Linder J, Hruza GJ. Enhanced cosmetic outcome with running horizontal mattress sutures. *Dermatol Surg.* 2005;31(10):1313-1316.

INDEX

Figures are indicated by an italic *f* and tables by a *t* following the page number.